The Point of Care Ultrasound Handbook

The Point of Care Ultrasound Handbook

Editor: Horton Green

AMERICAN
MEDICAL PUBLISHERS
www.americanmedicalpublishers.com

AMERICAN
MEDICAL PUBLISHERS
www.americanmedicalpublishers.com

Cataloging-in-Publication Data

The point of care ultrasound handbook / edited by Horton Green.
p. cm.
Includes bibliographical references and index.
ISBN 979-8-88740-501-8
1. Diagnostic ultrasonic imaging. 2. Ultrasonic imaging. 3. Point-of-care testing.
4. Diagnostic imaging. 5. Ultrasonics in medicine. I. Green, Horton.
RC78.7.U4 P65 2023
616.075 43--dc23

American Medical Publishers,
41 Flatbush Avenue,
1st Floor, New York,
NY 11217, USA

ISBN 979-8-88740-501-8 (Hardback)

Contents

Preface

This book has been an outcome of determined endeavour from a group of educationists in the field. The primary objective was to involve a broad spectrum of professionals from diverse cultural background involved in the field for developing new researches. The book not only targets students but also scholars pursuing higher research for further enhancement of the theoretical and practical applications of the subject.

Ultrasound refers to high frequency sound waves which are higher than the upper audible limit of human hearing. These sound waves are used in a variety of fields, such as diagnostic imaging, ultrasonic devices and non-destructive testing of structures and products. In clinical use, ultrasound is used to capture live images of internal structures of the body. The point of care ultra sound is the use of ultrasound in an emergency situation, for making decisions regarding immediate patient care. It is used to diagnose medical conditions and injuries, where diagnostic methods that are utilized conventionally would consume more time and increase the risk to the health of the patient. The point of care ultrasound is also helpful in monitoring the patient's response to the therapeutic interventions. This book provides significant information of point of care ultrasound to help develop a good understanding of this diagnostic method. A number of latest researches have been included to keep the readers up-to-date with the global concepts in this area of medical imaging.

It was an honour to edit such a profound book and also a challenging task to compile and examine all the relevant data for accuracy and originality. I wish to acknowledge the efforts of the contributors for submitting such brilliant and diverse chapters in the field and for endlessly working for the completion of the book. Last, but not the least; I thank my family for being a constant source of support in all my research endeavours.

Editor

1

Common pitfalls in point-of-care ultrasound: a practical guide for emergency and critical care physicians

Pablo Blanco[1,2*] and Giovanni Volpicelli[3]

Abstract

Background: Point-of-care ultrasonography (POCUS) is a widely used tool in emergency and critical care settings, useful in the decision-making process as well as in interventional guidance. While having an impressive diagnostic accuracy in the hands of highly skilled operators, inexperienced practitioners must be aware of some common misinterpretations that may lead to wrong decisions at the bedside.

Objectives: This article provides a revision list of common POCUS misdiagnoses usually found in practice and offers useful tips to recognize and avoid them.

Discussion: The following aspects were selected and reviewed: pericardial effusion vs. pleural vs. ascites vs. epicardial fat; right ventricle dilation in acute pulmonary embolism and inferior vena cava for volume status assessment in cardiac ultrasound; lung point and lung pulse misinterpretations and mirror artifacts vs. lung consolidations in lung ultrasound; peritoneal fluid vs. the stomach and a critical appraisal of gallbladder signs of acute cholecystitis in abdominal ultrasound; the rouleaux phenomenon vs. deep vein thrombosis or acute right strain in vascular ultrasound.

Conclusions: Following some rules in technique and interpretation, and always integrating POCUS findings into the broader clinical context, most POCUS misdiagnosis can be avoided, and thus patients' safety can be enhanced. Being aware of a list of common pitfalls may help to avoid misdiagnoses.

Keywords: Ultrasonography, Point-of-care, Injuries, Critical care

Introduction

Point-of-care ultrasonography (POCUS) is living a gold era in emergency and critical care medicine, because it is now widely recognized its usefulness in complementing the physical examination and serving as a safe interventional guidance at the bedside [1, 2]. Moreover, an ultrasonography-supported paradigm is gradually becoming a routine approach when caring for critically ill patients [3, 4]. However, it is important to highlight some rising concerns regarding provoked patients' injuries that can result when POCUS is used inappropriately by novice or inexperienced practitioners. POCUS misdiagnoses due to inexperience may lead to errors in the treatment that may worsen patients' outcomes or even be fatal. It is important to remind that before taking any action and being independent in the decision-making process, practitioners must be properly trained and well prepared to the possibility of misinterpretations. Nowadays, POCUS competences are covered in many curricula [1, 5–8] and included in most hands-on training programs, which represent the best way to teach properly POCUS and train new operators. Here, we report a revision of some common POCUS misdiagnoses that may be encountered in the common clinical practice. We will highlight the potential impact of these mistakes on patient outcome,

*Correspondence: ohtusabes@gmail.com
[1] Intensive Care Unit, Hospital Dr. Emilio Ferreyra, 4801, 59 St., 7630 Necochea, Argentina
Full list of author information is available at the end of the article

and finally we will list several tips that may be of help for a correct interpretation of POCUS imaging.

Cardiac ultrasound

Pericardial effusion versus other diagnosis

Pericardial effusion (PEF) is often found in critically ill patients and is defined by transthoracic echocardiography (TTE) as a diastolic fluid-filled space located within the two layers of the pericardium. Pericardial fluid is usually anechoic but sometimes can show a complex echotexture as, for instance, when it contains clots, pus or fibrin. PEF can be circumferential or regional. Even when circumferential, PEF not always is easy to visualize because it may distribute irregularly, and thus several TTE views are needed to demonstrate its presence and real amount. Magnitude and short time of collection are the two main characteristics that influence the possibility of tamponade. The most important tips to recall regarding PEF recognition at POCUS are:

- Tracking anterior to descending aorta in parasternal long axis and apical 4-chamber views (Fig. 1a, b) [9, 10].
- PEF is always present in dependent segments (posterior wall, lateral wall, inferior wall).
- Checking diastolic collapse of cardiac chambers that is a sign of hemodynamically significant PEF: characteristically, the right ventricle outflow tract and the right atrium (RA) are the first parts of the cardiac chambers that collapse under the external pressure of PEF, followed next by the right ventricle (RV) with further increase in the pericardial pressure; diastolic collapse of the left atrium (LA) and left ventricle (LV) can be observed only in the most extreme cases [9, 10]. Right chambers will be fairly resistant to collapse in severe pulmonary hypertension, when abnormal high intracavitary pressure is opposed to the high intra-pericardial pressure [11]. Of note, diastolic collapse of both atriums in significant PEF occurs in ventricular systole (i.e., atrial diastole), and thus one can determine its presence when the atrioventricular valves are closed. This allow for distinction between diastolic collapses in PEF from the normal atrial systole which occurs when the atrioventricular valves are opened.
- Checking dilated (more than 2 cm diameter in long axis) and reduced or absent collapsibility (less than 20% collapse) of the inferior vena cava (tamponade) in spontaneously breathing patients [9, 10].

In case of hypovolemic patients with small, under-filled cardiac chambers, even a mild PEF may be overestimated because the hyper contractile heart could simulate a diastolic collapse of the right chambers. In these cases, the observation of a depleted inferior vena cava (more than 50% or complete collapse during respiration) is a key finding, allowing to rule out a significant role of PEF in the hemodynamic instability.

The most common problematic differential diagnosis of PEF are represented by pleural effusion, peritoneal free-fluid (ascites) and epicardial and/or mediastinal fat. In addition, a large hiatal hernia, pericardial or other mediastinal cysts or left ventricle pseudoaneurysm may sometimes be hardly differentiated but more rarely.

Pleural effusion is defined as a fluid-filled space located within the pleural space. When not directly investigated by lung ultrasound but incidentally detected during TTE, pleural effusion is usually present in a significant amount. Characteristically, left sided pleural effusion appears posterior and lateral to the descending aorta in parasternal long axis and apical 4-chamber views (Fig. 1b, c) [9, 10]. In subcostal views, a right pleural effusion can also be visualized besides the right cardiac chambers, extending over the bare area of the liver (Fig. 1d). When observed in detail, a mobile and consolidated lung is visualized into the pleural fluid (Fig. 1b–d). Additionally, lung ultrasound in coronal views will also show this effusion.

Ascites appears invariably in subcostal views, anterior to the right cardiac chambers. In these cases, the falciform ligament is observed within the fluid, which in addition with the visible diaphragmatic movement, allows to confirm the diagnosis (Fig. 2a) [12]. Moreover, extending the examination to the rest of the abdomen will easily demonstrate the presence of ascites to complete the diagnosis.

Epicardial fat is the adipose tissue accumulated between the visceral pericardium and the myocardium (i.e., epicardial region) [13, 14]. It is slightly isoechoic and is best observed in systole (obliterates completely in diastole) and exclusively in anterior regions. Thus, it is commonly visualized in parasternal long and short axis views (Fig. 2b) as well as in the subcostal 4-chamber view [13]. Mediastinal fat is located anterior to the pericardium and is best observed also in parasternal views (short and long axis) during systole (Fig. 2b) [13].

Error implication An erroneously diagnosed PEF in the unstable patient may lead to undue pericardiocentesis with the strong possibility of cardiac chamber perforation, pericardial tamponade, and eventually, death.

How to avoid this error It is essential to integrate the US findings in the clinical context and consider all the infor-

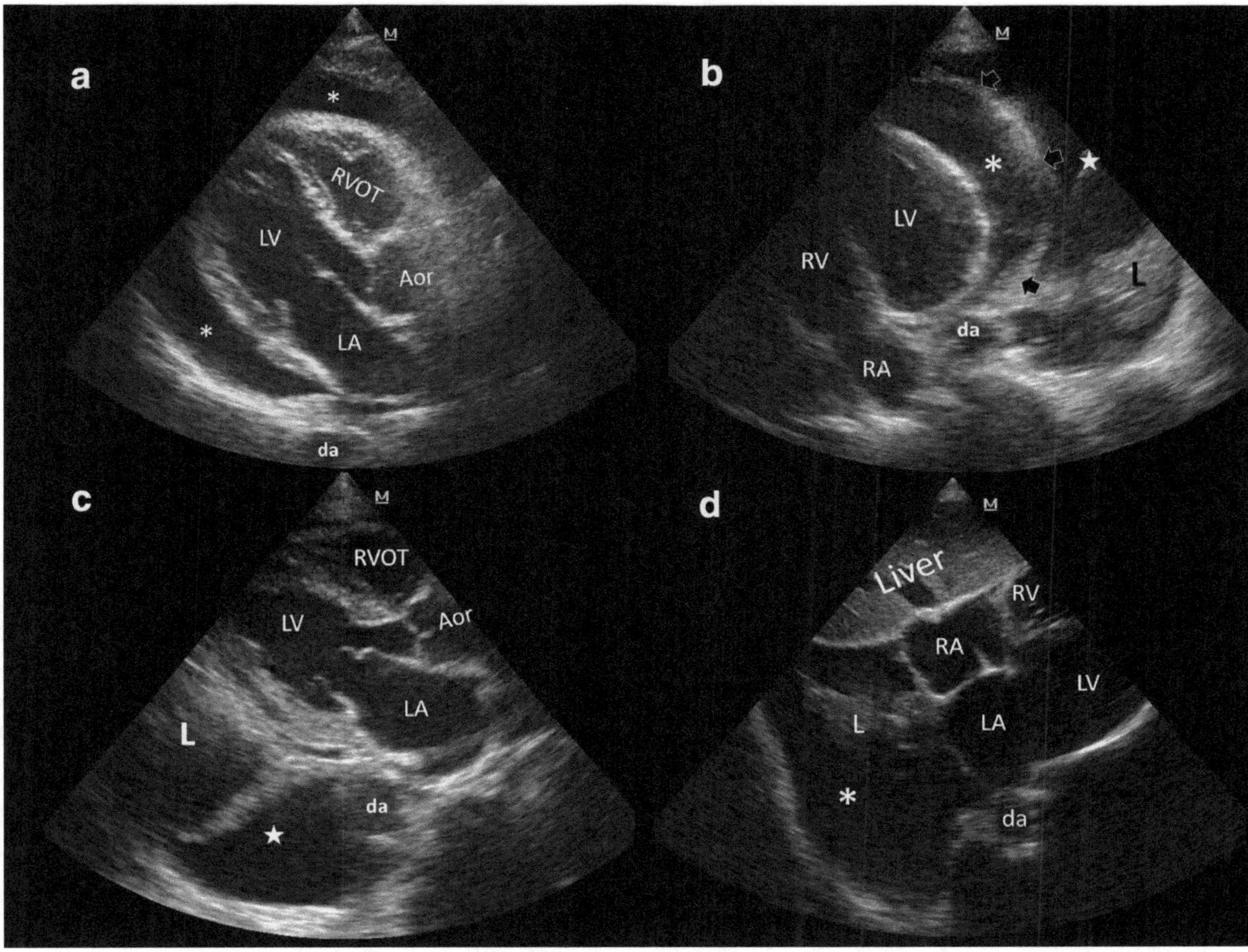

Fig. 1 Pericardial versus pleural effusion. **a** Parasternal long axis view. Pericardial effusion (*asterisks*) tracks anterior to the descending aorta (da); *LV* left ventricle, *LA* left atrium, *RVOT* right ventricle outflow tract, *Aor* aortic root. **b** Apical 4-chamber view. Pericardial effusion (*asterisk*) tracks anterior to the descending aorta (da); pleural effusion (*white star*) tracks posterior and lateral to the da. *Arrows* pericardial delineation, *L* lung consolidation, *LV* left ventricle, *RV* right ventricle, *RA* right atrium. **c** Pleural effusion (*white star*) tracks posterior and lateral to the da; *L* lung consolidation, *LV* left ventricle, *LA* left atrium, *RVOT* right ventricle outflow tract, *Aor* aortic root. **d** Right pleural effusion (*asterisk*) extending into the bare area of the liver, besides the heart in subcostal 4-chamber view; *L* lung consolidation, *RA* right atrium, *RV* right ventricle, *LA* left atrium, *LV* left ventricle, *da* descending aorta

mation on the patient condition, signs and symptoms; tamponade is a clinical diagnosis, which is supported by a compatible POCUS scan. Eventually, in doubtful cases it may be considered draining other effusions if these are well demonstrated and reevaluate thereafter the magnitude of a PEF. If PEF is still present but is not large and shows no hemodynamic consequences on the motility of the right cardiac chambers, drainage should be avoided unless an infectious PEF is suspected. In case of unusual regional location of PEF with intuitive difficulties in the procedure for draining, as it may be a posterior PEF, a surgical consult should be considered. In difficult cases, eventually, the correlation with other imaging methods (e.g., CT) is required.

Right ventricle dilation and acute pulmonary embolism

The diagnosis of right ventricle dilation is of paramount importance in the bedside diagnosis of pulmonary embolism in emergency situations and unstable patients. However, not always the dilation is clearly visible and many possibilities of error should be considered. The diagnosis of dilation basically relies on a comparison between the end-diastolic diameters of the RV and LV. A wrong and incomplete visualization of the cardiac chambers may lead to misdiagnosis. Moreover, the possibility of a chronic dilation not linked to acute right overload may induce further errors. This possibility may be encountered in case of evaluation of patients with chronic volume overload status (e.g., chronic significant

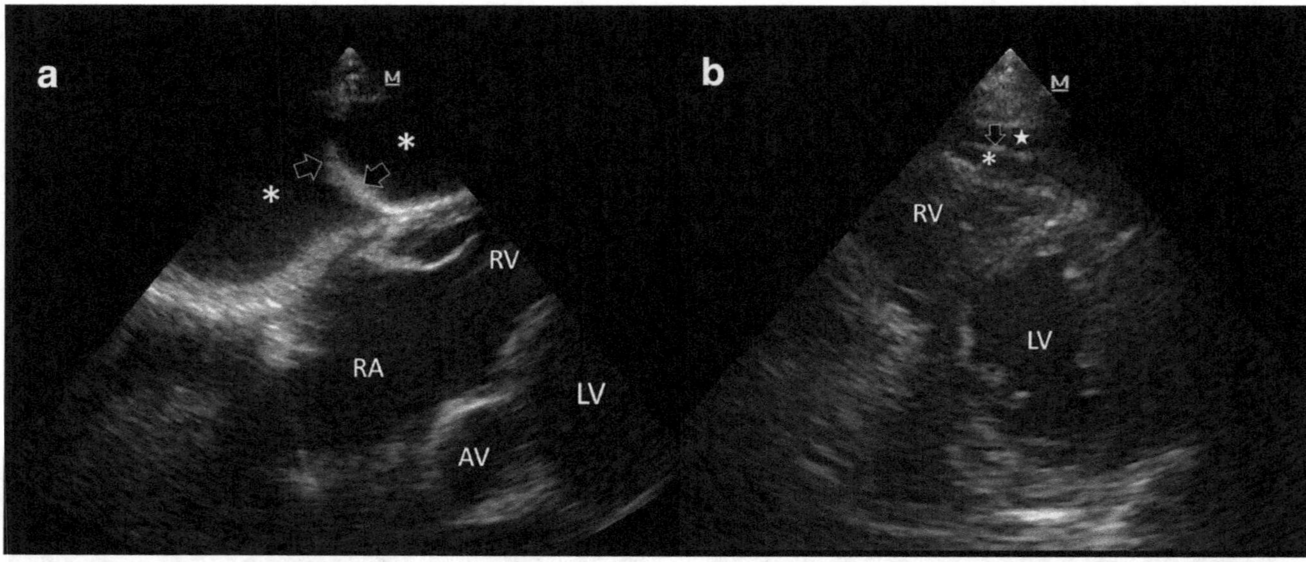

Fig. 2 **a** Pericardial effusion versus ascites. Ascites (*asterisks*) is shown anterior to the heart in subcostal 4-chamber view. The falciform ligament (*arrows*) is depicted, confirming this effusion. *LV* left ventricle, *AV* aortic valve, *RV* right ventricle, *RA* right atrium. **b** Epicardial (*asterisk*) and mediastinal fat (*white star*), demonstrated in parasternal short-axis view, in systole; *LV* left ventricle, *RV* right ventricle, *arrow* pericardium

tricuspid or pulmonary regurgitation) and chronic pressure overload conditions (e.g., chronic pulmonary hypertension) [15]. RV infarction is another condition coursing with RV dilation and impairment of RV function and sometimes hardly to differentiate from pulmonary embolism. In patients with cardiac arrest from any cause, ventricular chambers tend to equalize in short time, and thus applying RV dilation criteria may not be accurate for RV strain.

Error implication A wrong diagnosis of RV dilation in the extreme emergency may lead to the erroneous conclusion of a state of acute right pressure overload (massive pulmonary embolism) that may induce undue thrombolysis or more invasive treatments (e.g., thrombectomy). On the other hand, missing the visualization of real RV dilation from an acute status may delay proper treatment and be harmful for the patient.

How to avoid this error To diagnose correctly RV dilation, the two ventricles should be clearly and fully visualized, preferably in the apical 4-chamber view, and the two end-diastolic diameters taken beside at the level of the atrioventricular valve plane. When this view is not fully demonstrative, a conclusion should never be drawn. A ratio of at least 0.9 is indicative of dilated RV [16–19]. When other views are chosen for difficulty in obtaining a clear apical 4-chamber, different cut-offs should be applied (Table 1). Along with RV dilation, other signs of RV pressure overload may be considered, such as systolic interventricular septal flattening with systolic D-shaped

Table 1 Criteria for diagnosing right ventricle dilation at point-of-care bedside echocardiography (Adapted from [16]–[19])

Echocardiography view	Criteria for right ventricle dilation
4-Chamber apical view	Right/left ventricular end-diastolic diameter ratio >0.9
Parasternal long axis view	Right ventricular end-diastolic diameter >30 mm
Subcostal view	Right/left ventricular end-diastolic diameter ratio >0.7 or 0.9

For the evaluation of the dimension of the right ventricle the preferred view should be the apical 4-chamber. The other views should be used as second choice in case of doubtful measure or impossibility to obtain a clear image

RV (observed in short-axis views), impairment of RV systolic function (e.g., low TAPSE, RV free wall and RV inferior wall hypokinesia) as well as a RV-RA peak pressure gradient higher than 30 mmHg [15, 16, 19]. However, these additional signs are more laborious and need an advanced skill to be evaluated. Moreover, they are not sufficiently sensitive and specific when considered alone [15–17]. Finally, in cases of dilated RV, adjunctive signs of chronic dilation should be considered, like the thickness of the RV wall (superior to 5 mm), LV status, regional impairments, together with clinical history when available.

RA thrombus in transit and thrombus located between both atriums in the foramen ovale are specific signs of pulmonary embolism, and thus should always be considered.

Inferior vena cava and fluid status

The inferior vena cava (IVC) is responsible for lower body systemic blood returning towards the heart. Thus, it is a common practice to consider that volemic status and/or fluid responsiveness may be in someway related to ultrasound measurement of the IVC diameter and its dynamics during the respiratory cycles, which allows a rough estimation of the right atrial pressure. While a depleted IVC is often observed in hypovolemic patients, typically the IVC is dilated in a hypervolemic condition with a less pronounced or null respiratory collapse [20]. However, some gray-zone conditions that alter this supposed linear relationship between the size of the vein and the actual volume status can be easily encountered and observed in practice. For instance, patients with high left ventricle filling pressures and normal IVC [21], potentially fluid responsive patients with physiologically dilated IVC [22], cases of acute right ventricular infarction, pericardial tamponade, acute massive pulmonary embolism, intraabdominal hypertension, asthma/COPD exacerbations and mechanically ventilated patients with positive pressures, all represent conditions where the IVC measurement may fail in indicating reliably the volume status. In addition, acute or chronic cor pulmonale, severe tricuspid regurgitation and pericardial constriction may show highly variable IVC dynamics, independent from the real volume status of the patient [23]. A further possibility of misinterpretation of the ultrasound study of the IVC may happen when the technique is not correctly applied. For a correct measure, the IVC should be visualized in long axis and the inner walls clearly imaged. In M-mode, the movement of the vessel under the probe may erroneously give the impression of a respiratory collapse that is not real. This must be checked observing simultaneously the M-mode with two dimensional imaging (Additional file 1: Video S1, Additional file 2: Video S2, Additional file 3: Video S3). Other phenomena observed is the inspiratory lateral translation of the IVC, producing a misalignment between the IVC and the US scanning plane, and thus simulating an inspiratory collapse [23]. These are common pitfalls that may trick even expert operators.

Error implications These misinterpretations may lead to avoid fluid treatment and even using undue diuretics in patients who are volume depleted and potentially fluid responsive (e.g., in cases of patients mechanically ventilated, or in some emergencies like myocardial infarction of the right ventricle and obstructive causes of shock). On the other hand, errors in the IVC ultrasound may lead to erroneous administration of fluid challenges in patients with high left sided cardiac pressures or conditions of non-responsiveness to volume load, sometimes inducing pulmonary congestion, worsening hemodynamic status and even delaying proper administration of vasopressors and inotropes.

How to avoid this error It is essential to integrate the IVC analysis with a comprehensive multi-organ ultrasound approach that should include a basic focused evaluation of the dimensions, ratio and function of the right and left cardiac chambers, a basic evaluation of the pulmonary congestion by assessing lung ultrasound for B lines, and of course, a full consideration of all the available clinical information. A correct interpretation of the volume status through the IVC assessment should always combine the respiratory variation of the IVC with its absolute size. In mechanically ventilated patients without inspiratory efforts and tidal volume >8 ml/kg (predicted body weight), IVC variation (distensibility index) distinguished fairly accurately the fluid responsive from non-responsive patients [23–25]. In patients with non-invasive ventilation, the interplay between the active respiratory efforts of the patient (negative pressure inducing an inspiratory flattening of the IVC) and the machine (positive pressure inducing an inspiratory engorgement of the IVC) has unpredictable effects on the inferior vena cava [23]. In spontaneously breathing patients with hypovolemia, a IVC collapsibility >42% may predict fluid responsiveness with high specificity (97%) [26]; however, normovolemic patients with large respiratory efforts may simulate this IVC dynamics [23]. Patients with shallow respiratory efforts may induce the opposite changes in the IVC collapsibility.

Other conditions affecting the transmural pressures between the thorax and the abdomen (e.g., asthma/COPD exacerbations, active expiratory efforts, patients with invasive mechanical ventilation and inspiratory efforts) may preclude the use of the IVC for volume assessment, as well as other situations that can induce high RA pressures (e.g., RV infarction, tamponade).

Lung ultrasound

Lung sliding, lung point, B lines and lung pulse in the diagnosis of pneumothorax

The lung point is a fundamental ultrasonographic sign highly specific for confirming pneumothorax [27]. Two other equivalent signs are also highly specific for diagnosing pneumothorax [27]: the hydro-point [28] and the heart-point sign [29]. However, some normal physiological conditions can be misdiagnosed for false lung points [30, 31]. The requirement necessary to define the real lung point is an absent lung sliding with absent subpleural parenchymal ultrasound signals (B-lines or consolidations) and the lung point as the contact between the aforementioned region and the sliding lung (or pleural fluid as in hydro-pneumothorax) [32]. Indeed, some similar ultrasound patterns representing the interphases between the expanding lung and the diaphragm (Additional file 4: Video S4) and between the expanding lung and the heart (Additional file 5: Video S5), may be misdiagnosed for false lung points, especially when observed with high frequency probes, sometimes inducing the operator to wrong conclusions.

A complex situation can also be encountered in patients with pulmonary peripheral blebs. These patients commonly have structural lung parenchymal alterations that sometimes are at risk to develop a secondary pneumothorax in a background of chronic obstructive pulmonary disease [33]. Thus, differential diagnosis with pneumothorax may be crucial. In these cases, sometimes a regular lung sliding can be demonstrated in large peripheral blebs even if with some difficulty [34]. However, very often, the presence of pleural adhesions precludes the visualization of the respiratory movement of the lung and may induce erroneous interpretation. In stable patients absence of sliding should never be considered enough to finalize the diagnosis of pneumothorax. Especially, in patients with complex pulmonary disorders (large blebs and adhesions), a more detailed chest CT study may be required.

Pneumomediastinum may mimic a left sided pneumothorax, producing air artifacts during the chest ultrasound examination and even obscuring a regular parasternal and apical echocardiographic views. Correlation with chest X-ray or CT is usually required to confirm the diagnosis and exclude a pneumothorax [35].

While a false pattern of absence of sliding may contribute to misdiagnose pneumothorax, sometimes a respiratory or cardiac movement of the lung image at ultrasound may be misinterpreted for a false lung sliding (Additional file 6: Video S6). Even the beat of an intercostal artery or the thoracic internal artery in parasternal region may simulate a false lung pulse (Additional file 7: Video S7), thus inducing the operator to misdiagnose the absence of pneumothorax. Similarly, in complex cases of recurrence of pneumothorax after abrasion pleurodesis, the visualization of B lines due to multiple septa still connecting the lung to the chest wall may induce to erroneously rule out the condition (Additional file 8: Video S8) [36].

Error implications The misdiagnosis of the absence of sliding or a false lung point may lead to an unnecessary pleural drainage. Furthermore, in doubtful cases, higher costs and irradiation exposure may arise if other unnecessary diagnostic imaging methods are ordered. In case of false sliding, false pulse or multiple septa, the diagnosis of pneumothorax may be dangerously delayed or even missed.

How to avoid these errors Use a set of criteria to define pneumothorax by combining the four basic signs: abolished lung sliding, absent parenchymal signs (B lines and consolidations), absent lung pulse and look for the lung point for final confirmation in stable patients. Eventually, rule in a pneumothorax by chest CT if the patient is stable or correlate the ultrasound pattern with previous images, when available, in case of history of blebs or previous abrasion pleurodesis. In complicated cases, like secondary pneumothorax, recurrences, post-procedural pneumothorax, and trauma, a complex pattern should always be considered a strong possibility and induce the caring physician to carefully scan the whole chest to improve the accuracy of lung ultrasound.

Mirror artifact vs. lung consolidation

Mirror artifacts consist in the repetition of a false image resulting from the ultrasound beam hitting against a highly reflective surface [37], such as the diaphragm. Most frequent in the right side, this artifact can simulate a lung consolidation by the repetition of the liver tissue pattern above the diaphragm (Fig. 3a).

Error implications This misdiagnosis may lead to higher costs and adverse effects derived from indications of antibiotics as well as unneeded chest X-ray or CT.

How to avoid this error Along with integration into the clinical picture, observing the same tissue pattern of the liver or spleen is usually enough to rule in this artifact. The presence of pleural effusion that invariably accompanies lung consolidations and sonographic air or fluid bronchograms (Fig. 3b) is never observed in mirror image artifacts, and thus may aid in differentiating real lung diseases.

Abdominal ultrasound

Peritoneal fluid versus the stomach

Peritoneal fluid recognition is recommended during the first evaluation of trauma patients [38] as well as in patients presenting with several abdominal complaints and shock [39, 40]. When the abdomen is evaluated in left coronal views, a full stomach appearing below the diaphragm may mimic a condition of peritoneal fluid

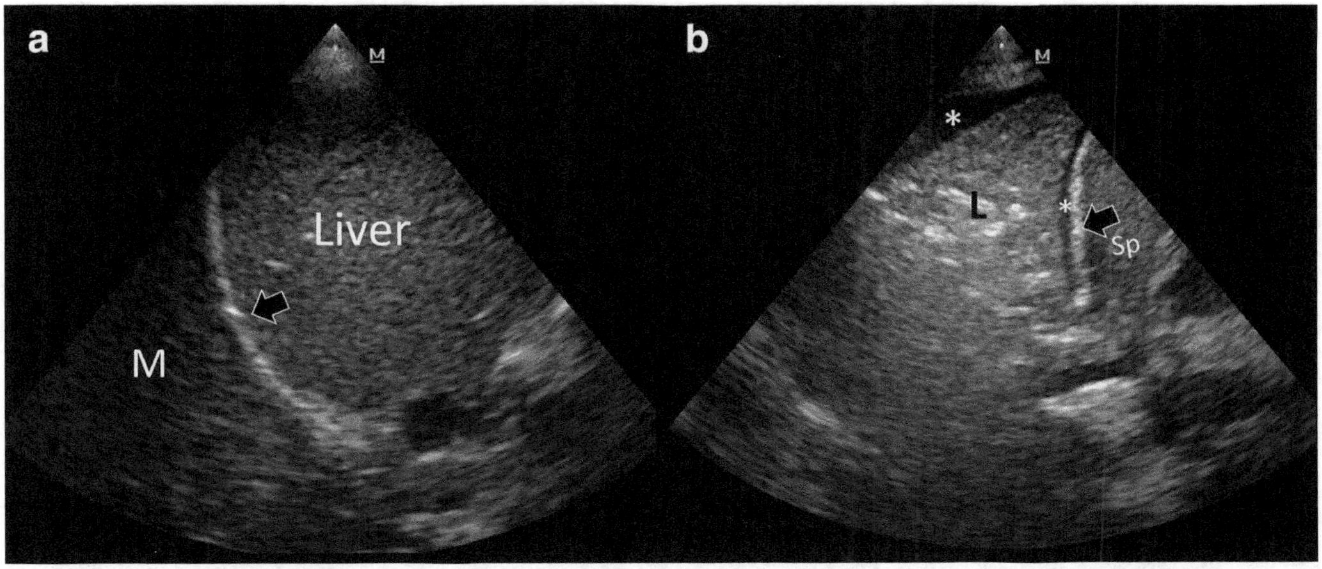

Fig. 3 **a** Mirror image artifact (M), showing a similar tissue-like pattern in comparison with the liver; *arrow*: diaphragm. **b** Lung consolidation (L). Distinctively, it is shown a tissue-like pattern, sonographic air bronchogram and pleural fluid (*asterisks*); *arrow* diaphragm, *Sp* spleen

(Fig. 4a). In other situations, the stomach may even appear in epigastric subcostal views and may simulate a fluid abdominal collection (Fig. 4b). Depending on gastric contents (fluid, air, food), the appearance of the stomach may vary, ranging from simple anechoic fluid up to a heterogeneous ultrasound pattern.

Error implications A misdiagnosis of false peritoneal fluid may lead to undue ultrasound-guided puncture and subsequent intraabdominal organ damage (i.e., spleen, diaphragm and stomach perforation), and eventually involving the pleural space causing pneumothorax. Furthermore, higher costs and undue irradiation may arise from confirmatory CT studies. Eventually, this misinterpretation may lead to laparotomy, and thus adjunctive surgical risks.

How to avoid this error First, it is important to consider the possibility of a full stomach since it is visible in most non-fasted patients as well as in patients with delayed gastrointestinal emptying, which is a common condition in the critically ill. In doubtful cases and when the patients are able to take oral fluids, a possibility for differential diagnosis consists in observing bubbles appearing after having asked to the patient to drink some water. In unconscious patients or in extreme emergency situations, such as in postoperative abdominal patients with sepsis of unknown origin or in trauma patients, the opposite may be done by using the nasogastric or orogastric tube and evaluating if the image persists after gastric drainage. Moreover, the gastric tube can be also visualized by ultrasound coming down to the stomach during the maneuver, confirming the location of the organ (Fig. 4c).

Distended gallbladder, thickened gallbladder walls and acute cholecystitis

Along with a compatible clinical picture, ultrasonographic criteria of acute cholecystitis are a distended gallbladder, thickened walls, biliary sludge and lithiasis (calculus type), pericholecystic fluid and sonographic Murphy's sign [41, 42].

Gallbladder distension and wall thickening, although important signs, are not specific for acute cholecystitis when considered alone (Tables 2, 3). For example, thickened gallbladder walls are commonly observed in patients coursing with generalized edemas such as those with cardiac failure (Fig. 5a, b), pre-eclampsia or renal failure. In non-fasted patients, the gallbladder is physiologically contracted, and thus may show thickened walls. In the presence of thickened walls, pericholecystic fluid and biliary sludge but the absence of clearly visible gallstones, acute cholecystitis during septic shock can be misdiagnosed [43].

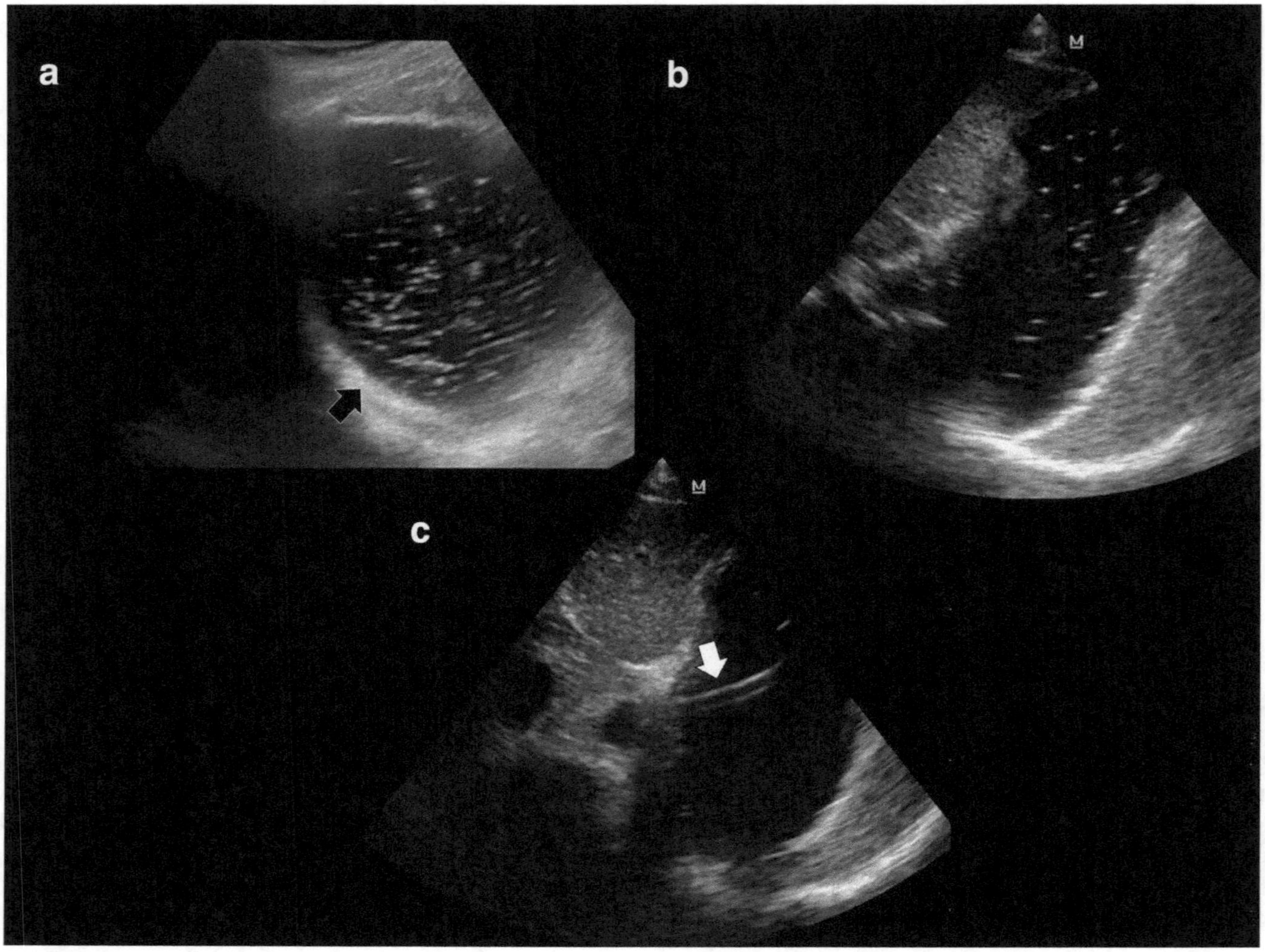

Fig. 4 **a** Stomach observed from the left coronal view. Note the fluid content and the echoes inside (air bubbles); *arrow* diaphragm. **b** Stomach observed from an epigastric view simulating a collection. **c** A gastric tube is observed confirming that it is the stomach (*white arrow*)

Table 2 Causes of gallbladder wall thickening (Modified from [39])

Generalized edematous states	Inflammatory conditions	Miscellaneous	Neoplastic	Physiological
Congestive heart failure	Acute and chronic cholecystitis	Adenomyomatosis	Gallbladder adenocarcinoma	Non-fasting patient (contracted gallbladder)
End-stage cirrhosis	Cholangitis	Cystic vein varices	Metastases	
Renal failure	Acute hepatitis	Malabsorption		
Hypoalbuminemia	Pancreatitis			
Pre-eclampsia	Perforated duodenal ulcer			

Table 3 Causes of gallbladder distension

Physiological	Obstruction
Fasting	Cystic duct (e.g., lithiasis) Common bile duct Pancreas

Error implications This misdiagnosis may lead to higher costs and adverse effects derived from the indications of antibiotics, and eventually, to cholecystectomy or cholecystotomy, and thus unnecessary surgery risks.

How to avoid this error It is essential to integrate ultrasound findings into the patient clinical context, always

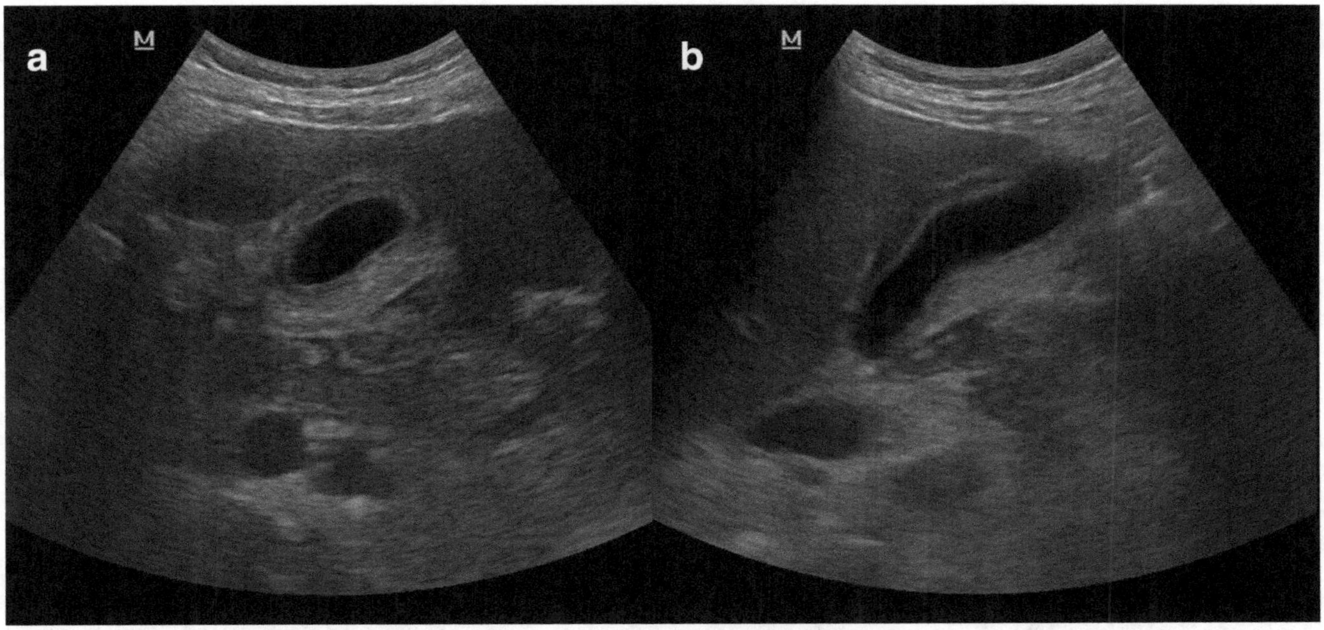

Fig. 5 Gallbladder wall thickening in short (**a**) and long (**b**) axis in a patient with severe heart failure, hepatomegaly and ascites

considering common underlying diseases resulting in morphological alterations of the gallbladder (e.g., cardiac failure). In the absence of clearly visible gallstones, the diagnosis of cholecystitis should always be confirmed by other methods [43].

Vascular ultrasound

Rouleaux vs. deep vein thrombosis

Most cases of deep vein thrombosis (DVT) are found in lower limbs, exposing patients to the risk of pulmonary embolism. A common differential diagnosis of DVT is the presence of "rouleaux formation" that is an accumulation of erythrocytes lying over the venous valves represented by spontaneously echogenic blood flow inside the vessel [44] (Fig. 6a; Additional file 3: Video S3). While rouleaux is a common finding and usually does not have a clinical impact, it is important to highlight that this can also be frequently observed when there is a proximal venous obstruction, and thus a more proximal DVT must be ruled out.

Error implications A misdiagnosis of DVT only based on rouleaux may lead to higher costs and unnecessary side-effects (bleeding) derived from unnecessary patient anticoagulation. However, depending on the setting, the vessel observed and the patient condition, the rouleaux (or sludge sign) should sometimes induce to extend the observation to the possibility of proximal obstruction. The sludge sign in the inferior vena cava during cardiac arrest with electrical activity and hyperkinetic left cardiac chambers may be a sign of acute right overload [45]. The same sign in the femoral vein, corroborated by asymmetric femoral veins waveforms at color Doppler analysis, may be a sign of isolated iliac thrombus [45].

How to avoid this error In contrast to a real condition of thrombosis, veins with rouleaux formation are compressible. Furthermore, distal compression allows to squeeze the blood and clear the rouleaux while thrombus cannot be released (Fig. 6b; Additional file 3: Video S3). To rule in or out a more proximal venous obstruction in the presence of rouleaux, the operator should look for direct visualization of a thrombus or examine compressibility of the proximal veins. In addition, the use of a spectral Doppler analysis to assess for respiratory flow variations of peripheral veins on both sides may be useful (Fig. 6c, d). More than a pattern of low intensity of the signal, especially, an asymmetric waveform obtained by comparing the two sides, indicates the possibility of a stop between the heart and the site of insonation and induces to extend the US venous study or use more advanced imaging for confirmation.

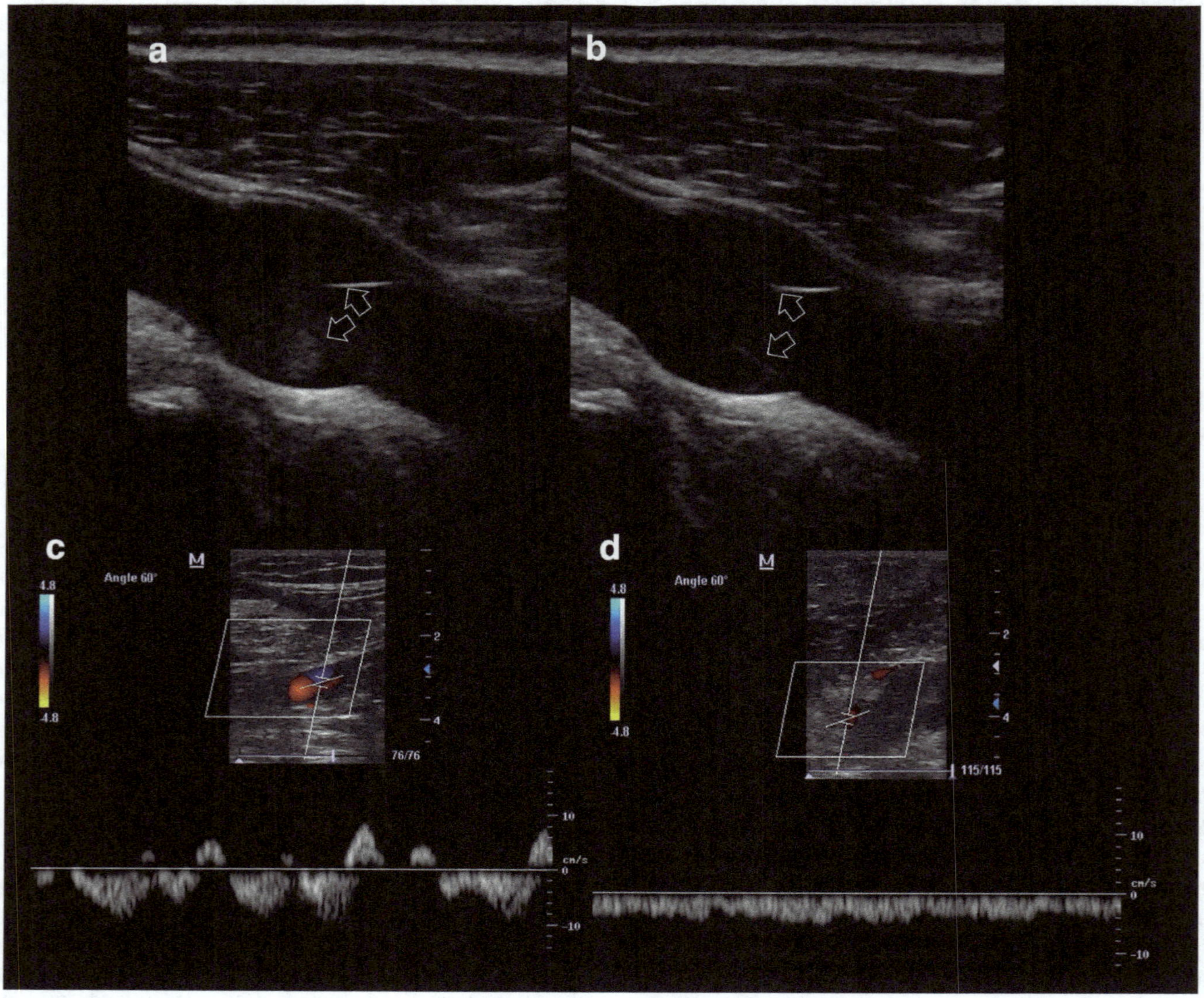

Fig. 6 **a** Rouleaux formation over the venous valves (*arrows*). **b** After distal compression, the blood was squeezed and the rouleaux are finally cleared. *Arrows* venous valves. **c** Normal phasic venous waveform, indicating a non-stopping flow between the heart and the site of insonation. **d** Abnormal non-phasic venous flow, indicating a stop between the heart and the site of insonation

Conclusions

There are some common misleading situations that critical care physicians may encounter in their sonography practice. Following some rules in technique and interpretation, the accuracy of POCUS can be improved and the possibility of dangerous misdiagnoses avoided. It is essential to remember that POCUS does not replace the clinical judgment, physical examination or common sense. POCUS must always be used in a holistic manner to improve the clinical accuracy and patient safety.

Additional files

Additional file 1: Video 1. The inferior vena cava (IVC) in long axis in a patient with massive acute pulmonary embolism (Videos 1 to 3). The view of video 1 shows a significant venous collapse during respiration that is predictive of low venous pressure.

Additional file 2: Video 2. The inferior vena cava (IVC) in long axis in a patient with massive acute pulmonary embolism (Videos 1 to 3). In video 2, the M-mode documents the collapse of IVC during respiration.

Additional file 3: Video 3. The inferior vena cava (IVC) in long axis in a patient with massive acute pulmonary embolism (Videos 1 to 3). The same view (video 3) in long axis performed with the correct technique shows the absence of collapse in the obvious clinical condition of acute right strain. The difference is the correct displaying of the IVC in video 3, which is based on the constant visualization of the inner walls of the vessel.

Additional file 4: Video 4. Normal interphase between the expanding lung and the diaphragm. Note the ultrasonographic tissue pattern of the liver as well as the lung sliding.

Additional file 5: Video 5. Normal interphase between the heart and the expanding lung.

Additional file 6: Video 6. Lung ultrasound in a condition of pneumothorax. The movement of the muscles of the chest wall during the respiratory effort gives the impression of lung sliding. However, the real sliding should be observed against the chest wall and independent from the movement of the intercostal muscles.

Additional file 7: Video 7. Lung ultrasound in a condition of pneumothorax. The pulsing movement of the image is due to an intercostal artery visualized in long axis, giving the impression of a false pulsation of the lung. The real lung pulse should be independent from the movement of the chest wall.

Additional file: Video 8. A case of recurrence of pneumothorax after pleurodesis abrasion. The septa still connecting the lung to the chest wall explain the coexistence of B lines and the absence of sliding in a condition of pneumothorax.

Additional file 9: Video 9. Wash out of rouleaux formation after distal compression, ruling out thrombosis at the site of insonation.

Abbreviations

POCUS: point-of-care ultrasonography; PEF: pericardial effusion; TTE: transthoracic echocardiography; RA: right atrium; RV: right ventricle; LV: left ventricle; LA: left atrium; IVC: inferior vena cava; CT: computerized tomography; DVT: deep vein thrombosis.

Authors' contributions

PB and GV contributed equally to this work. Both authors read and approved the final manuscript.

Author details

[1] Intensive Care Unit, Hospital Dr. Emilio Ferreyra, 4801, 59 St., 7630 Necochea, Argentina. [2] Intensive Care Unit, Clínica Cruz Azul, 2651, 60 St., 7630 Necochea, Argentina. [3] Emergency Medicine, San Luigi Gonzaga University Hospital, 10043 Turin, Italy.

Acknowledgements

PB would like to thank Mrs. Julieta Vigna for the language guidance.

References

1. Frankel HL, Kirkpatrick AW, Elbarbary M, Blaivas M, Desai H, Evans D, Summerfield DT, Slonim A, Breitkreutz R, Price S, Marik PE, Talmor D, Levitov A (2015) Guidelines for the appropriate use of bedside general and cardiac ultrasonography in the evaluation of critically ill patients-part I: general ultrasonography. Crit Care Med 43(11):2479–2502
2. Blanco P (2016) Physical examination along with point-of-care echocardiography: an indisputable right path. Am J Emerg Med 34(3):673
3. Blanco P (2015) A traditional paradigm vs. an ultrasound-supported paradigm in emergency and critical care medicine: a crisis of the mind is needed. J Emerg Med 49(2):e63–e64
4. Álvarez-Fernández JA, Núñez-Reiz A, en representación del Club de Ecografía UCI Madrid de la SOMIAMA (2015) Clinical ultrasound in the ICU: changing a medical paradigm. Med Intensiva 40(4):246–249
5. Ultrasound Certification Task Force on behalf of the Society of Critical Care Medicine. Recommendations for achieving and maintaining competence and credentialing in critical care ultrasound with focused cardiac ultrasound and advanced critical care echocardiography. http://journals.lww.com/ccmjournal/Documents/Critical%20Care%20Ultrasound.pdf. Accessed 02 Jan 2016
6. Via G, Hussain A, Wells M, Reardon R, ElBarbary M, Noble VE, Tsung JW, Neskovic AN, Price S, Oren-Grinberg A, Liteplo A, Cordioli R, Naqvi N, Rola P, Poelaert J, Gulič TG, Sloth E, Labovitz A, Kimura B, Breitkreutz R, Masani N, Bowra J, Talmor D, Guarracino F, Goudie A, Xiaoting W, Chawla R, Galderisi M, Blaivas M, Petrovic T, Storti E, Neri L, Melniker L, International Liaison Committee on Focused Cardiac UltraSound (ILC-FoCUS), International Conference on Focused Cardiac UltraSound (IC-FoCUS) (2014) International evidence-based recommendations for focused cardiac ultrasound. J Am Soc Echocardiogr 27(7):683.e1–683.e33
7. Volpicelli G, Elbarbary M, Blaivas M, Lichtenstein DA, Mathis G, Kirkpatrick AW, Melniker L, Gargani L, Noble VE, Via G, Dean A, Tsung JW, Soldati G, Copetti R, Bouhemad B, Reissig A, Agricola E, Rouby JJ, Arbelot C, Liteplo A, Sargsyan A, Silva F, Hoppmann R, Breitkreutz R, Seibel A, Neri L, Storti E, Petrovic T, International Liaison Committee on Lung Ultrasound (ILC-LUS) for International Consensus Conference on Lung Ultrasound (ICC-LUS) (2012) International evidence-based recommendations for point-of-care lung ultrasound. Intensive Care Med 38(4):577–591
8. Expert Round Table on Echocardiography in ICU (2014) International consensus statement on training standards for advanced critical care echocardiography. Intensive Care Med 40(5):654–666
9. Strony R, Linkenheil E (2016) How to delineate pericardial effusion from pleural effusion on bedside ultrasound. J Emerg Med 50(3):495–496
10. Goodman A, Perera P, Mailhot T, Mandavia D (2012) The role of bedside ultrasound in the diagnosis of pericardial effusion and cardiac tamponade. J Emerg Trauma Shock 5(1):72–75
11. Adams JR, Tonelli AR, Rokadia HK, Duggal A (2015) Cardiac tamponade in severe pulmonary hypertension. A therapeutic challenge revisited. Ann Am Thorac Soc 12(3):455–460
12. Cardello FP, Yoon DH, Halligan RE Jr, Richter H (2006) The falciform ligament in the echocardiographic diagnosis of ascites. J Am Soc Echocardiogr 19(8):1074.e3–1074.e4
13. Bertaso AG, Bertol D, Duncan BB, Foppa M (2013) Epicardial fat: definition, measurements and systematic review of main outcomes. Arq Bras Cardiol 101(1):e18–e28
14. Blaivas M, DeBehnke D, Phelan MB (2000) Potential errors in the diagnosis of pericardial effusion on trauma ultrasound for penetrating injuries. Acad Emerg Med 7(11):1261–1266
15. Grifoni S, Olivotto I, Cecchini P, Pieralli F, Camaiti A, Santoro G, Pieri A, Toccafondi S, Magazzini S, Berni G, Agnelli G (1998) Utility of an integrated clinical, echocardiographic, and venous ultrasonographic approach for triage of patients with suspected pulmonary embolism. Am J Cardiol 82(10):1230–1235
16. The Steering Committee (2012) Single-bolus tenecteplase plus heparin compared with heparin alone for normotensive patients with acute pulmonary embolism who have evidence of right ventricular dysfunction and myocardial injury: rationale and design of the pulmonary embolism thrombolysis (PEITHO) trial. Am Heart J 163(1):33.e1–38.e1
17. Nazerian P, Vanni S, Volpicelli G, Gigli C, Zanobetti M, Bartolucci M, Ciavattone A, Lamorte A, Veltri A, Fabbri A, Grifoni S (2014) Accuracy of point-of-care multiorgan ultrasonography for the diagnosis of pulmonary embolism. Chest 145(5):950–957

18. Volpicelli G, Lamorte A, Tullio M, Cardinale L, Giraudo M, Stefanone V, Boero E, Nazerian P, Pozzi R, Frascisco MF (2013) Point-of-care multiorgan ultrasonography for the evaluation of undifferentiated hypotension in the emergency department. Intensive Care Med 39(7):1290–1298
19. Becattini C, Agnelli G, Vedovati MC, Pruszczyk P, Casazza F, Grifoni S, Salvi A, Bianchi M, Douma R, Konstantinides S, Lankeit M, Duranti M (2011) Multidetector computed tomography for acute pulmonary embolism: diagnosis and risk stratification in a single test. Eur Heart J 32(13):1657–1663
20. Perera P, Mailhot T, Riley D, Mandavia D (2010) The RUSH exam: rapid ultrasound in SHock in the evaluation of the critically Ill. Emerg Med Clin North Am 28(1):29–56
21. Blanco P, Sasai T (2015) Assessment of left ventricle preload by transthoracic echocardiography: an easy task? J Intensive Care 3(1):23
22. Lang RM, Badano LP, Mor-Avi V, Afilalo J, Armstrong A, Ernande L, Flachskampf FA, Foster E, Goldstein SA, Kuznetsova T, Lancellotti P, Muraru D, Picard MH, Rietzschel ER, Rudski L, Spencer KT, Tsang W, Voigt JU (2015) Recommendations for cardiac chamber quantification by echocardiography in adults: an update from the American Society of Echocardiography and the European Association of Cardiovascular Imaging. J Am Soc Echocardiogr 28(1):1e14–39.e14
23. Via G, Tavazzi G, Price S (2015) Ten situations where inferior vena cava ultrasound may fail to accurately predict fluid responsiveness: a physiologically based point of view. Intensive Care Med 42(7):1164–1167
24. Zhang Z, Xu X, Ye S, Xu L (2014) Ultrasonographic measurement of the respiratory variation in the inferior vena cava diameter is predictive of fluid responsiveness in critically ill patients: systematic review and meta-analysis. Ultrasound Med Biol 40(5):845–853
25. Barbier C, Loubières Y, Schmit C, Hayon J, Ricôme JL, Jardin F, Vieillard-Baron A (2004) Respiratory changes in inferior vena cava diameter are helpful in predicting fluid responsiveness in ventilated septic patients. Intensive Care Med 30(9):1740–1746
26. Airapetian N, Maizel J, Alyamani O, Mahjoub Y, Lorne E, Levrard M, Ammenouche N, Seydi A, Tinturier F, Lobjoie E, Dupont H, Slama M (2015) Does inferior vena cava respiratory variability predict fluid responsiveness in spontaneously breathing patients? Crit Care 19:400
27. Lichtenstein D, Mezière G, Biderman P, Gepner A (2000) The lung point: an ultrasound sign specific to pneumothorax. Intensive Care Med 26:1434–1440
28. Volpicelli G, Boero E, Stefanone V, Storti E (2013) Unusual new signs of pneumothorax at lung ultrasound. Crit Ultrasound J 5(1):10
29. Stone MB, Chilstrom M, Chase K, Lichtenstein D (2010) The heart point sign: description of a new ultrasound finding suggesting pneumothorax. Acad Emerg Med 17(11):e149–e150
30. Gillman LM, Alkadi A, Kirkpatrick AW (2009) The "pseudo-lung point" sign: all focal respiratory coupled alternating pleural patterns are not diagnostic of a pneumothorax. J Trauma 67(3):672–673
31. Zhang Z, Chen L (2015) A physiological sign that mimics lung point in critical care ultrasonography. Crit Care 19:155
32. Moreno-Aguilar G, Lichtenstein D (2015) Lung ultrasound in the critically ill (LUCI) and the lung point: a sign specific to pneumothorax which cannot be mimicked. Crit Care 19:311
33. Gelabert C, Nelson M (2015) Bleb point: mimicker of pneumothorax in bullous lung disease. West J Emerg Med 16(3):447–449
34. Campione A, Luzzi L, Gorla A, Terzi A (2010) About ultrasound diagnosis of pulmonary bullae vs. pneumothorax. J Emerg Med 38(3):384–385 **(author reply 385)**
35. Saracino C, Tessaro M (2015) Pneumomediastinum as a sonographic mimic of pneumothorax. J Ultrasound Med 34(8):1521–1522
36. Volpicelli G, Garofalo G, Lamorte A, Frascisco MF (2012) Young man with left thoracic pain. Ann Emerg Med 60(2):e3–e4
37. Malhotra R, Bramante RM, Radomski M, Nelson M (2014) Mirror image artifact mimicking heterotopic pregnancy on transvaginal ultrasound: case series. West J Emerg Med 15(6):712–714
38. Nural MS, Yardan T, Güven H, Baydin A, Bayrak IK, Kati C (2005) Diagnostic value of ultrasonography in the evaluation of blunt abdominal trauma. Diagn Interv Radiol 11(1):41–44
39. Coppolino F, Gatta G, Di Grezia G, Reginelli A, Iacobellis F, Vallone G, Giganti M, Genovese E (2013) Gastrointestinal perforation: ultrasonographic diagnosis. Crit Ultrasound J 5(Suppl 1):S4
40. Mouaqit O, Hibatallah A, Oussaden A, Maazaz K, Taleb KA (2013) Acute intraperitoneal rupture of hydatid cysts: a surgical experience with 14 cases. World J Emerg Surg 8:28
41. Gore RM, Thakrar KH, Newmark GM, Mehta UK, Berlin JW (2010) Gallbladder imaging. Gastroenterol Clin North Am 39(2):265–287
42. Khalili K, Wilson SR (2011) The biliary tree and gallbladder. In: Rumack CM, Wilson SR, Charboneau JW, Levine D (eds) Diagnostic ultrasound, 4th edn. Elsevier Mosby, Philadelphia
43. Volpicelli G, Balik M, Georgopoulos D (2014) Echography is mandatory for the initial management of critically ill patients: no. Intensive Care Med 40(11):1766–1768
44. Charlotte H, Kuntz K, Youngs D (2013) Leg Pain. In: Charlotte H, Kuntz K, Youngs D (eds) Clinical guide to sonography: exercises for critical thinking, 2nd edn. Elsevier Mosby, St Louis
45. Volpicelli G, Mussa A, Frascisco MF (2012) Sonographic diagnosis of pulmonary embolism with cardiac arrest without major dilation of the right ventricle or direct sign of lower limb venous thrombosis. J Clin Ultrasound 40(8):529–533

2

Improving hospital-based point-of-care ultrasound cleaning practices using targeted interventions: a pre–post study

Daniel Van Kalsbeek[1*], Karl Enroth[1], Elizabeth Lyden[2], Mark E. Rupp[3] and Christopher J. Smith[4]

Abstract

Background: Point-of-care ultrasound (POCUS) devices are becoming more widely used in healthcare and have the potential to act as fomites. The objective of this project was to study the thoroughness of cleaning of POCUS machines before and after a quality improvement initiative. We designed a mixed-methods, pre/post study which took place over the course of one year at a university-affiliated health center. Cleaning rates of four ultrasound machines used by hospital medicine and critical care medicine services were evaluated using fluorescent marking. Interventions targeted physicians' knowledge of best practices and improved access to cleaning supplies. Pre- and post-intervention cleaning rates were compared using a generalized linear model. The impact of the corona virus disease of 2019 (COVID-19) pandemic on baseline cleaning rates was also evaluated. Physicians' attitudes and knowledge of cleaning practices were evaluated via unpaired pre/post surveys.

Results: There was significant improvement in thoroughness of cleaning following intervention (pre 0.62, SE 0.05; post 0.89, SE 0.07), $p < 0.0001$). There was no difference in baseline cleaning rates before (0.63, SE 0.09) and after (0.61, SE 0.1) the onset of the COVID-19 pandemic ($p = 0.78$). Post-intervention surveying found improved understanding of guideline-based cleaning practice, better performance on knowledge-based questions, and fewer reported barriers to machine cleaning.

Conclusion: Thoroughness of cleaning of POCUS machines can be improved with practical interventions that target knowledge and access to cleaning supplies.

Keywords: Point-of-care ultrasound (POCUS), Infection control, Cleaning, Disinfection, Quality improvement

Background

Over the past three decades, the use of point-of-care ultrasound (POCUS) has been increasingly integrated into routine clinical practice, including critical care and hospital medicine [1–3]. Recently the Alliance for Academic Internal Medicine has advocated for POCUS training across all levels of medical education [3]. Advances in technology have allowed ultrasound machines to become more portable and user-friendly, making it possible to perform exams on multiple patients in a relatively short time frame [2, 4]. Clinically relevant infectious organisms have been cultured from ultrasound probes and gels, even when they are not visibly soiled, including methicillin-resistant *Staphylococcus aureus*, *Pseudomonas aeruginosa* and vancomycin-resistant enterococci [5–9]. Additionally relevant to the present time, it has been discovered that SARS-CoV-2 may remain viable on plastic surfaces for up to 72 h [10]. Thus, POCUS has the potential to act as a fomite for pathogens which are known to prolong hospital stays, escalate healthcare costs, and increase mortality [11].

Cleaning and disinfection of ultrasound equipment has been shown to significantly reduce microbiological

*Correspondence: vankalsbeek@live.com
[1] Department of Internal Medicine, 982055 Nebraska Medical Center, Omaha, NE 68198-2055, USA
Full list of author information is available at the end of the article

burden [12, 13]. Multiple professional groups have published guidelines for cleaning and disinfecting POCUS machines, and, though difficult to prove due to study design, adherence to these guidelines should reduce the risk of transmitting clinically relevant pathogens [14–21]. Unfortunately, surveys suggest suboptimal cleaning practice and a perceived lack of guidance among ultrasound users [22–24]. Hospital-based studies have shown that environmental cleaning performance can be improved using education and feed-back, leading to reduced likelihood of culturing clinically relevant organisms [20, 21, 25–27]. Similar studies pertaining to point-of-care ultrasound are lacking. To address this, we designed a project with the goal of identifying barriers to guideline-based cleaning of POCUS devices and improving cleaning practices using targeted interventions.

Methods

Design and setting

A mixed-methods, pre/post-study of POCUS machine cleaning practices was conducted over a 1-year period at a 718-bed academic health center. This project was considered quality improvement by the local institutional review board and therefore did not require approval as human subject research. Two Philips SPARQ (Andover, MA) and 2 GE Healthcare Venue (Chicago, IL) machines were included in the study. SPARQ machines were primarily used by hospital medicine (HM) faculty and internal medicine (IM) residents. One SPARQ machine was stored on an inpatient medical-surgery unit and the other was stored in a HM work room. Venue machines were used primarily by IM residents, pulmonary/critical care medicine (PCCM) fellows, and PCCM faculty, but they were also accessible to surgical and anesthesia critical care providers. One Venue was stored in a neuro-critical care unit and the other was stored in a medical critical care unit. All machines were outfitted with linear, convex, and phased array transducers.

The IM residency program has approximately 95 house officers, including categorical, preliminary, primary care, and medicine-pediatric residents. The residency program has a longitudinal POCUS curriculum, including workshops, lectures, and a dedicated POCUS rotation. There are 13 PCCM fellows, who also have a dedicated POCUS curriculum and rotation. POCUS training and clinical use is variable for HM and PCCM faculty, with some high-frequency users and some non-users.

Intervention

Interventions were guided by a targeted needs assessment. To better educate physicians, we created a website that outlined best practices for POCUS cleaning and disinfection [28]. The website included a 3-min instructional video, a summary of cleaning steps, and links to best-practice guidelines from our institution and relevant professional societies. The website was distributed via email to all resident, fellow, and faculty physicians targeted by our survey. The instructional video was also integrated into training sessions for the IM residents and PCCM fellows. Placards were placed on POCUS machines which included a summary of cleaning steps and a QR code to access the website for just-in-time training.

The educational intervention promoted a 2-step cleaning and disinfection process based on American Institute of Ultrasound in Medicine guidelines [14]. First, users were instructed to remove all visible soiling with a disinfecting wipe or soapy washcloth. Then, using a fresh disinfecting wipe, all high-use areas (touch screen, keyboard, handles, probes, and cords) were wiped thoroughly. PDI Sani-Cloth® AF-3 disinfecting wipes were used throughout the study. This product is a quaternary ammonium-containing, low-level disinfectant, which is appropriate for disinfecting medical equipment that contacts intact skin [29].

We improved access to cleaning materials by ensuring that each machine always had a dedicated container of disinfecting wipes. Machines with inadequate space for wipes were equipped with commercially available canister caddies (Fig. 1). Wipes were restocked by researchers twice weekly, as needed, during study periods. Providers were also encouraged to replace wipes when necessary.

Data collection

A fluorescent marking gel (DAZO, ECOLAB) was used to monitor POCUS machine cleaning practices. The use of these gels is a well-established method for monitoring environmental cleaning practices in infection control research [25–27, 30, 31]. Circular marks roughly 2.54 cm in diameter were placed on 12 high-touch areas on each machine including probes, cords, and user-interface surfaces (Figs. 1 and 2). The marking sites were determined based on best practice recommendations [14, 15] and guidance from our infection control department. The size of gel markings were informed by pilot testing which revealed this pattern allowed the most consistent application of gel. Gel markings were evaluated twice per week during the first two weeks of each month during the study period by members of the research team (DV and KE). The absence of fluorescence under UV light was classified as cleaned. The presence of any visible fluorescence was classified as dirty. This was done to minimize subjectivity when interpreting partially cleaned marks and because residual fluorescence was felt to indicate poor cleaning technique. The presence of gross debris, defined as the presence of soiling that was visible to the naked eye, was also documented. The machines were

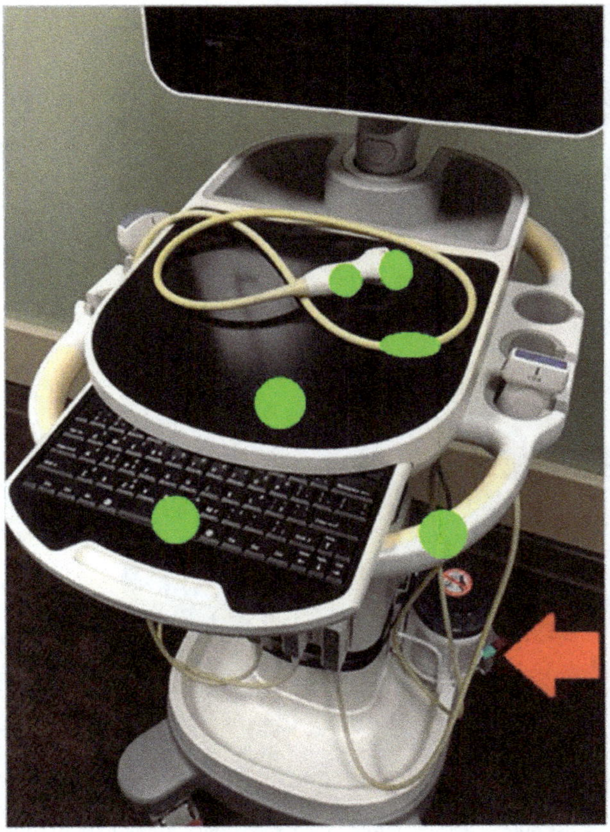

Fig. 1 Locations of fluorescent marks. A Phillips SPARQ model ultrasound machine is pictured to demonstrate marking locations. Green circles represent the areas marked with fluorescent gel during the study (size exaggerated for clarity). For simplicity, only one probe and cord is displayed, but all probes and cords were marked in this fashion during the study. Also pictured is the disinfecting wipe caddie that was added to these models to improve access to cleaning supplies (red arrow)

thoroughly cleaned per institutional guidelines and evaluated with UV light to ensure no remaining fluorescence remained prior to re-marking. Prior to the start of the project, researchers met to ensure machine marking and data collection procedures were consistent between team members. Machine use was tracked via a dedicated sign-out sheet for each machine.

The pre-intervention data collection occurred from November 2019 to January 2020. Before implementation of the planned intervention, the COVID-19 pandemic spread rapidly across the United States. The heightened awareness around infection control during this time had the potential to confound post-intervention data. To address this possibility, the research team collected an additional 2 months of baseline data from May to June 2020. During this time only three of the four POCUS machines were available for data collection. Interventions were implemented in July 2020. Post-intervention data were collected from August to October 2020.

Survey

A 16-question survey was created to assess participants' demographics, POCUS experiences, and attitudes and knowledge towards machine cleaning (Additional file 1). The survey was created through an iterative process with input from a survey design expert within the institution. It was pilot tested by three members of a POCUS interest group (one faculty, two residents) to ensure clarity, ease of use, and face validity. The survey was distributed to all IM residents; fellows from PCCM & Rheumatology; and faculty from HM, PCCM, and Rheumatology with POCUS training. Rheumatology physicians were included as they routinely use POCUS in clinical practice at our institution. A link to the anonymous, online survey was distributed via institutional email in April 2020 (pre-intervention) and October 2020 (post-intervention).

Analysis

The primary outcome was the composite machine cleaning rates in the pre-intervention phase compared to the post-intervention phase. Secondary outcomes included comparison of cleaning rates based on primary machine ownership (HM vs PCCM) and marking site groups (transducers vs. cords vs. touch surfaces). Cleaning rates were analyzed using a generalized linear mixed model (GLMM) which accounted for the correlation of cleaning rates for each machine. Model-adjusted mean percentages and standard errors of cleaned components by phase were used to summarize the data. To account for occasions when a machine was not used between sampling periods, data were excluded when there was no documentation of use on the machine's sign-out sheet and there was no evidence of use (i.e., all gel marks remained intact and no gross debris was present). This was done to avoid falsely under-estimating cleaning rates. Unpaired pre- and post-intervention survey results were compared using descriptive statistics. All analyses were done using SAS version 9.4, and a p-value of less than 0.05 was considered statistically significant.

Results

There was no difference in pre-intervention cleaning rates before (0.63, SE 0.09) and after (0.61, SE 0.1) the COVID-19 outbreak ($p=0.78$). These data were, therefore, combined to form an aggregate baseline cleaning rate that was used in the final analysis. Pre- and post-intervention cleaning rates are displayed in Table 1. A total of 768 surfaces were evaluated in the pre-intervention phase (504 pre-COVID, 264 post-COVID) and 504 surfaces in the post-intervention phase. There was a significant improvement in the thoroughness of cleaning following intervention (pre 0.62, SE 0.05; post 0.89, SE 0.07; $p<0.0001$),

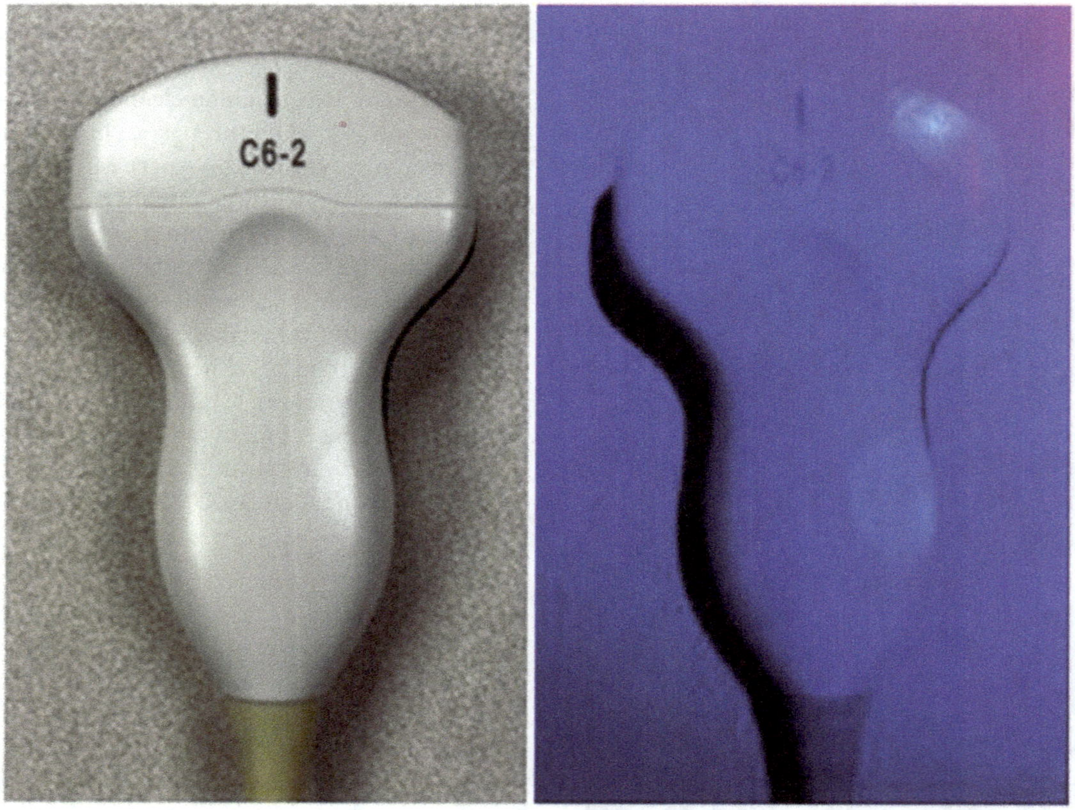

Fig. 2 Fluorescent gel marks. Pictured is a curvilinear probe used to exemplify the size and location of fluorescent marks under ambient room light (left) and UV light with room lights turned off (right)

Table 1 Model-adjusted ultrasound machine cleaning rates before and after quality improvement interventions

	Before (SE)	After (SE)	*p*-value
All machines combined	0.62 (0.05)	0.89 (0.07)	$p<0.0001$
Primary machine usage sub-groups			
Hospital medicine machines	0.50 (0.08)	0.91 (0.14)	$p<0.0001$
Critical care machines	0.74 (0.04)	0.87 (0.05)	$p=0.075$
Surface category sub-groups			
Probe lens and handles	0.74 (0.06)	0.96 (0.07)	$p<0.0001$
Probe cords	0.40 (0.06)	0.78 (0.10)	$p<0.0001$
High-touch surfaces	0.63 (0.06)	0.88 (0.08)	$p=0.011$

representing a 44% relative improvement. In a sub-group analysis, the HM-based machines (pre 0.50, SE 0.08; post 0.91, SE 0.14; $p<0.0001$) demonstrated greater improvement in the thoroughness of cleaning than the CCM-based machines (pre 0.74, SE 0.04; post 0.87, SE 0.04; $p=0.075$). All surface category sub-groups showed significant improvement in cleaning rates ($p\leq 0.01$ for all groups), with probe cords showing the largest improvement (Table 1). During the pre-intervention phase there were 12 instances where gross debris was found on the machines, while there was a single instance in the post-intervention phase. All instances of gross debris were found on probe lenses and/or handles. While not specifically analyzed, the gross debris visually appeared to be an accumulation of dried gel, often associated with a designed crevice such as the probe orientation marker. There was a single instance where blood appeared to be intermixed in the gross debris.

Table 2 displays the pre- and post-intervention survey results. The response rates for the pre- and post-intervention surveys were 54% (74/137) and 42% (58/139), respectively. The majority of respondents were IM residents (66%). Roughly half of respondents used POCUS weekly or more. Lack of knowledge, limited access to cleaning supplies, and time constraint were identified as the most common barriers to guidelines-based POCUS cleaning and disinfection. Following the intervention, self-reported familiarity with machine cleaning best practices improved from 22 to 74%. The proportion of participants correctly answering knowledge-based questions related to disinfectant use (pre—59%, post—74%) and cleaning processes (pre—76%, post—93%) also improved. Participants reported fewer barriers related to

Table 2 Ultrasound machine cleaning survey results before and after quality improvement interventions

Survey topic	Before ($n=74$)	After ($n=58$)
Female sex, *n* (%)	35 (47%)	23 (40%)
Level of training, *n* (%)		
Internal medicine resident	51 (69%)	36 (62%)
Fellow	6 (8%)	7 (12%)
Faculty	17 (23%)	15 (26%)
Faculty/fellow area of practice, *n* (%)		
Hospital medicine/general internal medicine	9 (39%)	9 (41%)
Pulmonary/critical care	8 (35%)	4 (18%)
Rheumatology	6 (26%)	9 (41%)
Frequency of POCUS use, *n* (%)		
Weekly or more	34 (46%)	25 (43%)
Less than weekly	40 (54%)	33 (57%)
Respondents reporting familiarity with best practice guidelines for POCUS cleaning, *n* (%)	16 (22%)	43 (74%)
Respondents reporting they know where to find institutional guidelines for cleaning, *n* (%)	3 (4%)	33 (57%)
My cleaning practices follow best practice guidelines, *n* (%)		
Agree or strongly agree	12 (16%)	34 (76%)
Disagree or strongly disagree	4 (5%)	0 (0%)
I don't know	58 (78%)	14 (24%)
Correct response to objective knowledge questions, *n* (%)		
Appropriate use of disinfectants	44 (59%)	43 (74%)
Recommended steps of cleaning and disinfecting process	56 (76%)	54 (93%)
Barriers to cleaning, Median Likert (IQR)[a]		
Access to cleaning supplies	3 (2–3)	2 (1–3)
Time constraint	3 (2–3)	2 (1–3)
Lack of knowledge	3 (3–4)	2 (1–3)

[a] 5-point Likert scale: 1 = never, 2 = rarely, 3 = sometimes, 4 = often, 5 = always

cleaning supply access, time constraints, and knowledge deficits following the intervention.

Discussion

We were able to significantly improve the thoroughness of cleaning of POCUS machines by using targeted interventions. We identified lack of knowledge, inadequate access to cleaning supplies, and time constraint as primary barriers to guideline-based cleaning and disinfection. These findings support the concern raised by a global survey of ultrasound users which suggested that real-world cleaning practices are unsatisfactory and that users are unfamiliar with guidelines [22, 23]. Given the morbidity, mortality, and cost associated with nosocomial infection, preventative efforts should be pursued whenever feasible [32, 33]. The interventions we described are practical and could be readily implemented at other institutions. A review of guideline-based cleaning and disinfection practice should become a standard component of POCUS training. The effort and expense of such interventions is likely justified if they can prevent even a small number hospital acquired infection [32].

The spread of the COVID-19 pandemic during our pre-intervention phase had the potential to confound our results, for example, through heightened provider awareness of disinfecting practices or system-level interventions. However, we did not find any difference in cleaning rates following the first spike of COVID-19-related admission in our region of the country [34]. This finding is a powerful example of how difficult it can be to change clinical practices. We believe our project was successful because it identified specific physician-reported barriers allowing for tailored intervention [35].

When sub-grouped by area of use, the thoroughness of cleaning for machines used primarily for critical care approached, but did not meet, significance. These machines are shared with specialties that were not targeted by our interventions, providing a possible explanation for this finding. Of the surface category sub-groups, probe cords had the lowest baseline cleaning rate and the greatest relative improvement. While probe cords may not be thought of as a high-contact surface, they are frequently handled during exams or draped across the patient, and attention must be given to this area during cleaning. Though statistical analysis was not performed due to the unpaired nature of our survey, there was an improvement in all response categories following intervention, further supporting the efficacy of these actions.

Although our intervention focused on POCUS users, we would like to highlight an opportunity for manufacturers to improve device design to promote easier cleaning and better infection control. Specifically, there should be efforts to reduce the number of difficult-to-clean crevices, such as we encountered around probe orientation markers. These are in the highest-contact region and we consistently found them to be poorly cleaned. Additional areas of concern include the keyboard and control knobs/wheels.

There were limitations to our study. This was a single-center study, which may limit generalizability. The pre/post-intervention study design makes it possible that confounding variables influenced our findings. Our design allowed measurement of cleaning but not disinfection, although prior infection control studies demonstrated that improvement in thoroughness of cleaning correlated closely with microbiological assessment [20, 21, 26]. Additionally, thoroughness of cleaning was assessed twice per week, making it possible that machines were used multiple times between assessments. This could have falsely increased our cleaning rates, though should not affect the relative change. Despite these potential limitations, we feel our findings provide meaningful and useful data.

Based on the results of this study, guideline-based cleaning practices and education have been integrated into our POCUS curriculum. This includes ongoing use of the online resources created for the project and improved access to dedicated disinfecting wipes on POCUS machines. In the future, we would like to work with our infection control division to update institutional cleaning and disinfection policies so that they are more easily interpretable with regards to POCUS. An internal sustainability study would add important information, and we would be interested in the findings of a similar project carried out at other sites. Finally, demonstrating a correlation between improvement in point-of-care ultrasound cleaning and decreased patient acquisition of microbes or healthcare-associated infection is desirable.

Conclusion

We identified barriers to guideline-based cleaning and disinfection of point-of-care ultrasound machines: a lack of knowledge, time constraint, and inadequate access to cleaning supplies. By targeting these domains with practical interventions, we were able to significantly improve the thoroughness of cleaning of four point-of-care ultrasound machines used by internal medicine and critical care medicine providers.

Acknowledgements

The authors would like to thank Dr. Phil Carling for providing DAZO gel, Alisha Dorn for technical infection control expertise, Zachary Benton-Slocum for his work with website creation and design, and Dr. Derek Kruse and Dr. Amy Cannella for being delegates of their respective specialties.

Authors' contributions

DV: conceptualization, project administration, data collection, data interpretation, media design, media editing, survey design, survey distribution, writing—original draft, writing—review and editing. KE: conceptualization, data collection, data interpretation, media design, media editing, writing—review and editing. EL: statistical analysis, data interpretation, writing—review and editing. MR: conceptualization, data interpretation, writing—review and editing. CS: conceptualization, project administration, project supervision, survey design, survey distribution, data interpretation, writing—review and editing. All authors read and approved the final manuscript.

Author details

[1]Department of Internal Medicine, 982055 Nebraska Medical Center, Omaha, NE 68198-2055, USA. [2]Department of Biostatistics, 984375 Nebraska Medical Center, Omaha, NE 68198-4375, USA. [3]Department of Internal Medicine, Division of Infectious Diseases, 985400 Nebraska Medical Center, Omaha, NE 68198-5400, USA. [4]Department of Internal Medicine, Division of Hospital Medicine, 986430 Nebraska Medical Center, Omaha, NE 68198-6430, USA.

References

1. Beaulieu Y, Marik PE (2005) Bedside ultrasonography in the ICU: part 1. Chest 128(2):881–895
2. Campbell SJ, Bechara R, Islam S (2018) Point-of-care ultrasound in the intensive care unit. Clin Chest Med 39(1):79–97
3. Soni NJ, Schnobrich D, Mathews BK et al (2019) Point-of-care ultrasound for hospitalists: a position statement of the society of hospital medicine. J Hosp Med 14:E1–E6
4. Bhagra A, Tierney DM, Sekiguchi H, Soni NJ (2016) Point-of-care ultrasonography for primary care physicians and general internists. Mayo Clin Proc 91(12):1811–1827
5. Frazee BW, Fahimi J, Lambert L, Nagdev A (2011) Emergency department ultrasonographic probe contamination and experimental model of probe disinfection. Ann Emerg Med 58(1):56–63
6. Shokoohi H, Armstrong P, Tansek R (2015) Emergency department ultrasound probe infection control: challenges and solutions. Open Access Emerg Med 7:1–9
7. Marigliano A, D'Errico MM, Pellegrini I, Savini S, Prospero E, Barbadoro P (2010) Ultrasound echocardiographic gel contamination by Burkholderia cepacia in an Italian hospital. J Hosp Infect 76(4):360–361
8. Westerway SC, Basseal JM, Brockway A, Hyett JA, Carter DA (2017) Potential infection control risks associated with ultrasound equipment—a bacterial perspective. Ultrasound Med Biol 43(2):421–426
9. Lee AS, White E, Monahan LG, Jensen SO, Chan R, van Hal SJ (2018) Defining the role of the environment in the emergence and persistence of vanA vancomycin-resistant enterococcus (VRE) in an intensive care unit: a molecular epidemiological study. Infect Control Hosp Epidemiol 39(6):668–675
10. van Doremalen N, Bushmaker T, Morris D (2020) Aerosol and surface stability of SARS-CoV-2 as compared with SARS-CoV-1. N Engl J Med 382(16):1564–1567
11. Cosgrove SE, Qi Y, Kaye KS, Harbarth S, Karchmer AW, Carmeli Y (2005) The impact of methicillin resistance in Staphylococcus aureus bacteremia on patient outcomes: mortality, length of stay, and hospital charges. Infect Control Hosp Epidemiol 26(2):166–174

12. Mullins K, Burnham K, Henricson EK, Cohen S, Fair J, Ray JW (2020) Identification and analysis of bacterial contamination of ultrasound transducers and multiuse ultrasound transmission gel bottle tips before and after the aseptic cleansing technique. J Ultrasound Med 39(10):1957–1963
13. Mullaney PJ, Munthali P, Vlachou P, Jenkins D, Rathod A, Entwisle J (2007) How clean is your probe? Microbiological assessment of ultrasound transducers in routine clinical use, and cost-effective ways to reduce contamination. Clin Radiol 62(7):694–698
14. AIUM official statement: guidelines for cleaning and preparing external- and internal-use ultrasound transducers and equipment between patients as well as safe handling and use of ultrasound coupling gel. American Institute of Ultrasound in Medicine. Updated March 27, 2020. https://www.aium.org/officialStatements/57. Accessed 7 Dec 2020
15. ACEP Policy Statement: Guideline for Ultrasound Transducer Cleaning and Disinfection. Published June 2018. https://www.acep.org/globalassets/new-pdfs/policy-statements/guideline-for-ultrasound-transducer-cleaning-and-disinfection.pdf. Accessed 12 Dec 2020
16. ACEP guideline on COVID-19: ultrasound machine and transducer cleaning. Published March 2020. https://www.acep.org/globalassets/new-pdfs/policy-statements/guideline-on-covid-19--ultrasound-machine-and-transducer-cleaning.pdf. Accessed 12 Dec 2020
17. Basseal J, Westerway S, Juraja M et al (2017) Guidelines for reprocessing ultrasound transducers. Australas J Ultrasound Med 20:30–40
18. Koibuchi H, Kotani K, Taniguchi N (2013) Ultrasound probes as a possible vector of bacterial transmission. Med Ultrason 15(1):41–44
19. Suleyman G, Alangaden G, Bardossy AC (2018) The role of environmental contamination in the transmission of nosocomial pathogens and healthcare-associated infections. Curr Infect Dis Rep 20(6):12
20. Hayden MK, Bonten MJ, Blom DW, Lyle EA, van de Vijver DA, Weinstein RA (2006) Reduction in acquisition of vancomycin-resistant enterococcus after enforcement of routine environmental cleaning measures. Clin Infect Dis 42(11):1552–1560
21. Eckstein BC, Adams DA, Eckstein EC et al (2007) Reduction of *Clostridium Difficile* and vancomycin-resistant *Enterococcus* contamination of environmental surfaces after an intervention to improve cleaning methods. BMC Infect Dis 7:61
22. Westerway SC, Basseal JM (2017) The ultrasound unit and infection control—are we on the right track? Ultrasound 25(1):53–57
23. Westerway SC, Basseal JM, Abramowicz JS (2019) Medical ultrasound disinfection and hygiene practices: WFUMB global survey results. Ultrasound Med Biol 45(2):344–352
24. Hoyer R, Adhikari S, Amini R (2016) Ultrasound transducer disinfection in emergency medicine practice. Antimicrob Resist Infect Control 5:12
25. Carling PC, Parry MM, Rupp ME et al (2008) Improving cleaning of the environment surrounding patients in 36 acute care hospitals. Infect Control Hosp Epidemiol 29(11):1035–1041
26. Goodman ER, Platt R, Bass R, Onderdonk AB, Yokoe DS, Huang SS (2008) Impact of an environmental cleaning intervention on the presence of methicillin-resistant *Staphylococcus aureus* and vancomycin-resistant enterococci on surfaces in intensive care unit rooms. Infect Control Hosp Epidemiol 29(7):593–599
27. Carling PC, Briggs JL, Perkins J, Highlander D (2006) Improved cleaning of patient rooms using a new targeting method. Clin Infect Dis 42(3):385–388
28. Van Kalsbeek D, Enroth K, Benton-Slocum Z, Smith CJ. Cleaning and disinfection of point-of-care ultrasound machines. Published June 2020. https://www.unmc.edu/intmed/residencies-fellowships/cleaning_ultrasound.html. Accessed 24 Jan 2021
29. Rutala WA, Weber DJ (2008) Guidelines for disinfection and sterilization in healthcare facilities. Center for disease control and prevention
30. Rupp ME, Fitzgerald T, Sholtz L, Lyden E, Carling P (2014) Maintain the gain: program to sustain performance improvement in environmental cleaning. Infect Control Hosp Epidemiol 35(7):866–868
31. Carling P (2013) Methods for assessing the adequacy of practice and improving room disinfection. Am J Infect Control 41(5 Suppl):S20-25
32. Hassan M, Tuckman HP, Patrick RH, Kountz DS, Kohn JL (2010) Cost of hospital-acquired infection. Hosp Top 88(3):82–89
33. Westphal GA, Pereira AB, Fachin SM et al (2019) Characteristics and outcomes of patients with community-acquired and hospital-acquired sepsis. Rev Bras Ter Intensiva 31(1):71–78
34. Douglas County Health Department COVID-19 Dashboards (2020) Douglas county health department. https://www.douglascountyhealth.com/infectious-disease/diseases-and-conditions/2019-novel-coronavirus-2019-ncov. Accessed 7 Dec 2020
35. Grol R, Grimshaw J (2003) From best evidence to best practice: effective implementation of change in patients' care. Lancet 362(9391):1225–1230

3

Correlation of OSCE performance and point-of-care ultrasound scan numbers among a cohort of emergency medicine residents

Youyou Duanmu[1*], Patricia C. Henwood[2], Sukhjit S. Takhar[3], Wilma Chan[4], Joshua S. Rempell[5], Andrew S. Liteplo[6], Viktoria Koskenoja[7], Vicki E. Noble[8] and Heidi H. Kimberly[2]

Abstract

Background: Point-of-care ultrasound (POCUS) is an important clinical tool for a growing number of medical specialties. The current American College of Emergency Physicians (ACEP) Ultrasound Guidelines recommend that trainees perform 150–300 ultrasound scans as part of POCUS training. We sought to assess the relationship between ultrasound scan numbers and performance on an ultrasound-focused observed structured clinical examination (OSCE).

Methods: This was a cross-sectional cohort study in which the number of ultrasound scans residents had previously performed were obtained from a prospective database and compared with their total score on an ultrasound OSCE. Ultrasound fellowship trained emergency physicians administered a previously published OSCE that consisted of standardized questions testing image acquisition and interpretation, ultrasound machine mechanics, patient positioning, and troubleshooting. Residents were observed while performing core applications including aorta, biliary, cardiac, deep vein thrombosis, Focused Assessment with Sonography in Trauma (FAST), pelvic, and thoracic ultrasound imaging.

Results: Twenty-nine postgraduate year (PGY)-3 and PGY-4 emergency medicine (EM) residents participated in the OSCE. The median OSCE score was 354 [interquartile range (IQR) 343–361] out of a total possible score of 370. Trainees had previously performed a median of 341 [IQR 289–409] total scans. Residents with more than 300 ultrasound scans had a median OSCE score of 355 [IQR 351–360], which was slightly higher than the median OSCE score of 342 [IQR 326–361] in the group with less than 300 total scans ($p = 0.04$). Overall, a LOWESS curve demonstrated a positive association between scan numbers and OSCE scores with graphical review of the data suggesting a plateau effect.

Conclusion: The results of this small single residency program study suggest a pattern of improvement in OSCE performance as scan numbers increased, with the appearance of a plateau effect around 300 scans. Further investigation of this correlation in diverse practice environments and within individual ultrasound modalities will be necessary to create generalizable recommendations for scan requirements as part of overall POCUS proficiency assessment.

Keywords: Education, Point of care, Ultrasound, Competency

*Correspondence: youyou.duanmu@gmail.com
[1] Department of Emergency Medicine, Stanford University School of Medicine, 900 Welch Road Suite 350, Palo Alto, CA 94304, USA
Full list of author information is available at the end of the article

Background

Point-of-care ultrasound (POCUS) has become an important clinical tool across a variety of medical specialties [1–5]. Proficiency in POCUS is especially vital to the practice of emergency medicine (EM) [6–11]. Since 2012, the Accreditation Council for Graduate Medical Education (ACGME) has designated the use of ultrasound for diagnosing emergent medical conditions, critical care and trauma resuscitation, and procedural guidance as 1 of 23 milestone competencies for EM residents [8]. The 2016 American College of Emergency Physicians (ACEP) policy statement on emergency ultrasound advises that a trainee should perform 25–50 ultrasounds in each of the core applications and a total of 150–300 scans as part of POCUS training [9].

It has been suggested that the completion of a predetermined number of ultrasounds correlates with proficiency in clinical practice; however, there remains significant variability in the number of scans required by different training programs [12, 13]. There are data showing that residents who performed greater than 150 ultrasounds scored significantly higher on a written ultrasound examination [14]. However, a more recent consensus statement recommended that 150 scans may not be sufficient as a competency benchmark, but should be regarded as a minimum standard beyond which other measures of competency should be assessed [15]. A 2017 survey of 539 EM residents found that residents believed an average of 325 scans is required for proficiency [16].

Medical training programs have adapted the observed structured clinical examination (OSCE) to evaluate competency in a variety of applications [17–21]. The OSCE is an especially useful tool for medical skills that involve a combination of technical and knowledge-based aptitude. Its use is recommended by the ACEP policy statement to assess for ultrasound competency, but to our knowledge there is no prior data comparing OSCE performance to overall scan numbers [9].

Ultrasound is a multi-modal skill set requiring complex methods of competency assessment. In this study, we sought to assess whether there was a relationship between the number of ultrasounds previously performed by senior EM residents and their performance on a standardized ultrasound OSCE.

Methods

This was a cross-sectional cohort study in which the number of ultrasound scans residents had previously performed was obtained from a prospective database and compared to total scores on an ultrasound OSCE. A modified version of a previously published ultrasound OSCE was given to all 29 postgraduate year (PGY)-3 and PGY-4 residents at a single academic emergency medicine residency program that spans two institutions [17, 22, 23]. The OSCE took place in a simulation center using standardized patients as models. It consisted of standardized questions testing image acquisition and interpretation with points for technique, image quality, and correct interpretation of anatomy. Twelve ultrasound fellowship trained emergency physicians served as evaluators. Residents were observed performing aorta, biliary, cardiac, deep vein thrombosis, Focused Assessment with Sonography in Trauma (FAST), pelvic, and thoracic ultrasounds, which are included in the ACEP core emergency ultrasound applications. The total possible score for the OSCE was 370. Based on the total OSCE score and overall evaluator impression, residents were given an OSCE general competency score from 1 to 5 and those with a score of 2 or below were provided individualized remediation. To assess inter-rater reliability, 11 residents had two evaluators independently grade their OSCE performance. For those 11 subjects, the mean of their two OSCE scores was used in the general analysis.

The number of ultrasound scans the residents had performed was obtained from a prospective database and included ultrasounds performed clinically and during the 1-week PGY-1 and 2-week PGY-2 ultrasound rotations. Scans were evaluated in total and by application type. None of the residents had participated in an outside ultrasound rotation. The scans logged in the database had all been reviewed for quality assurance by ultrasound-trained faculty.

Data were analyzed using Stata 14.2 (Stata Corporation, College Station, TX). A locally weighted scatter plot smoothing (LOWESS) method was used to visually estimate the trend between OSCE score and previously performed ultrasound scan numbers. A Wilcoxon rank-sum test was used to assess for differences in OSCE score by PGY year. A two-sample t test was used to assess for differences in OSCE score at a scan number cutoff of 300, because this appeared to be the region of plateau of the LOWESS curve as well as the upper range of recommended scan numbers based on the ACEP guidelines. Intraclass correlation (ICC) with one-way random effects was used to assess inter-rater reliability for those OSCEs that had two evaluators. The study was deemed exempt from review by the Partners Healthcare Institutional Review Board.

Results

All 29 senior residents in our program participated in the OSCE, including 15 PGY-3 and 14 PGY-4 residents. The median OSCE score for all participants was 354 [interquartile range (IQR) 343–361]. Residents had performed a median of 341[IQR 289–409] total scans, including 105 [IQR 87–120] cardiac, 79 [IQR 65–96] FAST, 48 [IQR

36–64] thoracic, 15 [IQR 12–10] pelvic, 16 [IQR 10–21] biliary, 15 [IQR 13–19] aorta and 3 [IQR 1–5] deep vein thrombosis. The LOWESS smoother curve suggested a pattern of increase and then a plateau in OSCE total score as total scan numbers increased (Fig. 1). Residents who had previously performed more than 300 scans had a slightly higher median OSCE score (355 [IQR 350–360]) than residents who had performed fewer than or equal to 300 scans (342 [IQR 326–361]), $p=0.04$. The median OSCE score for PGY-3 residents was 354 [IQR 346–364], while the median score for PGY-4 residents was 352 [IQR 335–359], which was not significantly different ($p=0.43$). There was a moderate ICC of 0.61 [CI 0.08–0.88], $p=0.01$, for the 11 residents who had two evaluators.

Discussion

Ultrasound is a multi-faceted skill that involves acquisition of images, interpretation of scans, and knowledge of how to incorporate findings into clinical practice. The evaluation of ultrasound competency also requires a multi-modal approach. OSCEs have been found to be a useful tool for measuring ultrasound proficiency, as both scanning technique and interpretation can be assessed in real time [17–20].

The results of this small single residency program study demonstrate that a higher number of scans performed were associated with higher performance on the OSCE with graphical review of the data suggesting a plateau around 300 scans. Defining a minimum number of scans required to attain competency can be challenging, and the current ACEP recommendation of 150–300 scans is a wide target. Our data intimates that within the suggested range of ultrasounds recommended by ACEP, there may be a plateau effect at the higher range of this requirement, but further investigation should be aimed at determining whether this plateau is consistent in different cohorts or rather may be institutionally dependent and vary with training methodologies. We found that in our cohort, a cutoff of 300 overall scans showed a small division in OSCE performance between residents, although it is unclear if this is clinically significant.

A recent study by Blehar et al. suggested that ultrasound image accuracy improved with the number of scans performed up to a "plateau" point where additional scan numbers did not greatly increase accuracy [24]. Our LOWESS curve of OSCE score and prior scan numbers also suggests an asymptotic pattern. This is similar to the concept outlined in the Pusic et al. paper on learning curves, in which medical training is correlated with rising skill level until competence is gained, after which

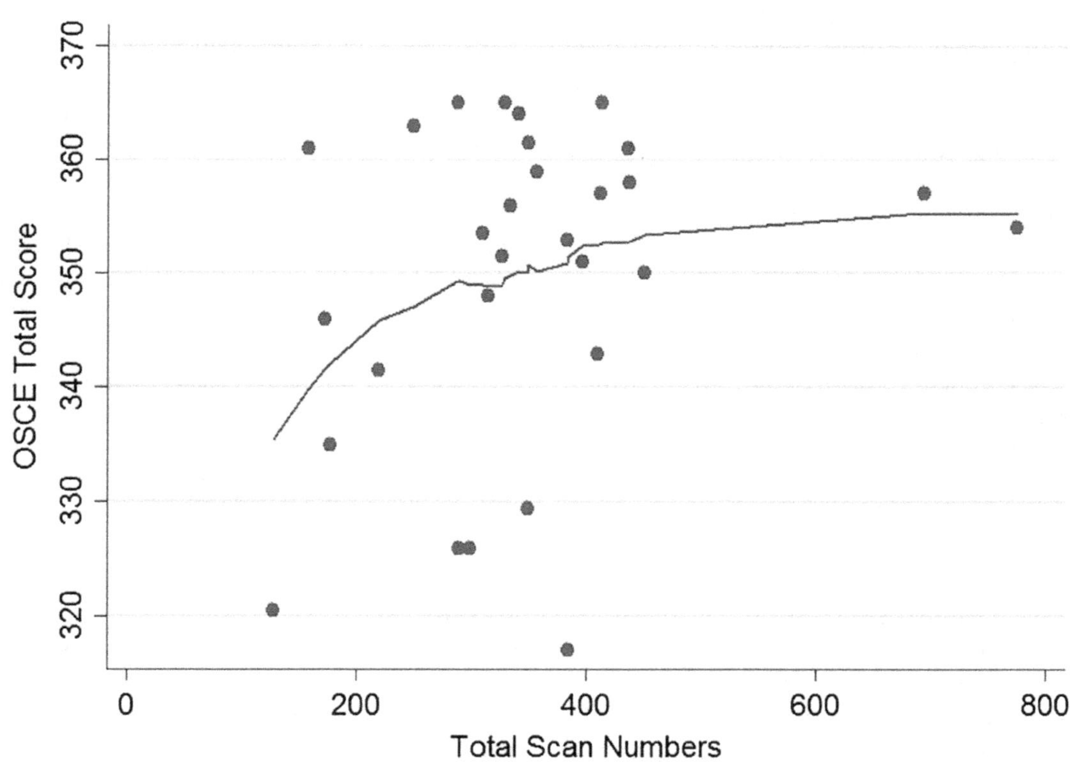

Fig. 1 Scatter plot of observed structured clinical exam (OSCE) total score vs. total ultrasound scan numbers fit with locally weighted scatter plot smoothing (LOWESS) curve

increasing proficiency becomes more subtle despite additional practice [25]. Due to the varied complexity of ultrasound modalities, Blehar et al. found that proficiency for different ultrasound applications plateaued at different scan numbers [24]. We assessed scan proficiency as an aggregate, but were unable to analyze separate proficiency for each modality due to limited sample size.

It would also be valuable to identify a scan number requirement for credentialing physicians who are currently practicing. However, it is unclear if data obtained from emergency medicine residency training programs would be applicable to physicians who did not have structured ultrasound teaching during residency, or whether the plateau effect would differ based on the practice setting. Further investigation to examine the performance of competency assessment tools in a multi-center observational study across a variety of settings is indicated to better characterize the relationship between ultrasound numbers and observed performance in aggregate and within modalities.

This study has several limitations. It was performed at a single residency program with a small sample size and may not be generalizable outside of our institution or beyond emergency medicine. Although OSCE performance visually appeared to plateau around 300 scans, the clinical significance of this number is unclear. Only one resident had less than 150 scans and thus we did not evaluate a cutoff value of 150 scans. Residents had performed a larger percentage of cardiac and FAST examinations than the other modalities. The pattern of OSCE performance and plateau as an aggregate may be affected by this uneven scan number distribution, which included several modalities with median scan numbers below the ACEP-recommended benchmark for individual ultrasound applications [9]. Absolute number of ultrasounds performed may not be a reliable measure of a resident's comprehensive ultrasound education, as it does not include instruction during the ultrasound elective, informal clinical teaching or exposure to a variety of pathology. Furthermore, residents' ultrasounds were completed under the supervision of ultrasound-certified attending physicians and were often accompanied by real-time teaching and quality assurance review. There is a possibility that the database underrepresents actual scanning activity considering scans performed outside of the emergency department or those not properly documented would not have been captured.

The OSCE was created by the ultrasound faculty at our institution and has not been independently validated, although it had gone through an iterative process of improvement and has been used in multiple different clinical contexts over the past 4 years [17, 22, 23]. There was only moderate reliability between faculty who administered OSCE to the same resident, which indicates that the OSCE may require additional standardization to be a reliable measure of ultrasound proficiency. Small sample size precluded sub-group analysis of correlation between OSCE score and prior scan numbers for the individual ultrasound applications.

Conclusion

The results of this small single residency program study suggest a pattern of improvement in OSCE performance as scan numbers increased, with the appearance of a plateau effect around 300 scans. While these are interesting findings for the assessment of ultrasound competency, additional investigation of this correlation in diverse practice environments and within individual ultrasound modalities will be necessary to create generalizable recommendations for scan requirements needed as part of overall POCUS competency assessment.

Abbreviations

POCUS: point-of-care ultrasound; EM: emergency medicine; OSCE: observed structured clinical exam; FAST: Focused Assessment with Sonography in Trauma; PGY: postgraduate year; IQR: interquartile range; ACEP: American College of Emergency Physicians; ACGME: Accreditation Council for Graduate Medical Education; LOWESS: locally weighted scatter plot smoothing; ICC: intraclass correlation; CI: confidence interval.

Authors' contributions

YD contributed to the data analysis and was the major contributor in writing the manuscript. PCH was involved in study design, data collection and in writing the manuscript. SST assisted with statistics and manuscript revisions. WC was involved in study design, data collection and review of the manuscript. JSR, ASL, VK and VEN were involved in data collection and manuscript revisions. HHK was responsible for project design, data collection and was a major contributor in writing the manuscript. All authors read and approved the final manuscript.

Author details

[1] Department of Emergency Medicine, Stanford University School of Medicine, 900 Welch Road Suite 350, Palo Alto, CA 94304, USA. [2] Department of Emergency Medicine, Brigham and Women's Hospital, Boston, MA, USA. [3] Department of Emergency Medicine, Mills-Peninsula Medical Center, Burlingame, CA, USA. [4] Department of Emergency Medicine, Hospital of the University of Pennsylvania, Philadelphia, PA, USA. [5] Department of Emergency Medicine, Cooper University Hospital, Camden, NJ, USA. [6] Department of Emergency Medicine, Massachusetts General Hospital and Harvard Medical School, Boston, MA, USA. [7] Department of Emergency Medicine, UP Health System-Marquette, Marquette, MI, USA. [8] Department of Emergency Medicine, University Hospitals-Cleveland Medical Center, Cleveland, OH, USA.

Acknowledgements

Not applicable.

References

1. Schnobrich D, Gladding S, Olson A et al (2013) Point-of-care ultrasound in internal medicine: a national survey of educational leadership. J Grad Med Educ. 5(3):498–502
2. Meineri M, Bryson GL, Arellano R et al (2018) Core point-of-care ultrasound curriculum: what does every anesthesiologist need to know? Can J Anesth/Journal canadien danesthésie. 65(4):417–426
3. Bornemann P (2017) Assessment of a novel point-of-care ultrasound curriculums effect on competency measures in family medicine graduate medical education. J Ultrasound Med 36(6):1205–1211

4. Beal EW, Sigmond BR, Sage-Silski L et al (2017) Point-of-care ultrasound in general surgery residency training: a proposal for milestones in graduate medical education ultrasound. J Ultrasound Med 36(12):2577–2584
5. Strony R, Marin J, Bailitz J et al (2018) Systemwide clinical ultrasound program development: an expert consensus model. West J Emerg Med 19(4):649–653
6. Reardon R, Heegaard B, Plummer D et al (2006) ultrasound is a necessary skill for emergency physicians. Acad Emerg Med 13(3):334–336
7. Moore C, Gregg S, Lambert M (2004) Performance, training, quality assurance, and reimbursement of emergency physician-performed ultrasonography at academic medical centers. J Ultrasound Med 23(4):459–466
8. Accreditation Council for Graduate Medical Education, American Board of Emergency Medicine. The Emergency Medicine Milestone Project. https://www.acgme.org/Portals/0/PDFs/Milestones/EmergencyMedicineMilestones.pdf. Accessed 12 June 2017
9. American College of Emergency Physicians (2017) Ultrasound guidelines: emergency, point of care, and clinical ultrasound guidelines in medicine. Ann Emerg Med 69(5):e27–e54
10. Akhtar S, Theodoro D, Gaspari R et al (2009) Resident training in emergency ultrasound: consensus recommendations from the 2008 council of emergency medicine residency directors conference. Acad Emerg Med 16:S32–S36
11. Lewiss R, Pearl M, Nomura J et al (2013) CORD-AEUS: consensus document for the emergency ultrasound milestone project. Acad Emerg Med 20(7):740–745
12. Costantino T, Burton J, Tayal V (2015) Ultrasound competency and practice: what's in a number? Acad Emerg Med 22(5):597–599
13. Ahern M, Mallin MP, Weitzel S et al (2010) Variability in ultrasound education among emergency medicine residencies. West J Emerg Med. 11(4):314–318
14. Costantino TG, Satz WA, Stahmer SA et al (2003) Predictors of success in emergency medicine ultrasound education. Acad Emerg Med 10(2):180–183
15. Nelson M, Abdi A, Adhikari S et al (2016) Goal-directed focused ultrasound milestones revised: a multiorganizational consensus. Acad Emerg Med 23(11):1274–1279
16. Stolz LA, Stolz U, Fields JM et al (2017) Emergency medicine resident assessment of the emergency ultrasound milestones and current training recommendations. Acad Emerg Med 24(3):353–361
17. Henwood P, Mackenzie D, Rempell J et al (2016) Intensive point-of-care ultrasound training with long-term follow-up in a cohort of Rwandan physicians. Trop Med Int Health 21(12):1531–1538
18. Hofer M, Kamper L, Sadlo M et al (2011) Evaluation of an OSCE assessment tool for abdominal ultrasound courses. Ultraschall Med 32(02):184–190
19. Sisley A, Johnson S, Erickson W et al (1999) Use of an objective structured clinical examination (OSCE) for the assessment of physician performance in the ultrasound evaluation of Trauma. J Trauma 47(4):627
20. Sornsuphalimchareon S, Puwichcharoenchue P, Jitrapornintrarak J (2018) Factors affecting objective structured clinical examination scores of final year medical students in the evaluation of focused assessment with sonography for Trauma. J Contemp Med Educ 7(2):42
21. Amini R, Adhikari S, Fiorello A (2014) Ultrasound competency assessment in emergency medicine residency programs. Acad Emerg Med 21(7):799–801
22. Henwood P, Mackenzie D, Rempell J et al (2014) A practical guide to self-sustaining point-of-care ultrasound education programs in resource-limited settings. Ann Emerg Med 64(3):277–285.e2
23. Bell G, Wachira B, Denning G (2016) A pilot training program for point-of-care ultrasound in Kenya. Afr J Emerg Med. 6(3):132–137
24. Blehar D, Barton B, Gaspari R (2015) Learning curves in emergency ultrasound education. Acad Emerg Med 22(5):574–582
25. Pusic MV, Boutis K, Hatala R et al (2015) Learning curves in health professions education. Acad Med 90(8):1034–1042

4

Evaluation of a short formation on the performance of point-of-care renal ultrasound performed by physicians without previous ultrasound skills: prospective observational study

François Javaudin[1], François Mounier[1], Philippe Pes[1], Idriss Arnaudet[1], Frédéric Vignaud[1], Eric Frampas[2], Philippe Le Conte[1*] and Winfocus-France study group

Abstract

Background: Point-of-Care Ultrasound (PoCUS) is recommended by emergency medicine societies for the detection of hydronephrosis. Training of certified Emergency Physicians (EP) without prior ultrasound experience remains debated. We investigate performance of a brief training session for the detection of hydronephrosis with PoCUS performed by EP without previous ultrasound experience.

Patients and methods: This was a prospective observational study of a convenience sample of patients older than 18 years with presumed renal colic, acute pyelonephritis or documented acute renal failure. Exclusion criteria were pregnancy and documented end of life.After inclusion and informed consent, a PoCUS was performed. A radiologist's renal ultrasound (RRUS) was then conducted, the radiologist being blind to PoCUS result.The objective was to determine the diagnostic performance of PoCUS performed by EP for the detection of hydronephrosis using RRUS as gold standard.

Results: Six EP participated in this study. 55 patients were included, five secondary excluded for lack of RRUS. Age was 47 ± 22 years, sex ratio 1. Hydronephrosis prevalence was 38% (CI 95% [26–52%]). Sensitivity of PoCUS was 100% (CI 95% [82–100%]) while its specificity was 71% (CI 95% [52–86%]) with a NPV of 100% (CI 95% [85–100%]) and a 68% (CI 95% [48–84%]) PPV. Kappa coefficient was 0.65 (CI 95% [0.45–0.85]).

Discussion: We demonstrated that a short training program enables EP without previous ultrasound skills to rule out hydronephrosis with satisfactory performances. The main limitation was the absence of collection of the number of PoCUS by EP. After this didactic course, an experiential phase must be carried out.

Keywords: Point-of-care ultrasound, Hydronephrosis, Training, Evaluation

Introduction

A renal ultrasound (RUS) is mandatory in suspected renal colic (RC), acute pyelonephritis (AP) and acute renal failure (ARF) in search of hydronephrosis because management would be altered. A review on point-of-care ultrasound (PoCUS) found that sensitivity ranged from 72 to 97% and specificity from 73 to 83% for the presence of hydronephrosis [3]. Emergency Medicine Societies promote usage of PoCUS in suspected renal colic [1, 4, 10].

The training of certified Emergency Physicians (EP) with no prior ultrasound (US) experience remains debated.

*Correspondence: philippe.leconte@chu-nantes.fr
[1] Service des urgences, Centre Hospitalier Universitaire de Nantes, 44035 Nantes cedex, Nantes, France
Full list of author information is available at the end of the article

Philippe Pes, Idriss Arnaudet—Winfocus-France member
Philippe Pes—Winfocus international member

In our institution, such EP participates to a 16-h training program over a 2-day period (USLS-BL1 endorsed by WINFOCUS International). The program includes operation of ultrasound device, interpretation of normal and pathological images to assess hydronephrosis, free peritoneal and pericardial fluid, proximal deep venous thrombosis, pulmonary and first-grade cardiac ultrasound. Approximately half of the time is spent performing imaging under supervision. The aim of this prospective observational survey was to assess the accuracy of renal PoCUS after this course compared with radiologist's RUS (RRUS) as a gold standard.

Patients and methods

This was a prospective study of a convenience sample of patients with presumed RC, AP or documented ARF. It was undertaken in the ED of a tertiary teaching hospital with an annual census of 75,000 from August 2014 to March 2015. This study was approved by the Ethics Committee of Nantes University Hospital (reference RC15_0443).

The inclusion criteria for patients were a suspected RC, AP or documented ARF in patients older than 18 years of age. Exclusion criteria were pregnancy, RRUS nearly completed, documented end of life precluding further investigation. Patients for whom RRUS was not performed were secondarily excluded.

Participating EP were recruited in our ED. Inclusion criteria were the absence of previous POCUS exposure before participation to our study, in particular, no POCUS course during their medical school nor during their EM residency. They committed themselves to not follow another POCUS training until conclusion of the study.

After inclusion, information and consent to participate, a PoCUS was performed. A RRUS was then realized, the radiologist being blind to PoCUS result. Only the RRUS result was used for the management of the patients.

Using a Philips CX50 (Philips, Netherlands) with a 3.5–5 MHz curved array probe, EP obtained images of both kidneys. They completed a reporting form including demographic data, the presence or absence of hydronephrosis for each kidney. It was defined as a dilatation of the collective system. Finally, the difficulty for the PoCUS was assessed.

Formal RRUS was performed by radiologist with usual devices in the radiology department. A report was then filled with the same items.

The objective of this study was to assess the accuracy of renal PoCUS after a brief course compared with radiologist's RUS (RRUS) as a gold standard. As a part of our policy, computed tomography is not performed in this clinical setting. The main objective was sensitivity and negative predictive value (NPV) of PoCUS. Secondary objectives were concordance explored by Kappa coefficient, specificity, positive predictive value (PPV) and likelihood ratios. The required number of subjects for sensitivity 0.9 with alpha risk 0.05 and beta 0.10 was 38.

Values stored in Microsoft Excel™ were analyzed with Graphpad™. 95% confidence intervals were calculated for sensitivity, specificity, NPV, PPV, likelihood ratios and concordance.

Results

Six EP participated to this study, four women and two men, mean age 37 ± 7 years old. Mean time since their certification in Emergency Medicine was 7 ± 7 years. 55 patients were included, five secondarily excluded because of lack of RRUS (Fig. 1). Age was 47 ± 22 years, sex ratio 1. There were 31 RC, 9 AP and 10 ARF. Hydronephrosis prevalence was 38% [26–52%]. Sensitivity and NPV were 100% [79–100%] and 100% [81–100%], respectively. Specificity and PPV were 68% [47–83.4%] and 71% [53–81%], respectively. Positive likelihood ratio was 3.4 [2.0–6.0], negative likelihood ratio was 0.0 [0.0–NC] and Kappa coefficient was 0.65 [0.45–0.85] (Table 1). PoCUS difficulty was assessed as difficult (two patients, 4%), medium (13 patients, 26%) or easy (35 patients, 70%).

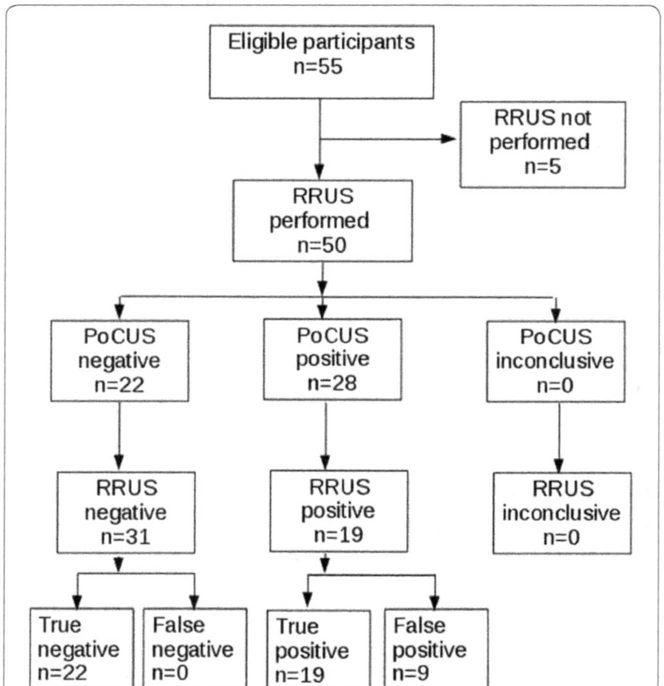

Fig. 1 STARD chart of patients included in a prospective study exploring PoCUS accuracy

Table 1 Results of PoCUS compared with RRUS for hydronephrosis in 50 patients

	RRUS +	RRUS −
PoCUS +	19 (38%)	9 (18%)
PoCUS −	0 (0%)	22 (44%)
	Sensitivity: 100% [82–100%] NPV: 100% [85–100%]	Specificity: 71% [52–86%] PPV: 68% [48–84%]

PoCUS point-of-care ultrasound; *RRUS* radiologist's renal ultrasound; *NPV* negative predictive value; *PPV* positive predictive value

Discussion

We found that this training enabled EP without previous US skills to exclude hydronephrosis with good performance. Indeed, all hydronephrosis on RRUS were detected by POCUS performed by EP ($n = 19$) and none ($n = 0$) was detected by RRUS when POCUS was negative. That is why sensitivity and NPV were 100%. However, specificity and PPV were not sufficient. Kappa value indicated a good strength of agreement.

Limitations were the absence of collection of the number of PoCUS by EP and the absence of collection of the delay between PoCUS and RRUS.

The choice of sensitivity as the primary objective was motivated by the fact that hydronephrosis is rare both in ARF [7], AP [2] and is present in only 18% in ED's acute flank pain patients [9]. Thus, the ability of an EP to rule out hydronephrosis should be more helpful than to confirm its presence. PoCUS might be seen as a screening tool with a high sensitivity and NPV.

Training in ultrasound of certified EP is a challenging problem since many physicians does not use it in every day practice. In USA, a survey performed in Connecticut in 2014 showed that 24% used PoCUS on a daily basis [5]. In Europe, there is a lack of such information but the situation might not be quite different. However, PoCUS is now strongly recommended by Emergency Medicine Societies [1, 4, 10] and is an integrate part of the Emergency medicine curriculum [10]. The American College of Emergency Physicians has formalized the training pathway for EP without previous ultrasound skills [1]. It begins with a didactic course followed by an experiential phase of supervised ultrasounds. A similar PoCUS training pathway is proposed in United Kingdom [10]. Performance of short training period has been investigated in a Spanish study [8] with similar results as ours. The learning curve in the detection of hydronephrosis has been evaluated, the best results were obtained after 30 exams [6].

In conclusion, we demonstrated that a short training program allows EP without previous US skills to rule out hydronephrosis with good performances. The experiential phase of supervised ultrasounds must be carried out.

Authors' contributions

PLC and FJ designed the study; FJ and FM retrieved and entered data; FM, PLC and PP analyzed data and wrote the article; IA, PP, and FV made the training session; EF was responsible for the radiology US. All authors read and approved the final manuscript.

Author details

[1] Service des urgences, Centre Hospitalier Universitaire de Nantes, 44035 Nantes cedex, Nantes, France. [2] Service de radiologie, Centre Hospitalier Universitaire de Nantes, Nantes, France.

Acknowledgements

We are indebted to Emmanuel Montassier, MD, Ph.D. for his English review of the paper.

References

1. ACEP (2016) Ultrasound Guidelines: emergency, point-of-care, and clinical ultrasound guidelines in medicine. Ann Emerg Med 69(5):e27–e54
2. Carnell J, Fischer J, Nagdev A (2011) Ultrasound detection of obstructive pyelonephritis due to urolithiasis in the ED. Am J Emerg Med 29:e1-843. https://doi.org/10.1016/j.ajem.2010.07.006
3. Dalziel PJ, Noble VE (2013) Bedside ultrasound and the assessment of renal colic: a review. Emerg Med J 30:3–8. https://doi.org/10.1136/emermed-2012-201375
4. Duchenne J, Martinez M, Rothmann C, Claret P-G, Desclefs J-P, Vaux J, Miroux P, Ganansia O (2016) First level of clinical ultrasound in emergency medicine. French Society of Emergency Medicine (SFMU) guidelines by formal consensus. Ann Fr Médecine Urgence 6(4):1–12. https://doi.org/10.1007/s13341-016-0649-5
5. Herbst MK, Camargo CA Jr, Perez A, Moore CL (2015) Use of point-of-care ultrasound in Connecticut emergency departments. J Emerg Med 48(191–196):e2. https://doi.org/10.1016/j.jemermed.2014.09.017
6. Jang TB, Jack Casey R, Dyne P, Kaji A (2010) The learning curve of resident physicians using emergency ultrasonography for obstructive uropathy. Acad Emerg Med 17:1024–1027. https://doi.org/10.1111/j.1553-2712.2010.00850.x
7. Skarupskiene I, Balciuviene V, Ziginskiene E, Kuz STARD, Diagram minskis V, Vaiciuniene R, Bumblyte IA (2016) Changes of etiology, incidence and outcomes of severe acute kidney injury during a 12-year period (2001–2012) in large university hospital. Nephrol Ther 12:448–453. https://doi.org/10.1016/j.nephro.2016.03.003
8. Torres-Macho J, Antón-Santos JM, García-Gutierrez I, de Castro-García M, Gámez-Díez S, de la Torre PG, Latorre-Barcenilla G, Majo-Carbajo Y, Reparaz-González JC, de Casasola GG, Working Group of Clinical Ultrasound, Spanish Society of Internal Medicine (2012) Initial accuracy of bedside ultrasound performed by emergency physicians for multiple indications after a short training period. Am J Emerg Med 30:1943–1949. https://doi.org/10.1016/j.ajem.2012.04.015
9. Westphalen AC, Hsia RY, Maselli JH, Wang R, Gonzales R (2011) Radiological imaging of patients with suspected urinary tract stones: national trends, diagnoses, and predictors. Acad Emerg Med 18:699–707. https://doi.org/10.1111/j.1553-2712.2011.01103.x
10. Ultrasound training. http://www.rcem.ac.uk/RCEM/Exams_Training/UK_Trainees/Ultrasound_Training/RCEM/Exams_Training/UK_Trainees/Ultrasound_Training.aspx?hkey=b0565712-6409-49b9-96c3-eafbda02a404. Accessed 5 Feb 2017

5

Point-of-care ultrasound diagnosis of stump appendicitis in the emergency department

Apichaya Monsomboon[1,2], Bret P. Nelson[1], Phillip Andrus[1] and James W. Tsung[1*]

Abstract

Background: Stump appendicitis (SA) is a rare entity in patients with a history of appendectomy and may result in missed or delayed diagnosis. We report a case of SA diagnosed by emergency department (ED) point-of-care ultrasound (PoCUS) in an elderly woman, thus expediting her care.

Case presentation: An elderly female patient with a history of appendectomy 27 years ago was referred by her physician to the ED with right lower quadrant pain for 2 days. Using PoCUS the emergency physician identified SA. This was confirmed by computed tomography (CT) scan. The patient was then successfully managed non-operatively using antibiotics.

Conclusions: Despite its rarity, it is feasible to diagnose SA using PoCUS, as patients presenting with right lower quadrant pain and history of appendectomy are at risk for delayed diagnosis, perforation, and poor outcome. PoCUS may reduce time to diagnosis, time to definitive operative or non-operative management, and minimize morbidity.

Background

Stump appendicitis (SA) is a rare long-term complication of appendectomy. It is defined as the interval development of inflammation of the remaining appendix after an appendectomy [1]. The signs and symptoms are the same as acute appendicitis, thus making the diagnosis difficult. History of past appendectomy often leads to delayed or missed diagnosis that can cause morbidity. Perforation rate of SA reportedly ranges from 40 to 70% [1, 2].

SA was first described by Rose in 1945 [3], with a reported incidence of 1 in 50,000 cases [1]. However, the exact prevalence is not known [4] and likely underreported as it may imply inadequate surgical technique [5]. Buttrick et al. [6] conducted a 5-year case review of 3252 appendectomies at our institution, which revealed only two cases of SA yielding a prevalence of approximately 0.06%. In a 60-year review by Subramanian and Liang, patients presented a mean of 108 ± 20 months after initial appendectomy [5]. It was unclear if there were specific high-risk features for the development of SA [5]. However, they noted in their review that SA occurred after both open and laparoscopic appendectomies. Additionally, they noted that the mean length of the residual stump was 3.3 cm (range 0.5–6.5 cm) with no patient reported to have SA with residual stump < 0.5 cm [5]. The most common presenting symptom was abdominal pain (93%) with 77% of patients having right lower quadrant pain [5]. Fifty-seven percent of patients presented with gastrointestinal symptoms, including nausea and vomiting [5]. The differential diagnoses of right lower quadrant abdominal pain in patients with history of appendectomy are listed in Table 1 [4].

We report the first case of SA identified by point-of-care ultrasound (PoCUS) and was successfully managed non-operatively.

Case report

A 69-year-old female was referred to the emergency department (ED) by her primary care physician with right lower quadrant abdominal pain for 2 days. She had nausea but no vomiting, fever, or diarrhea. She reported a history of appendectomy 27 years ago. Her past medical history included rheumatic heart disease with prolapsed mitral valve and hypothyroidism.

*Correspondence: jtsung@gmail.com
[1] Division of Emergency Ultrasound, Department of Emergency Medicine, Icahn School of Medicine at Mount Sinai, New York, NY, USA
Full list of author information is available at the end of the article

Table 1 Differential diagnosis of right lower quadrant pain after appendectomy

Meckel's diverticulitis	Psoas abscess
Cecal diverticulitis	Cholecystitis
Regional enteritis	PID
Leaking aneurysm	Torsion of ovarian cyst
Abdominal wall hematoma	Mittelschmerz
Ureteral stone	Endometriosis
Seminal vesiculitis	Mesenteric adenitis
Prostatitis	Right lower lobe pneumonia
Acute testicular disease	Appendiceal stump abscess

Physical examination revealed a temperature of 35.8 °C (96.4 °F), with otherwise stable vital signs. She had appendectomy scar and tenderness in the right lower quadrant without guarding or rebound tenderness. Her white blood cell count was 7.4×10^9/L with neutrophils 62.5%.

PoCUS demonstrated a non-compressible blind-ended tubular structure measuring 9.4 mm in diameter (Fig. 1a) connecting to cecum, surrounding with small amount of free fluid and fat stranding (Fig. 1b). Subsequent computed tomography (CT) scan of the abdomen and pelvis confirmed these findings (Fig. 2). Video link: https://youtu.be/BH5VrGYcfYc.

The patient was admitted and administered intravenous piperacillin–tazobactam. Given her history of rheumatic heart disease, non-operative management was chosen. One day after admission, her clinical examination significantly improved with no peritoneal signs. She was discharged with a 10-day course of oral levaquin and metronidazole. She had a follow-up CT scan 2 months later which was unremarkable.

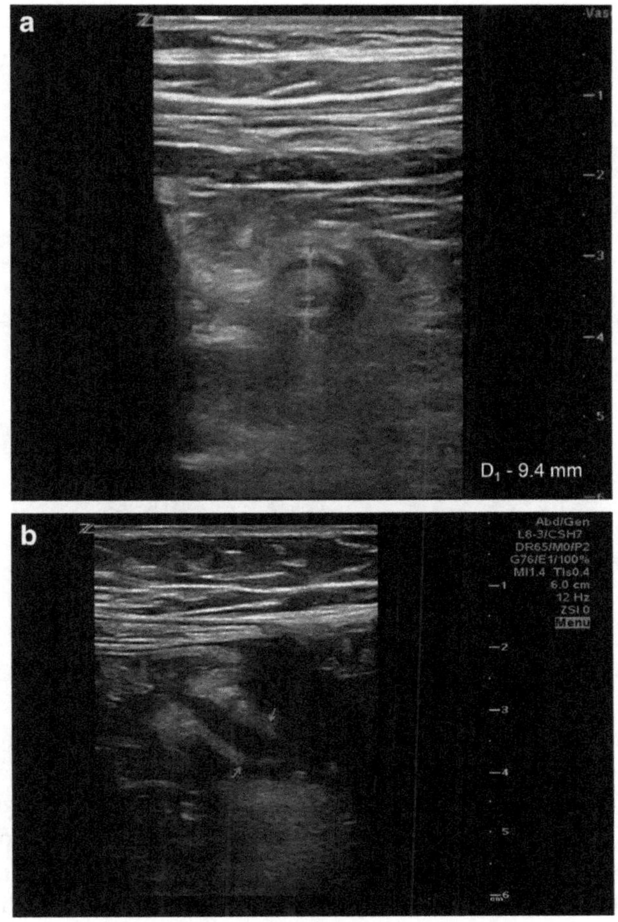

Fig. 1 **a** Transverse (short axis) ultrasound scan shows SA measuring 9.4 mm in diameter. **b** Longitudinal ultrasound scan shows tubular blind-ended structure with surrounding with free fluid

Procedure/technique

In patients who have localized right lower quadrant pain with high clinical suspicion for appendicitis, we recommend scanning the area of maximal tenderness and/or pain using a high-frequency (10–15 MHz) linear transducer. If the appendix is visualized, we try to identify the entire length of the appendix (abnormal cutoff diameter > 6 mm) from tip to base entering the cecum. We demonstrate the appendix in perpendicular orthogonal views (short and long axes). If the pain is non-localizing or more diffuse, we recommend starting at McBurney's point, visualizing the right psoas muscle, identifying a loop of ileum, and then following it to the ileocecal valve and cecum which is often adjacent to the appendix. An enlarged appendix with abnormal cutoff diameter > 6 mm suggests SA. Additionally, compressibility of the SA relative to adjacent bowel is assessed by graded compression [7] or sonopalpation with the ultrasound transducer [8, 9].

Discussion

To our knowledge, this is the first report of SA diagnosed with ED PoCUS. Before the advent of CT scan, definitive preoperative diagnosis of SA was not possible [10]. While CT scan may also diagnose other causes of abdominal pain (Table 1), it may prolong ED length-of-stay [8] and may not be available in low-resource settings. Since Puylaert et al. first described the graded compression technique for diagnosing appendicitis in 1986 [7], radiologist-performed ultrasound for SA, but not PoCUS, has been reported in the literature [5] as having the same as acute appendicitis. Published literature shows that PoCUS by emergency physicians has high specificity (97%) [11] and positive predictive value (91%) [11] to rule-in appendicitis [8, 11–13]. PoCUS can decrease ED length-of-stay compared to radiologist-performed ultrasound and CT scan, avoids radiation [8], and may be

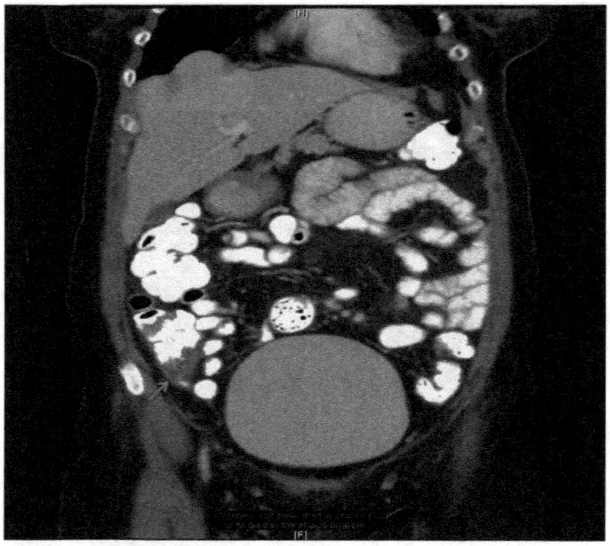

Fig. 2 CT scan shows thickening and inflammatory change of a tubular structure extending from the base of the cecum, surrounding with inflammatory change

performed serially in non-operative management. One literature review of 51 reported cases of SA indicated that radiologist-performed ultrasound may well have a high accuracy in establishing the diagnosis of SA as it does for acute appendicitis, but no studies on sensitivity and specificity for SA have been published [14]. Nevertheless, the choice between ultrasound and CT in this clinical setting is largely dependent on institutional preference and available expertise [5, 14, 15].

A treatment of choice for SA is completion appendectomy either by open or laparoscopic intervention [6, 16]. There is one reported SA case that was successfully treated with non-operative treatment [2] as was our case. However, Hendahewa et al. reported a case of SA which was managed operatively initially, but developed recurrent SA again 3 years later, and subsequently underwent laparoscopic appendectomy [17]. Non-operative management for SA may be suitable for some patients, especially in those patients having multiple comorbidities or at risk for poor outcomes during surgery. Close follow-up in these patients is warranted, as concern for recurrent SA may approach recurrence rates in non-operatively managed appendicitis.

Conclusion

Despite its rarity, it is feasible to diagnose SA using PoCUS, as patients presenting with right lower quadrant pain and history of appendectomy are at risk for delayed diagnosis, perforation, and poor outcome. PoCUS may reduce time to diagnosis, time to definitive operative or non-operative management, and minimize morbidity.

Abbreviations

SA: stump appendicitis; ED: emergency department; CT: computed tomography.

Acknowledgements

None.

Authors' contributions

AM performed the point-of-care ultrasound and acquired the images, conceptualized the case report, drafted the initial manuscript, and approved the final manuscript for publication. BPN and PA provided supervision, reviewed and revised the manuscript for critically important intellectual content, and approved the final manuscript for publication. JWT provided supervision and technical support, revised the manuscript for critically important intellectual content. All authors read and approved the final manuscript.

Author details

[1] Division of Emergency Ultrasound, Department of Emergency Medicine, Icahn School of Medicine at Mount Sinai, New York, NY, USA. [2] Present Address: Department of Emergency Medicine, Siriraj Hospital, Mahidol University, Bangkok, Thailand.

References

1. Liang MK, Lo HG, Marks JL (2006) Stump appendicitis: a comprehensive review of literature. Am Surg 72:162–166
2. Leff DR, Sait MR, Hanief M, Salakianathan S, Darzi AW, Vashisht R (2012) Inflammation of the residual appendix stump: a systematic review. Colorectal Dis 14:282–293
3. Rose TF (1945) Recurrent appendiceal abscess. Med J Aust 1(26):659–662
4. Harris CR (1989) Appendiceal stump abscess ten years after appendectomy. Am J Emerg Med 7:411–412
5. Subramanian A, Liang MK (2012) A 60-year literature review of stump appendicitis: the need for a critical view. Am J Surg 203(4):503–507
6. Buttrick SS, Choi JJ, Divino CM (2012) Stump appendicitis after open and laparoscopic appendectomies. Am Surg 78:143–144
7. Puylaert JB (1986) Acute appendicitis: US evaluation using graded compression. Radiology 158:355–360
8. Elikashvili I, Tay ET, Tsung JW (2014) The effect of point-of-care ultrasonography on emergency department length of stay and computed tomography utilization in children with suspected appendicitis. Acad Emerg Med 21:163–170
9. Faust JS, Tsung JW (2017) Eliciting renal tenderness by sonopalpation in diagnosing acute pyelonephritis. Crit Ultrasound J 9(1):1
10. Rao PM, Sagarin MJ, McCabe CJ (1998) Stump appendicitis diagnosed preoperatively by computed tomography. Am J Emerg Med 16:309–311
11. Fields JM, Davis J, Alsup C et al (2017) Accuracy of point-of-care ultrasonography for diagnosing acute appendicitis: a systematic review and meta-analysis. Acad Emerg Med 24(9):1124–1136
12. Fox JC, Solley M, Anderson CL, Zlidenny A, Lahham S, Maasumi K (2008) Prospective evaluation of emergency physician performed bedside ultrasound to detect acute appendicitis. Eur J Emerg Med 15:80–85
13. Mallin M, Craven P, Ockerse P (2015) Diagnosis of appendicitis by bedside ultrasound in the ED. Am J Emerg Med 33:430–432
14. Kanona H, Al Samaraee A, Nice C, Bhattacharya V (2012) Stump appendicitis: a review. Int J Surg 10:425–428
15. Kosaka N, Sagoh T, Uematsu H, Kimura H, Yamamori S, Miyayama S et al (2007) Difficulties in the diagnosis of appendicitis: review of CT and US images. Emerg Radiol 14:289–295
16. Martínez Chamorro E, Merina Castilla A, Muñoz Fraile B, Koren Fernández L, Borruel Nacenta S (2013) Stump appendicitis: preoperative imaging findings in four cases. Abdom Imaging 38:1214–1219
17. Hendahewa R, Shekhar A, Ratnayake S (2015) The dilemma of stump appendicitis—a case report and literature review. Int J Surg Case Rep 14:101–103

6

Point-of-care ultrasound evaluation and puncture simulation of the internal jugular vein by medical students

José Muniz Pazeli Jr.[1,2*], Ana Luisa Silveira Vieira[1,2], Rosimary Souza Vicentino[1], Luisa Jabour Pazeli[3], Bernardo Costa Lemos[1], Marinna Marques Rodrigues Saliba[1], Pedro Andrade Mello[1] and Maurício Dutra Costa[1]

Abstract

Objectives: To show that medical students can evaluate the internal jugular vein (IJV) and its anatomical variations after rapid and focused training. We also aimed to evaluate the success rate of IJV puncture in simulation following traditional techniques (TTs) and monitored via ultrasound (US).

Materials and methods: Six medical students without experience with US were given 4 h of theoretical–practical training in US, and then evaluated the IJV and common carotid artery (CCA) of 105 patients. They also simulated a puncture of the IJV at a demarcated point, where a TT was theoretically performed.

Results: Adequate images were obtained from 95% of the patients; the IJV, on the right side, was more commonly found in the anterolateral position in relation to the CCA (38%). On the left side, the most commonly position observed was the anterior (36%). The caliber of the IJV relative to the CCA greatly varied. The success rate in the IJV puncture simulation, observed with US, by the TTs was 55%.

Conclusion: The training of medical students to recognize large neck vessels is a simple, quick, and feasible task and that can be integrated into the undergraduate medical curriculum.

Keywords: Central venous catheterization, Medical education, Point-of-care ultrasound

Introduction

Central venous access is the cannulation of a central vein via percutaneous puncture [1]. It is indicated in certain medical situations such as the hemodynamic monitoring of critical ill patients and the infusion of medications, parenteral nutrition, or hemodialysis [2].

Central puncture is typically performed at the jugular, subclavian, or femoral vein [3]. In practice, the internal jugular vein (IJV) is a common site, but recent data show that subclavian puncture is associated with lower rates of infection and thrombosis [4].

Traditionally, puncture of a central vein is performed as the "blind" insertion of a needle following anatomical landmarks [5]. Puncture of the IJV for central venous access was first described in 1969 [6]. Since then, various other approaches have been proposed: anterior, central, and posterior approaches [7, 8].

While these traditional techniques (TTs) based on anatomical markers have been validated, they are associated with failure rates ranging from 5 to 40% [3] and complications such as pneumothorax, hematoma, hemothorax, lesions of nerves, and others. These occur at rates between 5 and 19% [9].

For these reasons, ultrasound (US) has been recommended since the 1980s to guide the procedure, optimizing successful cannulation and minimizing complications [10].

Over the last two decades, US equipment has become progressively more compact and accessible, facilitating its use at the point of care. Point-of-care ultrasound (POCUS) is performed and interpreted by the physician in charge wherever the patient is located [11]. Therefore,

*Correspondence: pazelijr@hotmail.com
[1] FAME - Barbacena's School of Medicina, Barbacena, Brazil
Full list of author information is available at the end of the article

US is actually an extension of the physical examination, offering the physician a valuable complement to the patient's propedeutic and monitoring in addition to guiding procedures, thus increasing their safety and efficacy [12, 13].

The use of US for central venous access can considerably reduce its risks and complications [5, 14].

Ultrasound-guided techniques (USGTs) can be quickly assimilated by professionals who have no previous experience. Moureau et al. suggested that supervised training ideally spans 16 to 18 h, although the technique has been mastered in less time [15, 16].

In this study, we aimed to show that medical students can evaluate the IJV and its anatomical variations after rapid and focused training. We also aimed to evaluate the success rate of IJV puncture in simulation following TTs and monitored via US.

Methods

Study design

This cross-sectional, observational study used humans and was approved by the Research Ethics Committee from Fundação Hospitalar do Estado de Minas Gerais (FHEMIG) under Protocol Number 59842616.0.0000.5119.

Study settings and population

From November 2016 to April 2017, we enrolled 105 patients hospitalized in the Clinic, Gynecology, and Obstetrics wards at Santa Casa de Misericórdia de Barbacena—Minas Gerais Brazil.

Patients aged at least 18 years of either sex were included. Each indicated agreement to participate in the study by providing their signature or their guardian's signature on the Informed Consent Form.

Excluded were patients with prior central venous access and those who did not agree to participate. Each patient was stable, without critical disease, and denied a prior central venous access.

Study protocol

Six 4th-year medical students without experience with US were selected from the Barbacena's School of Medicine and SUPREMA-Faculty of Medical Sciences and Health of Juiz de Fora. They were given 4 h of theoretical–practical training in US coordinated by an intensivist and nephrologist with extensive experience in TTs and USGTs.

The training included four 60-min stages: (a) a theoretical exposition including TTs, the physical principles of US, and USGTs; (b) a practical demonstration of anatomical markers and positioning the transducer; (c) practical training in ultrasonographic visualization of vessels and simulation of puncture via TTs, using each other as models; and (d) four supervised examinations per student and completion of the report.

Ultrasonographic evaluations were performed using a Sonosite Fujifilm MTurbo portable US (Bothell, WA, USA) equipped with a linear transducer with a frequency between 6 and 13 MHz.

Patients were placed in dorsal decubitus at 0°, and the cervical region was exposed via contralateral rotation of the neck. The apex of the triangle, composed of the clavicle and the two borders of the sternocleidomastoid muscle, was determined. The pulse at the common carotid artery (CCA) was verified, and immediately lateral to that point, the site chosen for the TT was marked with a pen (Fig. 1).

The US evaluation began by positioning the transducer at the marked point. Then, puncture via a TT was simulated by positioning a flexible cotton-coated rod at the marked point (Fig. 2). The artifact caused by the slight compression of this puncture point was visualized on the US screen and an imaginary line between that point and the position of the patient's ipsilateral nipple was drawn. This line corresponds to the path the needle would make in an actual puncture guided by anatomical landmarks. If this line passed through the IJV, it was understood that puncture via a TT would have been effective. If the traced line did not cross the vein path, the TT was deemed a failed attempt (Fig. 3). All exams and simulations were filmed and, shortly thereafter, they were analyzed by two physicians with extensive experience in both puncture techniques.

The evaluation was fully qualitative, and the following variables were obtained: IJV position relative to the

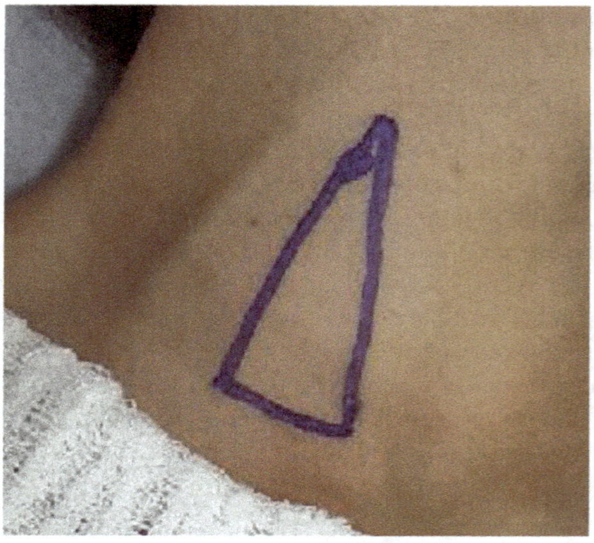

Fig. 1 Identification of the TT puncture point

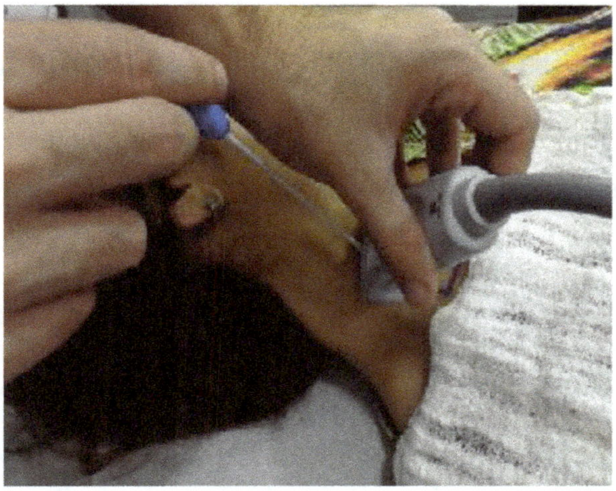

Fig. 2 Simulation of puncture

CCA (medial, anteromedial, lateral, anterolateral, posterior, or anterior); visual estimation of the IJV caliber relative to the CCA (less than 50%, between 50 and 100%, 101 and 150%, 150 and 200%, or greater than 200%); probability of reaching the IJV via the TT relative to the relative size and position of the IJV (success or failure).

Data analysis

Sample size was calculated based on an assumption that more than 12% of the Western population presents significant anatomical variations of the great vessels of the neck, as reported in the literature [17]. Thus, for a power of 80%, with a confidence index of 95%, the minimum sample was 63 individuals [18].

Relationships between studied variables were determined using the Fisher exact test and the Chi square test. Differences were considered significant when $p < 0.05$. Accuracies and their confidence intervals were calculated. Statistical analysis was performed using Stata software, version 9.2 (StataCorp, College Station, TX, USA).

Results

Of 105 patients ranging in age from 18 to 89 years, 82 were women.

Five were excluded because of poor image quality, leaving 100 patients included in the analysis.

On the right side, the IJV was most commonly found in the anterolateral position relative to the carotid artery (38% of the time) and was also found anterior (31%), anteromedial (21%), or lateral (10%) to that artery. In no case was it found in the medial position (Table 1).

On the left side, it was most commonly found in the anterior position (36%) and was also found in the anterolateral (31%), anteromedial (31%), lateral (1%), and

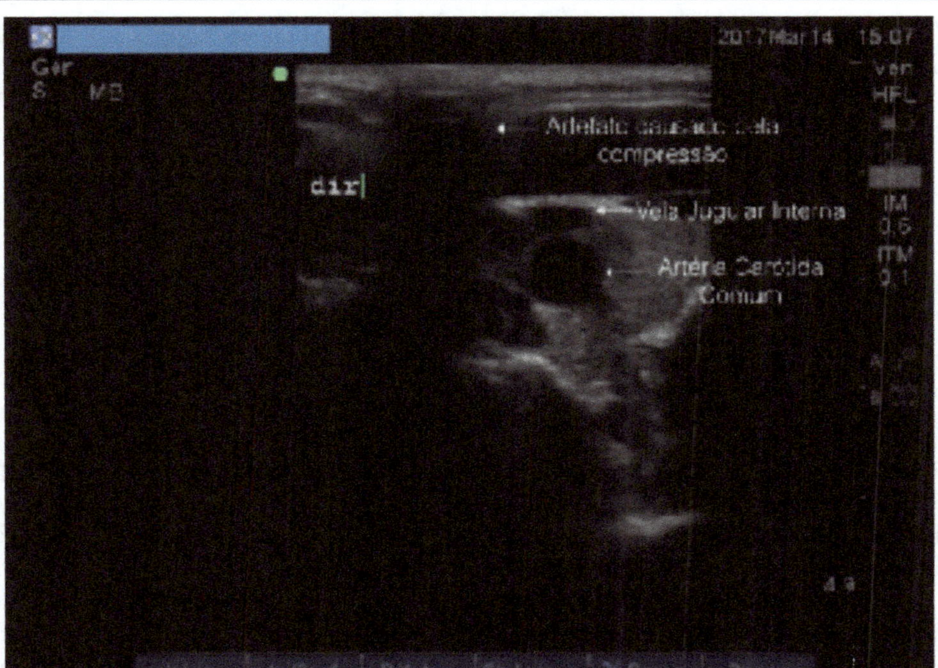

Fig. 3 Observation of the CCA, IJV and the artifact caused by the compression of the point where the puncture would be performed by the TT. In this case, the puncture would not reach the IJV

Table 1 Location of IJV in relation to CCA

	Right side of neck			Left side of neck		
	N	%	CI	*N*	%	CI
Anterior	31	31	(21.9–40.0)	36	36	(26.5–45.4)
Anterolateral	38	38	(28.4–47.5)	31	31	(21.9–40.0)
Lateral	10	10	(13.0–28.9)	1	1	(0.90–2.90)
Anteromedial	21	21	(4.1–15.80)	31	31	(21.9–40.0)
Medial	0			1	1	(0.90–2.90)
Posterior	0			0		

IJV internal jugular vein, *CCA* common carotid artery, *CI* confidence interval

Table 2 Size of IJV in relation to CCA

	Right side *n* = 100			Left side *n* = 100			Total *n* = 200		
	n	%	CI	*n*	%	CI	*n*	%	CI
Collapsed	20	20	(12.1–27.8)	18	18	(10.4–25.5)	38	19	(31.2–44.7)
< 50%	7	7	(1.9–12.0)	10	10	(4.1–15.8)	17	8.5	(11.7–22.2)
50–100%	28	28	(19.1–36.8)	27	27	(18.2–35.7)	55	27.5	(48.1–61.8)
101–150%	11	11	(4.8–17.1)	5	5	(0.7–9.2)	16	8	(10.9–21.0)
151–200%	12	12	(5.6–18.3)	10	10	(4.1–15.8)	22	11	(16.2–27.7)
> 200%	22	22	(13.8–30.1)	30	30	(21.0–38.9)	52	26	(45.0–58.9)
Total	100	100		100	100		200	100	

IJV internal jugular vein, *CCA* common carotid artery, *CI* confidence interval

Table 3 Probability of reaching IJV in relation to the relative size of IJV to CCA

	Yes		No	
	n	%	*n*	%
Collapsed	15	12	23	30.67
< 50%	10	8	7	7
50–100%	29	23.2	26	26
101–150%	13	10.4	3	4
151–200%	16	12.8	6	6
> 200%	42	33.6	10	10
Total	125	100	75	100

IJV internal jugular vein, *CCA* common carotid artery

Chi square = 21.723, $p = 0.001$

Table 4 Probability of reaching IJV in relation to its location in relation to CCA

	Yes		No	
	n	%	*n*	%
Anterior	42	62.69	25	37.31
Anterolateral	43	62.32	26	37.68
Anteromedial	35	67.31	17	32.69
Lateral	5	45.55	6	54.45
Medial	0	0	6	6
Total	125	100	75	100

IJV internal jugular vein, *CCA* common carotid artery

Fischer test $p = 0.478$

medial (1%) positions (Table 1). On both sides, the posterior position and its variables were not found.

The caliber of the IJV relative to the CCA greatly varied, as shown in Table 2.

The probability of reaching the IJV for puncture was related to its size and anatomical position relative to the CCA (Tables 3 and 4).

Several results were noted when the right and left sides of a given patient were compared. One was the number of times the IJV was in a position opposite to the anatomical (medial or anteromedial) position on one side yet in the anatomical (lateral or anterolateral) position on the opposing side. Of the 21 patients in which the vein was anteromedial to the artery on the right side, 19% of the time, it was in the anatomical position on the left side. Of the 32 patients in which the vein was anteromedial or medial on the left side, 28% of the time, it was in an anatomical position on the right side (Table 5).

Table 5 Relationship between anatomical position of IJV and CCA in the right side

Right/left	Anterior		Anterolateral		Anteromedial		Lateral		Medial		Total	
	n	%	*n*	%	*n*	%	*n*	%	*n*	%	*n*	%
Anterior	11	35.5	8	25.8	12	38.7	0	0	0	0	31	100
Anterolateral	16	42.1	15	39.5	6	15.8	1	2.6	0	0	38	100
Anteromedial	6	28.6	4	19.0	11	52.4	0	0	0	0	21	100
Lateral	3	30.0	4	40.0	2	20.0	0	0	1	10	10	100
Medial	0	0	0	0	0	0	0	0	0	0	0	0
Total	36		31		31		1		1		100	100

IJV internal jugular vein, *CCA* common carotid artery

Table 6 Relationship between size of the IJV in relation to CCA in the right (row) and in the left side (column) of the neck

Right/left	Collapsed		< 50%		50–100%		101–150%		151–200%		> 200%		Total	
	N	%	*N*	%	*N*	%	*N*	%	*N*	%	*N*	%	*N*	%
Collapsed	11	55	3	15.0	6	30.0	0	0.0	0	0.0	0	0.0	20	100
< 50%	3	42.8	3	42.8	1	14.3	0	0.0	0	0.0	0	0.0	7	100
50–100%	4	14.3	3	10.7	9	32.1	3	10.7	2	7.1	7	25.0	28	100
101–150%	0	0.0	0	0.0	3	27.7	2	18.9	3	27.3	3	27.3	11	100
151–200%	0	0.0	0	0.0	5	41.6	0	0.0	3	25.0	4	33.3	12	100
> 200%	0	0.0	0	0.0	3	13.6	0	0.0	2	9.1	16	72.7	22	100
Total	18		10		27		5		10		30		100	

IJV internal jugular vein, *CCA* common carotid artery

The size of the vein relative to the artery in the same patient was examined. Of 20 patients in which the IJV was collapsed on the right side, it was not collapsed on the left side 45% of the time. Similarly, of 18 patients in which it was collapsed on the left side, it was not collapsed on the right side 43% of the time (Table 6).

Discussion

These data show that medical students can be trained to recognize the anatomy of large vessels in the neck using US after rapid and focused training. Adequate images were obtained from 95% of the patients chosen for evaluation, reinforcing the simplicity and feasibility of the method.

Puncture of the IJV is a procedure often performed in hospitals, emergency departments, and during prehospital care for a wide range of indications. Although several studies have shown that USGTs are cost-effective, not only for reducing mechanical complications and infections, but primarily for increasing the success rate and reducing procedure time, it is not used routinely, especially in developing countries [14, 19], given the lack of equipment availability, lack of trained professionals, and other reasons [16].

As found by several others [20–23], great anatomical variability is found between the IJV and the CCA. Variability is also seen between the left and right sides of the same individual (Fig. 4). The IJV is in an anatomical position 48% of the time on the right side and 32% of the time on the left side. Use of TTs assumes that the IJV is in an anatomical position on both sides, but this was observed in fewer than 50% of our patients, combining anterolateral and lateral positions.

Additionally, great variability was found in the caliber of the IJV in our sample, and this is also supported by the literature [17, 21]. In our sample, the IJV was completely collapsed on the right and left sides 20% and 18% of the time, respectively (Fig. 5). Puncturing a collapsed vein is nearly impossible, even if the needle is directed correctly. Another complicating factor is that, in our sample, the IJV was anterior to the CCA 68% of the time. Attempting puncture in this condition can have disastrous consequences because of the risk of reaching the CCA, given that vein collapse amplifies this risk.

We emphasize that in our patients, examination was conducted in a supine position with 0° slope despite the recommendation to position the patient in a Trendelenburg, a suggestion that is not always feasible for a variety

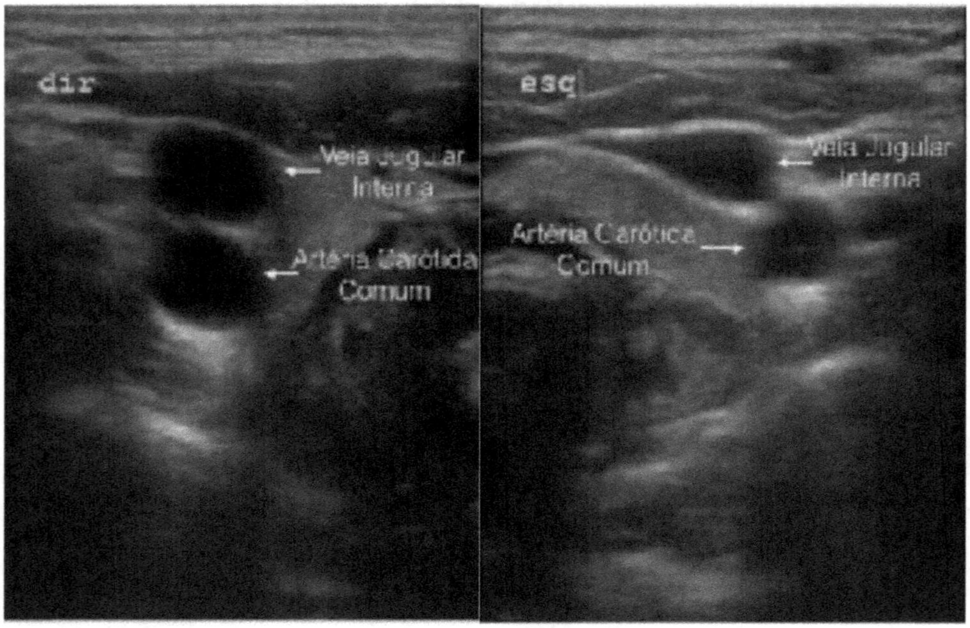

Fig. 4 Right and left IJV of a same patient, anterior and medial to the ACC, respectively

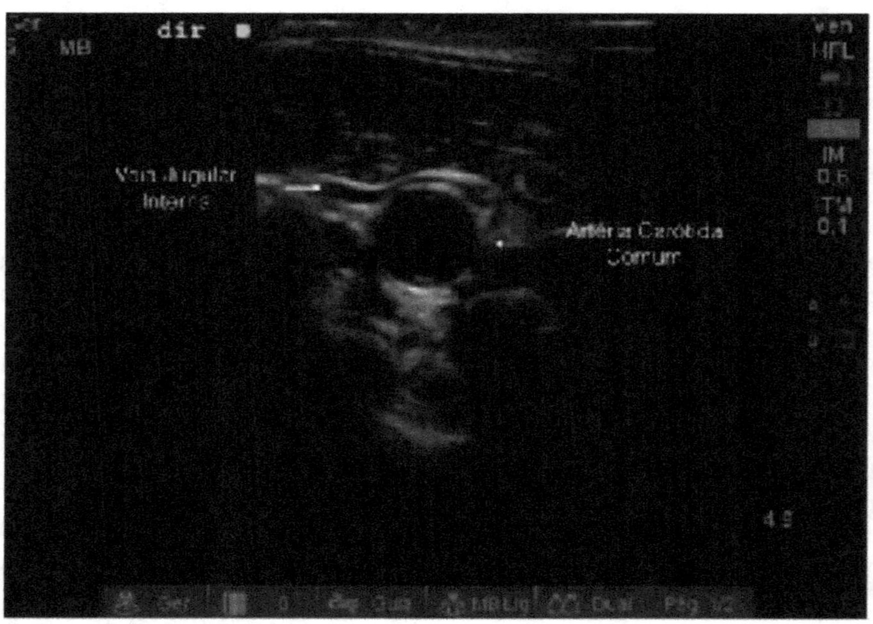

Fig. 5 Right IJV completely collapsed, anterolateral to CCA

of reasons. In this study, contralateral rotation of the neck was used because this position is most frequently recommended in IJV puncture by TTs. However, it has been shown that neck rotation does not interfere with the rate of success and/or reduction of complications when using USGTs [24].

In this study, puncture of the IJV was simulated at the demarcated point, where a TT was theoretically performed (Fig. 1). The success rate using US was determined as well (Fig. 3). Our data show that puncture could reach the IJV 62.5% of the time. Therefore, in 37.5% of the patients (75 of 200 simulations), more than one puncture attempt would be performed, increasing the possibility of complications [25]. The IJV was collapsed in 15 of 125 simulations in which the needle was supposed to reach that vein. Because it is unlikely that puncture is successful with a collapsed vein, we can conclude that the success rate would be 55% for the first attempt, confirming results from studies comparing TTs to USGTs [14, 19].

As suggested by Dinh et al. [26], incorporating training in USGTs in the curriculum for undergraduate medical students is highly desirable and feasible, and this is confirmed by our data. Implementing this and other applications of POCUS in medical schools would ensure that new generations of physicians are naturally empowered, increasing the resoluteness and safety of patient care.

This study is limited by the simulated nature of our procedures; however, actual puncture is not possible for ethical reasons. Also, students performed these procedures after training and without direct supervision, but our objective was to precisely verify the feasibility and simplicity of ultrasonographic visualization of the vessels of the neck after a short period of training. To avoid misinterpretation of the images, all were recorded and reviewed by physicians experienced in POCUS.

Conclusions

These data suggest that training medical students to recognize large neck vessels is a simple, quick, and feasible task and that can be integrated into the undergraduate medical curriculum.

Abbreviations

CCA: common carotid artery; IJV: internal jugular vein; POCUS: point-of-care ultrasound; TTs: traditional techniques; US: ultrasound; USGTs: ultrasound-guided techniques.

Author's contributions

Conceived the idea of the study: JMP Jr and ALSV; Designed the study: JMP Jr; Trained the medical students JMP Jr; Evaluated the patients: BCL; MMRS; MDC; PAM; RSV and LJP; Analysed the exams and simulations: JMP Jr and ALSV; Analysed the data: JMP Jr and ALSV; Wrote the manuscript: JMP Jr; ALSV and LJP; Translated the manuscript to English: JMP Jr; Formatted the manuscript to Critical Ultrasound: JMP Jr; Revised the manuscript: JMP Jr; ALSV; RSV; MMRS; BCL and PAM. All authors read and approved the final manuscript.

Author details

[1] FAME - Barbacena's School of Medicina, Barbacena, Brazil. [2] Federal University of Juiz de Fora, Juiz de Fora, Brazil. [3] SUPREMA - School of Medical Sciences and Health of Juiz de Fora, Juiz de Fora, Brazil.

References

1. Roldan CJ, Paniagua L (2015) Central venous catheter intravascular malpositioning: causes, prevention, diagnosis, and correction. West J Emerg Med 16:658–664
2. Simon PO Jr, Saad WE (2012) Ultrasound-guided vascular access. Ultrasound Clin 7:283–297
3. Maecken T, Grau T (2007) Ultrasound imaging in vascular access. Crit Care Med 35(5 Suppl):S178–S185
4. Parienti JJ et al (2015) Intravascular complications of central venous catheterization by insertion site. N Engl J Med 373:1220–1229
5. McGee DC, Gould MK (2003) Preventing complications of central venous catheterization. N Engl J Med 348:1123–1133
6. English I, Frew RM, Pigott JF, Zaki M (1969) Percutaneous catheterisation of the internal jugular vein. Anaesthesia 24(4):521–531
7. Mostert JW, Kenny GM (1970) Safe placement of central venous catheter into internal jugular veins. Arch Surg 101:431–432
8. Brinkman AJ, Costley DO (1973) Internal jugular venipuncture. JAMA 223(2):182–183
9. Moore CL (2014) Ultrasound first, second, and last for vascular access. J Ultrasound Med 33:1135–1142
10. Lamperti M, Bodenham AR, Pittiruti M et al (2012) International evidence-based recommendations on ultrasound-guided vascular access. Intensive Care Med 38:1105–1117
11. Moore CL, Copel JA (2011) Point-of-care ultrasonography. N Engl J Med 364:749–757
12. Solomon SD, Saldana F (2014) Point-of-care ultrasound in medical education-stop listening and look. N Engl J Med 370:1083–1085
13. Sekiguchi H (2016) Tools of the trade: point-of-care ultrasonography as a stethoscope. Semin Respir Crit Care Med 37:68–87
14. Karakitsos D, Labropoulos N, De Groot E et al (2006) Real-time ultrasound-guided catheterisation of the internal jugular vein: a prospective comparison with the landmark technique in critical care patients. Crit Care 10:R162
15. Moureau N et al (2013) Evidence-based consensus on the insertion of central venous access devices: definition of minimal requirements for training. Br J Anaesth 110:347–356
16. Nguyen BV, Prat G, Vincent JL et al (2013) Determination of the learning curve for ultrasound-guided jugular central venous catheter placement. Intensive Care Med 40:65–73
17. Prasad SR et al (2014) Ultrasonographic study of anatomical characteristics of internal jugular vein in relation to common carotid artery. J Dr NTR Univ Health Sci 3:97–101
18. Santos, Glauber Eduardo de Oliveira. Cálculo amostral on-line. Retrieved: 4 October 2018. http://publicacoesdeturismo.com.br/calculoamostral/
19. Rando K, Castelli J, Pratt JP, Scavino M, Rey G (2014) Ultrasound-guided internal jugular vein catheterization: a randomized controlled trial. Heart Lung Vessels 6(1):13–23
20. Lim CL, Keshava SN, Lea M (2006) Anatomical variations of the internal jugular veins and their relationship to the carotid arteries: a CT evaluation. Australas Radiol 50:314–318
21. Umaña M (2017) Variations in the anatomical relationship between the common carotid artery and the internal jugular vein: an ultrasonographic study. Colomb Med 46:54–57
22. Souza Neto EP, Grousson S, Duflo F, Tahon F, Mottolese C, Dailler F (2014) Ultrasonographic anatomic variations of the major veins in paediatric patients. Br J Anaesth 112:879–884
23. Maecken T, Marcon C, Bomas S, Zenz M, Grau T (2011) Relationship of the internal jugular vein to the common carotid artery: implications for ultrasound-guided vascular access. Eur J Anaesthesiol 28:351–355
24. Lamperti M et al (2012) Is a neutral head position safer than 45-degree neck rotation during ultrasound-guided internal jugular vein cannulation? Results of a randomized controlled clinical trial. Anesth Analg 114:777–784
25. Calvache JA, Rodríguez MV, Trochez A, Klimek M, Stolker RJ, Lesaffre E (2015) Incidence of mechanical complications of central venous catheterization using landmark technique. J Intensive Care Med 31:397–402
26. Dinh VA et al (2016) Medical student core clinical ultrasound milestones. J Ultrasound Med 35:421–434

7

A road map for point-of-care ultrasound training in internal medicine residency

Charles M. LoPresti[1,2], Daniel J. Schnobrich[3], Renee K. Dversdal[4*] and Frank Schembri[5]

Abstract

Background: Ever-expanding uses have been developed for ultrasound, including its focused use at the bedside, often referred to as point-of-care ultrasound (POCUS). POCUS has been well developed and integrated into training in numerous fields, but remains relatively undefined in internal medicine training. This training has been shown to be desirable to both educators and trainees, but has proven difficult to implement. We sought to create a road map for internal medicine residency programs looking to create a POCUS program.

Results: Four internal medicine residency programs that have successfully integrated POCUS training describe their programs, as well as the principles and concepts underlying program development and execution. Review of educational teaching and assessment methods is outlined, as well as suggestions for integration into an already busy residency curriculum. Commonly reported barriers to POCUS implementation such as faculty development, equipment purchasing, resident supervision and quality assurance are addressed. Specific POCUS applications to target are touched upon, and a comparison of applications taught within these four programs suggest that there may be enough similarities to suggest a common curriculum. Finally, future needs are discussed.

Conclusions: POCUS can be successfully taught to internal medicine residents as a part of internal medicine training. Many common elements and principles are evident on review of these four described successful programs. Future support, in the form of endorsed medical society guidelines, will be needed before POCUS is universally incorporated across internal medicine residency training programs.

Keywords: Point-of-care, Education, Internal medicine, Residents

Background

Since it first came into use in the 1960s, medical ultrasound has undergone innumerable improvements and evolutions that have created a tremendously versatile and powerful technology. In addition to its uses by sonographers to create comprehensive images for radiologists, obstetricians, and cardiologists, it is also heavily utilized to increase the safety of procedures, and over the past several decades, point-of-care ultrasound (POCUS) has become increasingly popular. POCUS refers to a focused, often dichotomous use by the treating provider at the bedside, which can be immediately integrated into management decisions. First popularized in emergency medicine, more recently there has been uptake of POCUS in both general and subspecialty internal medicine.

Despite these trends, structured POCUS curricula have only recently started coming into existence in internal medicine residency training [1]. Many IM program directors feel that formal POCUS education should be included in IM residency training, and many learners desire training, but numerous barriers exist including both a lack of formal guidelines and experience by most programs in teaching these skills [2]. In this document, we will outline what is needed to set up and execute a POCUS program to teach a foundational set of skills to internal medicine residents based upon the experience of four successful programs.

*Correspondence: dversdar@ohsu.edu
[4] Department of Medicine, Oregon Health & Science University, 3181 SW Sam Jackson Park Road, Portland, OR 97239-3098, USA
Full list of author information is available at the end of the article

Results

Training in point-of-care ultrasound

A comprehensive training program in POCUS should ideally be competency based and parallel training of other bedside evaluations and diagnostics. Such a program may involve a pre-course need and knowledge assessment, a variety of teaching methods, a post-course evaluation and mechanisms to assess continued competency and quality assurance.

Timing and length of training

Adding POCUS education to an already dense IM curriculum can be a challenging task, and its timing and length may be influenced by the extent of the curriculum to be delivered as well as practical considerations such as the number of available trained faculty, amount of time learners are accessible, and access to resources such as simulation for task training and scanning practice. While some programs have described their brief experiences teaching one discrete POCUS application, numerous IM programs teaching more comprehensive skills have dedicated roughly a 1- to 2-week period to introductory training followed by intermittent reinforcing sessions [3, 4]. In one report, Schnobrich et al. described a 30-h introductory course delivered over 5 days during intern orientation in which learners showed a statistically improved subjective and objective assessment of their ultrasound knowledge and skills in a wide range of skills [5]. Similarly, programs affiliated with Case Western Reserve, Boston University and Oregon Health & Science University have briefer introductory components of ultrasound use during or after intern orientation, but offer subsequent PGY2/3 electives. In all four programs, resident response to these formal curricula have been very positive and demands for more further formal instruction have been universally very strong.

A more frequent longitudinal component to didactic instruction may be beneficial, if sometimes more challenging to implement. Kelm et al. described IM-based training with a shorter initial training period (~ 4 h), but with a subset of residents participating in a longitudinal component involving monthly ultrasound-based morning reports and afternoon ultrasound rounds [6]. The authors found that the group participating in the ongoing training was more likely to correctly identify ascites, renal pathology and pleural effusion on static ultrasound images, and concluded that the addition of a longitudinal component to ultrasound education may result in improved knowledge retention. Regardless of how introductory and basic didactics are delivered, subsequent opportunities to scan patients on the ward or in clinic, integrate findings into management, and receive feedback are highly important to all programs.

Educational methods

A comprehensive POCUS program can be most effective when involving a variety of teaching methods. Many programs utilize some combination of online/in person didactic lectures, pre- or post-course quizzes, live models, simulation task trainers, dedicated ultrasound trainers, and direct patient scanning (Table 1). In several studies, residents were asked to rate the helpfulness of each of the above teaching modalities. IM residents found scanning live models and/or hospitalized or clinic patients, along with didactic lectures to be most helpful. Interestingly, taking and reviewing quizzes were rated as a less effective educational strategy [1, 5].

Table 1 Educational methods in POCUS training

Educational method	Utility
Didactic lectures	Effective for new learners to process the basics of ultrasound, knobology, introductions to specific applications. An interactive approach is helpful, with immediate demonstration of concepts on an ultrasound machine. Online didactics may be used to save instructor time
Procedural task trainers	Individual procedure-oriented trainers such as central line, thoracentesis and paracentesis mannequins, as well as ultrasound-compatible gel-blocks for IV placement
Ultrasound trainers	More costly, comprehensive ultrasound models manufactured by several companies capable of replicating the scanning experience, image acquisition and interpretation. Ultrasound trainers can be used to display idealized normal anatomy, or a variety of expandable pathologies
Live models	Represent a good resource, especially for students immediately after initial didactics. These can be standardized patients or individual learners who are part of the course (if comfort level permits) and are usually used to achieve standard views with normal anatomy. Often rated highly by students
Direct patient scanning	A powerful way for learners to solidify their knowledge. Usually positioned after learners acquire basic image acquisition and interpretation skills, it can be structured as a known or unknown assessment to increase challenge. Often very highly rated by students
Individual portfolio creation	A method to allow continued, independent learning. The learner acquires a collection of saved exams, which is later reviewed and appraised by an instructor

Resident supervision/continued quality assurance

Many medical specialties perform POCUS tailored to their practices, and each is responsible for defining adequate training, competency, and quality assurance in their fields. The American Medical Association (AMA) policy H-230.960 specifically states that the use of ultrasound is not the intellectual property of any one specialty, and each specialty must define for themselves their scope of practice. With this guidance, a comprehensive ultrasound program for IM residencies should include defined, IM-specific competencies with subsequent regular assessment. Like other ACGME patient care-related milestones, this should involve direct trainee assessment, often including the creation of a portfolio for image review and approval. In its current state, many programs will "sign off" on resident ability to use POCUS for procedural guidance, however, diagnostic POCUS is more nuanced, and rigorous quality assurance systems need to be in place prior to granting residents the ability to make clinical decisions on their own.

It is the responsibility of all teaching programs to provide adequate supervision to medical trainees for all of their professional activities. This supervision may be direct or indirect, and is ideally tailored to the learners' demonstrated proficiency, the activity being performed, and institutional resources. This supervision may often be quite challenging for internal medicine training programs, as the majority of teaching faculty are not likely to be proficient themselves. We are aware of a variety of mechanisms employed by teaching programs including partial delegation of supervisory roles to chief residents or other trained educators, the use of image review middleware to provide learners rapid feedback away from patient care, and formalization of entrustment using tools such as the CLUE-CEX exam or a formal entrustable professional activity [7].

Table 2 Core skills taught with emphasis in each residency program

	CWRU	UMN	OHSU	BU
Procedural guidance				
Central venous catheterization	+	+	+	+
Paracentesis	+	+	+	+
Thoracentesis	+	+	+	+
Arthrocentesis	+	–	–	–
Lumbar puncture	#	–	#	–
Peripheral access	+	–	–	+
Peripherally inserted central catheter (PICC)	–	–	–	–
Cardiac				
Pericardial effusion	+	+	+	+
Left ventricular contractility	+	+	+	+
Right ventricular enlargement	+	+	+	+
Chamber size/wall thickness	#	+	#	+
Severe valvular abnormalities	#	–	–	+
Other valvular abnormalities	–	–	–	–
Right atrial pressure (IVC)	+	+	+	+
Wall motion abnormalities	#	–	–	#
Pulmonary				
Pleural effusions	+	+	+	+
Pulmonary edema	+	+	+	+
Consolidation	+	+	#	+
Pneumothorax	+	+	+	+
Abdomen				
Ascites	+	+	+	+
Bladder volume	+	+	+	+
Hydronephrosis	+	+	+	+
Organomegaly	#	+	#	–
AAA	+	–	#	#
Gallbladder	#	–	–	#
Vascular				
Lower extremity DVT	+	–	#	+
Musculoskeletal				
Cellulitis/abscess	+	+	+	+
Muscle/tendon tears	–	–	–	–
Joint effusions	+	–	–	–
Fracture	#	–	–	–
Ophthalmologic				
Optic nerve sheath diameter	–	–	–	–

Additional skills may be presented as time and interest allows

CWRU Case Western Reserve University, *UMN* University of Minnesota, *OHSU* Oregon Health & Science University, *BU* Boston University

"+": Skill taught. "-": Skill not addressed. "#": Skill is demonstrated, but not with the intent for resident use

Point-of-care ultrasound applications

Several factors should be considered when choosing which POCUS applications to teach internal medicine residents. These include the amount of curricular time available, perceived usefulness of the applications, ability of the program to provide opportunities to learn these skills, and evidence that POCUS users can attain these skills in the time available. While no standard curriculum yet exists to guide which application or guidelines should be taught to IM residents, we note a striking agreement amongst the programs at each of our institutions despite being developed independently (Table 2).

Literature and precedent from emergency medicine (EM) are useful in determining the didactic time needed to teach various applications. Simple applications, such as evaluation for abscess, may be taught in as little as 30 min, while more complicated ones, such as cardiac or gallbladder, may take 4–6 h, plus significant additional time for mentored scanning [8, 9]. Notably, EM guidelines specify 16–25 h of didactic time followed by mentored and supervised scanning to teach 6–10 core applications, which has become an accepted standard for demonstrating experience and for credentialing [10]. EM guidelines also note that skills sets may transfer from one application to another, and thus there may be some benefit to teaching multiple skills [9].

Despite the many career paths of IM residents, most programs agree that a core of predominantly cardiac, pulmonary, and abdominal applications should be taught, and may additionally serve as a platform to build advanced skills upon. This is supported by surveys of internal medicine program directors [11], practicing internists [12], and internal medicine residents [2] which suggest that these skills are generally considered the most useful.

A final major consideration is to choose applications that the literature supports can be accomplished by most or all learners. For example, it is generally agreed that POCUS users with core training and 25–50 mentored scans can sufficiently evaluate for pericardial effusions, left ventricular contractility, and right heart function [10]. Other findings, such as most non-severe valvular abnormalities and wall motion abnormalities appear to be detected much less reliably at this level of training. While there may be value in demonstrating more advanced skills, it should be clear to all learners which skills can be reliably acquired during the training the residency can offer to prevent inappropriate use. The optimal ultrasound skill set is likely to further evolve as internists further develop its use in internal medicine practice, and should be continuously re-evaluated.

Resources and interdepartmental collaboration

To build a successful POCUS curriculum, IM residency programs require several categories of resources including equipment, faculty expertise, didactic content, hands-on teaching personnel, and a means of formative and summative assessment.

Equipment

As technology has evolved, POCUS equipment options have increased. Lower priced units have become available, including hand-held units to purchase or lease. These hand-held units are popular for their ease of transportation and use, however, present challenges for early learners given reduced screen size. Many suggest machines designed specifically for POCUS clinicians, as they often have a more approachable interface while losing little important functionality compared to machines designed for sonographers. Many manufacturers offer discounted educational pricing for educational-designated machines.

At a minimum, each program needs one dedicated machine configured with a linear, phased array and, if cost permits, a curvilinear probe. Maximizing access to POCUS machines encourages more frequent use, for example providing a cart-based unit for each floor and a hand-held for each resident team.

Some programs have access to simulation centers or ultrasound labs with machines that can be used by all learners. These spaces, when available, provide an arena for alternating didactics and hands-on sessions with normal models for the early learning phases. As learners progress, access to machines in clinical spaces is paramount for ongoing image acquisition and interpretation skill development, as actual patients provide both technical practice and the benefit of developing clinical integration skills.

Finances are often a limitation, and various methods have been used to acquire machines, including using medical school or hospital simulation centers (CWRU, UMN, OHSU, BU), noting the necessity of equipment if residents are expected to perform procedures (CWRU, UMN, OHSU, BU), quality improvement grant awards (UMN), use of machines destined for surplus from other divisions, group purchasing discounts when large departments/divisions are buying new machines, and making a return on investment (ROI) business case for ultrasound training later producing increases in billing or savings from enhanced patient safety (CWRU, BU).

Once machines are accounted for, there are other equipment considerations. If the assessment or quality assurance plan includes image portfolio collection and review, there should be a process to offload images in a HIPAA compliant fashion. Many machines come capable of connecting via wireless internet and archiving directly to image archival systems or the electronic medical record, however, others are not and require a "middleware" solution to sync images/clips to a secure on-site or cloud-based server. Some sites with student and resident learners decide not to have every educational image uploaded to the clinical spaces, and instead use "middleware" to differentiate between clinical and educational images. To save images, on-site requires the existence of a secure and sizeable server, which may already exist in other departments. Alternatively, a cloud-based server option can be added along with the "middleware" as a monthly operational cost.

Faculty

The availability of ultrasound-skilled faculty to lecture provides hands-on education and creates ongoing curricula which can be a challenge. It is imperative to have a faculty "champion" who leads the development and maintenance of the program. Several successful programs have appointed a "Director of IM Ultrasound Education" or similar role with protected time, averaging 0.15–0.25 FTE.

Besides having a faculty champion, other faculty must become involved to continuously promote the program. Reaching out to other willing educators is critical as hands-on scanning sessions require at most 5 learners per teacher, and ideally 3–4. Interdepartmental and interprofessional collaboration have been invaluable at each of our institutions in this effort. Sonographers and echocardiographers have been excellent teachers for image acquisition skills. Several universities have found dedicated Educational Sonographers to be a core asset for their programs. In addition, we encourage growing programs to collaborate with other POCUS users within their institutions, in departments such as EM, Pulmonology/Critical Care, Cardiology, Family Medicine, Rheumatology and Anesthesiology, amongst others.

Discussion

While some programs have quickly adapted POCUS training into traditional IM residency training, it remains relatively new, and there are many areas where growth and development are needed. Existing IM POCUS curricula are influenced heavily by well-documented EM training curricula. While this provides a good starting point, there are significant differences that make this extrapolation from EM to IM training less than ideal. IM residents see less unique patients per week than EM residents do, which inherently provides fewer opportunities to use POCUS, and may affect learning curves. Adding to the challenge, internal medicine residents typically learn from a much larger pool of faculty than many emergency medicine residents, making the direct training to proficiency of all teaching faculty difficult. Outcome data will be needed on the effectiveness of curricula to ensure that residents are learning, and effectively retaining this knowledge, and applying it correctly to real-world patient care. Given the already dense curriculum and time limitations of IM residency, innovative curriculum will need to be developed that works synergistically with what is already in place.

Further demonstration of techniques for supervision of resident POCUS use after initial training is needed, as residents are unlikely to be ready for completely independent practices after their initial training programs. Solutions to these issues are likely to need to be customized by each institution, and may overlap somewhat with those offered to attending physicians seeking to gain proficiency.

We feel that it is important to note that what we have outlined above amounts to opinion on what makes for a foundational POCUS program. The actual scope of practice for POCUS has not been defined, and outcomes research may help more accurately establish the appropriateness of various POCUS applications for the IM community.

Additionally, to make high-quality POCUS training more generalizable to all IM residency programs, it will be crucial that there is formal support and guidance from major medical societies governing internists. This was found to be a crucial catalyst for education, research, quality assurance and scholarship when undertaken by the American College of Emergency Physicians during emergency ultrasound's POCUS infancy. Formal support with guidelines on POCUS programs will allow individual programs to overcome many of the barriers they currently face.

Finally, it is important to note that the POCUS movement is not limited to the GME community. POCUS training is flourishing in the undergraduate medical education community as well. These POCUS-trained medical school graduates contend with entering an IM GME world currently unprepared to support their continued POCUS growth and use. It is imperative that the internal medicine community continues to develop POCUS curriculum and move towards standardization of POCUS training to ensure safe and high-quality use in the years to come.

Conclusions

POCUS can be successfully taught to internal medicine residents as a part of internal medicine training. Many common elements and principles are evident on review of these established programs (Table 3).

Table 3 Outline of POCUS program components at 4 institutions

	CWRU	UMN	OHSU	BU
Timeline of curriculum	PGY-1: 2 half day mixed didactic and hands-on sessions *Implemented 2013* PGY-2/3: optional 2-week elective (30 h/week) *Implemented 2015* ALL: interspersed hour long didactics throughout the 3 years of training (based on faculty availability) *Implemented 2015*	PGY-1: 25 h of training during intern orientation (all interns) *Implemented 2012* PGY-2/3: optional 40 h "advanced course" *Implemented 2014* Procedural service also available as a 2-week elective *Implemented 2016*	PGY-1: 3 half day mixed didactic and hands-on sessions *Implemented 2014* PGY-2/3: optional 2 to 3-week elective (30 h/week) *Implemented 2014*	PGY 1: ultrasound-guided procedural training during orientation (8 h) plus several sessions throughout the year (6 h) + OSCE *Implemented 2012* PGY-2/3: optional 1 week elective (36 h) *Implemented 2014* Procedural service which relies heavily on ultrasound also available as elective (40 h/week) *Implemented 2007*
Primary educational methods	Combination of didactics with supervised scanning using task trainers, ultrasound simulators and live ultrasound models For optional advanced elective, direct scanning of hospitalized patients	Intro course: largely web-based video didactics with quizzes, extensively uses of scanning of models, use of ultrasound simulators, and procedural task trainers Advanced course uses similar techniques, with addition of 25 h of scanning patients on wards	Didactic lectures alternating with hands-on scanning practice. Uses ultrasound simulators, and procedural task trainers	Didactic lectures followed by task trainers for procedures. Practice scanning on learners and ultrasound simulator followed by bedside patient scanning
Equipment	Multiple dedicated laptop and hand-held machines on wards and in simulation center available for resident use (hospital funded)	Multiple dedicated laptop machines on wards (hospital funded) and in simulation center (university funded)	Multiple dedicated laptop machines on wards (some hospital, some university funded) and simulation center (university funded). Have not yet received requested funding for hand-held units	Multiple laptop and larger machines based in ICU with loans to floor, and simulation center (all hospital funded)
Image management	Images uploaded to a dedicated network drive	Residents may keep portfolios and submit interpretations submitted manually starting with advanced course Process to use PACS and EMR in development	Middleware (see resources paragraph)	Locally stored on machines Residents may keep portfolios and submit manually as part of 1 week ultrasound elective
Quality assurance	Resident image review occurs from faculty supervision at the time of image acquisition	No formal system specific to residents. Exists in many clinical departments that residents rotate through	Weekly image review sessions for residents on elective, clinical image QA varies by department	No formal system. Confirmatory studies highly encouraged/stressed during didactics
Primary faculty involved	Hospitalists	Hospitalists, critical care	Hospitalists, emergency medicine, anesthesia	Critical care, cardiology, ER staff (case review during elective), internists at early stages

CWRU Case Western Reserve University, *UMN* University of Minnesota, *OHSU* Oregon Health & Science University, *BU* Boston University

Authors' contributions
CML, DJS, RKD, and FS contributed to the concept design, writing, editing and approving the final manuscript. All authors read and approved the final manuscript.

Author details
[1] Division of Medicine, Louis Stokes Cleveland Veterans Affairs Medical Center, 10701 East Boulevard, Cleveland, OH 44106, USA. [2] Case Western Reserve University School of Medicine, 2109 Adelbert Rd, Cleveland, OH 44106, USA. [3] Department of Medicine, University of Minnesota, 401 East River Parkway, Variety Club Research Center, Suite 131, Minneapolis, MN 55455, USA. [4] Department of Medicine, Oregon Health & Science University, 3181 SW Sam Jackson Park Road, Portland, OR 97239-3098, USA. [5] Department of Medicine, Boston Medical Center, 715 Albany St. E-113, Boston, MA 02118, USA.

Acknowledgements
The authors would like to thank Kevin Piro, M.D. (Oregon Health & Science University) for providing review and input of this manuscript. No compensation was provided for his contribution.

References

1. Keddis MT, Cullen MW, Reed DA, Halvorsen AJ, McDonald FS, Takahashi PY et al (2011) Effectiveness of an ultrasound training module for internal medicine residents. BMC Med Educ 28(11):75
2. Kessler C, Bhandarkar S (2010) Ultrasound training for medical students and internal medicine residents—a needs asssessment. J Clin Ultrasound 38(8):401–408
3. Hellmann DB, Whiting-O'Keefe Q, Shapiro EP, Martin LD, Martire C, Ziegelstein RC (2005) The rate at which residents learn to use hand-held echocardiography at the bedside. Am J Med 118(9):1010–1018
4. Riegert-Johnson DL, Bruce CJ, Montori VM, Cook RJ, Spittell PC (2005) Residents can be trained to detect abdominal aortic aneurysm using personal ultrasound imagers: a pilot study. J Am Soc Echocardiography. 18(5):394–397
5. Schnobrich DJ, Olson AP, Broccard A, Duran-Nelson A (2013) Feasibility and acceptability of a structured curriculum in teaching procedural and basic diagnostic ultrasound skills in internal medicine residents. J Grad Med Educ. 5(3):493–497
6. Klem DJ, Ratelle JT, Azeem N, Bonnes SL, Halvorsen AJ, Oxentenko AS et al (2015) Longitudinal ultrasound curriculum improves long-term retention among internal medicine residents. J Grad Med Educ. 7(3):454–457
7. Kimura BJ, Amundson SA, Phan JN, Agan DL, Shaw DJ (2012) Observations during development of an internal medicine residency training program in cardiovascular limited ultrasound examination. J Hosp Med. 7(7):537–542
8. Berger T, Garrido F, Green J, Lema PC, Gupta J (2012) Bedside ultrasound performed by novices for the detection of abscess in ED patients with soft tissue infections. Am J Emerg Med 30(8):1569–1573
9. American College of Emergency Physicians (2009) Emergency ultrasound guidelines. Ann Emerg Med 53(4):550–569
10. American College of Emergency Physicians (2017) Ultrsaound guidelines: emergency, point-of-care and clinical ultrasound guidelines in medicine. Ann Emerg Med 69(5):e27–e54
11. Schnobrich DJ, Gladding S, Olsen AP, Duran-Nelson A (2013) Point-of-Care ultrasound in internal medicine: a national survey of educational leadership. J Grad Med Educ. 5(3):498–502
12. Ma IWY, Arishenkoff S, Wiseman J, Desy J, Ailon J, Martin L, Otremba M, Halman S, Willemot P, Blouw M, Canadian Internal Medicine Ultrasound (CIMUS) Group (2017) Internal medicine point-of-care ultrasound curriculum: consensus recommendations from the canadian internal medicine ultrasound (CIMUS) group. J Gen Intern Med 32(9):10527

8

Point-of-care ultrasound in primary care: a systematic review of generalist performed point-of-care ultrasound in unselected populations

Bjarte Sorensen[1*] and Steinar Hunskaar[2,3]

Abstract

Background: Both the interest and actual extent of use of point-of-care ultrasound, PoCUS, among general practitioners or family physicians are increasing and training is also increasingly implemented in residency programs. However, the amount of research within the field is still rather limited compared to what is seen within other specialties in which it has become more established, such as in the specialty of emergency medicine. An assumption is made that what is relevant for emergency medicine physicians and their populations is also relevant to the general practitioner, as both groups are generalists working in unselected populations. This systematic review aims to examine the extent of use and to identify clinical studies on the use of PoCUS by either general practitioners or emergency physicians on indications that are relevant for the former, both in their daily practice and in out-of-hours services.

Methods: Systematic searches were done in PubMed/MEDLINE using terms related to general practice, emergency medicine, and ultrasound.

Results: On the extent of use, we identified 19 articles, as well as 26 meta-analyses and 168 primary studies on the clinical use of PoCUS. We found variable, but generally low, use among general practitioners, while it seems to be thoroughly established in emergency medicine in North America, and increasingly also in the rest of the world. In terms of clinical studies, most were on diagnostic accuracy, and most organ systems were studied; the heart, lungs/thorax, vessels, abdominal and pelvic organs, obstetric ultrasound, the eye, soft tissue, and the musculoskeletal system. The studies found in general either high sensitivity or high specificity for the particular test studied, and in some cases high total accuracy and superiority to other established diagnostic imaging modalities. PoCUS also showed faster time to diagnosis and change in management in some studies.

Conclusion: Our review shows that generalists can, given a certain level of pre-test probability, safely use PoCUS in a wide range of clinical settings to aid diagnosis and better the care of their patients.

Keywords: General practice, Family medicine, Emergency medicine, Point-of-care ultrasound, Ultrasound

Background

Point-of-care ultrasound, PoCUS, can be defined as the use of an image-producing ultrasound device for diagnostic and procedural guidance, by the clinician himself, at the point of care, in real time allowing for direct correlation with signs and symptoms [1]. It is integrated in the clinical work, and may increase accuracy of diagnoses or aid procedures, as well as reduce time spent to diagnoses and decreased overall costs [2].

General practitioners (GPs), or family physicians, work in a range of settings and levels of urgencies, from daytime run clinics, through out-of-hours (OOH) services such as primary care urgent care centres, to the provision of undifferentiated emergency medicine in rural and

*Correspondence: bjarte.sorensen@gmail.com
[1] Hjelmeland General Practice Surgery, Prestagarden 13, 4130 Hjelmeland, Norway
Full list of author information is available at the end of the article

remote regions. Globally, there are many different organisational models for OOH services, often running in parallel, including GP rota groups, cooperatives, primary care centres, as well as in-hospital emergency departments [3].

General practitioners are trained to manage both chronic conditions as well as acute emergencies, often within the same session, seeing women and men, young and old. In many countries, such as Australia [4] and Canada [5], general practitioners in rural and remote areas are expected to handle all emergencies and are often the only physicians available for initial diagnosis, management, and stabilisation within several hours of travel by road, water, or air. In countries such as Norway [6] and New Zealand [7], GPs are organised as part of the emergency response chain acting as a first responder and a team member to the ambulance services. Skills such as obtaining peripheral venous access and diagnosing life-threatening medical and traumatological conditions are expected [8, 9].

There are, therefore, many settings where the GP could potentially benefit from her own use of PoCUS. Both the interest and actual extent of use among GPs are increasing and PoCUS training is also increasingly implemented in residency programs [10]. However, the amount of research on PoCUS performed by GPs is still rather limited compared to other specialties in which it has become more established, such as in the specialty of emergency medicine [11, 12].

A recently published systematic review of PoCUS in general practice, identifying articles where the operators were GPs, concluded that it has the potential to be an important tool for the GP and possibly reduce health costs, but emphasises the need for further research [12]. Meanwhile, we think that it may be useful to also review studies where the setting is similar and the PoCUS operators also are, like GPs, physicians with a generalist training and perspective. We made the assumption that findings from studies where the operator is an emergency physician (EP) working in an unselected emergency department population also will be relevant for GPs.

The aim of this systematic review is thus twofold: first, to examine the extent of use among both GPs and EPs; second, to identify primary clinical research articles or meta-analyses on PoCUS for indications relevant for GPs in which the population is unselected (open GP practice or emergency departments) and the operators are either GPs or EPs.

Methods

Systematic searches were performed in the PubMed databases. Indexed MEDLINE-articles were identified by medical subject headings' (MeSH) keywords describing ultrasound, general practice, and emergency medicine (Table 1). Non-indexed PubMed articles were identified by corresponding keywords (Appendix 2 shows the exact search algorithm). The reference lists of included articles were also reviewed.

Only studies involving the clinical use of two-dimensional image-producing ultrasound at the point of care were included. Studies on hospitalised inpatients were excluded, as well as studies where the operator was a non-generalist, non-physician, or prehospital emergency medical service personnel. Case studies or case series were excluded, as were the use of ultrasound on hyperacute indications or for procedures less likely to be of relevance to most general practitioners (Appendix 1). Meta-analyses where the majority of the included articles fit our inclusion criteria were included, and the individual studies analyzed by these meta-analyses were excluded from our review to avoid double treatment. Articles published after the latest meta-analyses were included, as were articles outside the scope of the meta-analyses identified. Articles in other languages than English, German, Spanish, or any of the Scandinavian languages were excluded. The search was last performed on 1 June 2019.

Results

We identified 15,745 articles which were screened for eligibility, and after screening, 1413 full text articles we were left with 213 articles for inclusion, as shown in Fig. 1. Out of these, 19 were articles about the extent of use, while 26 were meta-analyses, and 168 primary research studies on PoCUS.

Table 1 Search algorithms

MeSH terms	Ultrasonography (included echocardiography)	Primary health care General practice (included family practice) General practitioners Physicians, primary care Physicians, family	Emergency medical services (included emergency service, hospital) Emergency medicine Emergency treatment Emergencies
Additional keywords used for search in non-indexed articles	Ultrasound POCUS Echocardiography	General practitioner Primary care physician Family physician	Emergency physician Prehospital medicine

The extent of use

There is great variation in the extent of use of PoCUS among GPs in Europe. In Norway, 23% of emergency primary care centres had access to their own ultrasound machines in 2015. However, only 1 of 15 of the GPs working there used ultrasound ever and only 0.3% of billings included an ultrasound item [13]. Ultrasound was in 2014 commonly used in Germany (about 45%) and Greenland (about two-thirds), while it was less commonly used in Sweden, Denmark, Austria, and Catalonia (< 1%) [14]. GPs, and EPs, working in emergency departments in rural Canada had good access to ultrasound equipment already in 2013 and increasingly until today (60–95%), while between 44 and 76% reported, they used ultrasound, a third of these on every shift [15–17].

Among EPs, ultrasound was used in 5% of the consultations in emergency departments in France in 2014 [18]. French emergency departments (EDs) have seen an increase in the availability of ultrasound equipment from 52 to 71% between 2011 and 2016 [19]. EPs had access to ultrasound equipment in 89% of Danish emergency departments in 2013 [20]. In China, 54% of EPs reported having access to equipment in 2016, and 43% of respondents reported using PoCUS in their clinical work [21]. In South Korea, it was available in 2014 in all surveyed EDs and 82.7% of respondents used PoCUS daily on adult patients, but only 23.6% performed

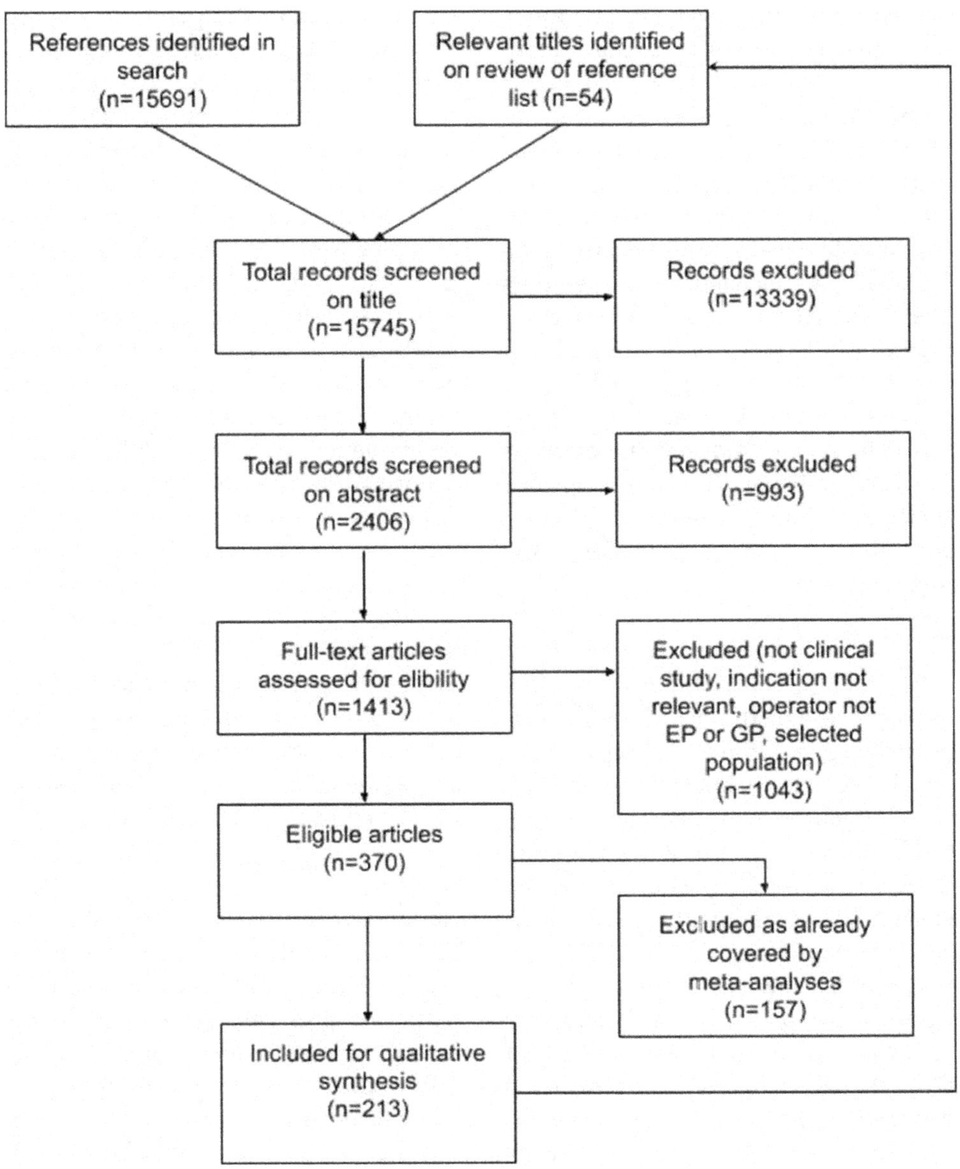

Fig. 1 Study selection flow diagram

paediatric PoCUS daily [22]. In Colombia, 57% of all emergency medicine residents responded that they lacked equipment, while 52% responded that they had used ultrasound during their training [23]. The use of PoCUS is integrated in the emergency physician training in the USA [24], and from 2004 to 2015, the access to equipment in emergency departments has risen from 19% to between 66 and 96%, and the lack of physician training is now seen as the major barrier rather than the lack of available technology [25–30].

Relevant indications

We found 26 meta-analyses and 168 primary studies on PoCUS used by generalists on a wide range of indications that we deemed relevant for the general practitioner, and they have been sorted according to the relevant organ systems: heart, lungs, vessels, abdomen, obstetric ultrasound, the eye; soft tissue, and musculoskeletal system.

The most studied parameter was diagnostic accuracy, and Tables 2, 3, 4, 5, 6, 7 and 8 show the test characteristics of a multitude of examinations. The sensitivities and specificities are displayed, and 95% confidence intervals are included where available. Positive and negative likelihood ratios (LR+/LR−) have been listed rather than positive and negative predictive values, as the former are prevalence independent, while the latter is only valid for the given prevalence in the studied population. Where either of the tabulated parameters was not available, we calculated these from the given data and indicated as such in the tables. Where available, the amount of time spent on specific didactic teaching is listed.

To the extent any other parameters than diagnostic accuracy were studied, this is presented narratively in the below text.

Heart

Studies on indications relating to the heart are summarized in Table 2. Even though a GP in a Norwegian pilot study from 1985 concluded that "echocardiography will not have any diagnostic significance in general practice in the foreseeable future" [31], a similar UK study was more positive in 1998 where one found GP performed evaluation of left-ventricular function frequently altered management [32].

Three studies from the last few years evaluated GPs' use of echocardiography compared to cardiologist as the reference, all of which found that, after 4–28 h of instruction, the GP could assess left-ventricular form and function with an accuracy high enough to impact management [33–35]. GPs have been found to reliably measure the mitral annular plane systolic excursion (MAPSE) through the use of pocket ultrasound after an 8 h teaching program with a sensitivity of 83% and a specificity of 78% [33]. A Spanish study found high accuracy for detecting left-ventricular hypertrophy (LVH) with GP operated pocket ultrasound in hypertensive patients in general practice, with a LR+ of 56 and a LR− of 0.1 [34]. They also found clinically useful test accuracy for other abnormalities. Another Spanish study found that GPs using pocket echocardiography on several indications had a very high specificity (93–100%) for a range of diagnoses, including LVH and valvular pathologies, but a rather low sensitivity (41–72%) [35].

Nine studies showed that EPs of varying experience could estimate left-ventricular ejection fraction (LVEF) and showed an overall agreement with cardiologists of between 84 and 93%, both on visual estimation and calculated values using, e.g., E-point septal separation [36–44]. Another study showed good agreement between EPs and cardiac sonographers on obtaining windows for left-ventricular outflow tract for velocity time integral studies [45], and it has been shown that EPs were able to obtain those windows for more than half of their ED patients [46]. Three studies identified high sensitivities and moderate-to-very good agreement with cardiologists for detection of diastolic dysfunction [47–49], while an Italian study found a high correlation between EP findings of restrictive mitral pattern and the presence of left-ventricular heart failure, with an LR+ of 8.27 [50]. EPs have also been shown to have good inter-rater agreement for the assessment of overall diastolic function [51].

Emergency physicians ability to detect wall motion abnormalities showed very good agreement with cardiologists in two studies [43, 52], while a 2018 US study sought to find whether EPs could use speckle tracking software to identify wall motion abnormalities and found that the sensitivity was low at 29%, but specificity high at 88% [53].

The ability to detect pericardial fluid by EPs was studied in four studies which all found sensitivities from 60 to 96% and specificities from 96 to 100% despite short training periods. False-negative findings were more likely for smaller effusions [39, 42, 43, 54].

Lungs

Findings from studies on lung ultrasound are detailed in Table 3. Lung ultrasound (LUS) can be used to detect diffuse interstitial syndrome (bilateral B lines), which, in the setting of suspected acute decompensated heart failure (ADHF), likely signifies pulmonary oedema. We identified five meta-analyses on this utility of LUS in the emergency department, all concluding that both the sensitivity and specificity are very high [55–59], and indeed the one test with the best test characteristics compared to all

Table 2 Summary of test accuracy findings in echocardiography

Test	Author	Op.	Year	Country or MA (studies)	Train.	*n*	Prev (%)	Age (years)	Criterion standard	Sn. (%) (95% CI)	Sp. (%) (95% CI)	LR+ (95% CI)	LR− (95% CI)
MAPSE < 10 mm	Mjølstad et al. [33]	GP	2012	Norway	8 h.	92	NR	73	Cardiologist echo.	83.3 (66.4–92.7)	77.6 (64.1–87.1)	3.72[a]	0.746[a]
LVH (ventricular wall > 13 mm)	Evangelista et al. [34]	GP	2013	Spain	NR	393	46	71	Cardiologist echo.	89.8 (NR)	98.4 (NR)	56.1[a]	0.114[a]
	Evangelista et al. [35]	GP	2016	Spain	NR	1312	16	67	Cardiologist echo.	71.4 (63.1–79.7)	97.4 (96.7–98.6)	27.5[a]	0.29[a]
LVEF < 50–55%	Unlüer et al. [41]	EP	2014	Turkey	NR	133	56	70	Cardiologist echo.	98.7 (91.8–99.9)	86.2 (74.1–93.4)	7.15 (3.76–13.6)	0.015 (0.002–0.109)
	Martindale et al. [55]	*EP*	*2016*	*MA (3)*	*NR*	*325*	*41*	*NR*	*Final diagnosis*	*80.6 (72.9–86.9)*	*80.6 (74.3–86.0)*	*4.1 (2.4–7.2)*	*0.24 (0.17–0.35)*
	Shah et al. [42]	EP	2016	Haiti	30 h.	117	40	36	Cardiologist echo.	93.6 (81.4–98.3)	100 (93.5–100)	∞[a]	0.064[a]
	Farsi et al. [43]	EP	2017	Iran	10 h.	205	51	61	Cardiologist echo.	89 (81–99)	96 (90–99)	22 (8–58)	0.12 (0.07–0.20)
LVEF < 40%	Dehbozorgi et al. [44]	EP	2019	Iran	NR	100	28	58	Final diagnosis (AHF)	100 (88–100)	88 (78–94)	8 (4.34–14.74)	0
LV dysfunction	Evangelista et al. [35]	GP	2016	Spain	NR	1312	4	67	Cardiologist echo.	50.0 (30.4–69.6)	92.7 (91.3–94.2)	6.85[a]	0.539[a]
LA dilatation	Evangelista et al. [35]	GP	2016	Spain	NR	1312	4	67	Cardiologist echo.	41.5 (25.2–57.8)	97.7 (96.8–98.6)	18.0[a]	0.701[a]
RVD	Evangelista et al. [34]	GP	2013	Spain	NR	393	22	71	Cardiologist echo.	80.2 (NR)	98.9 (NR)	73.9[a]	0.200[a]
	Farsi et al. [43]	EP	2017	Iran	10 h.	205	16	61	Cardiologist echo.	98 (94–99)	87 (69–96)	41 (15–109)	0.07 (0.02–0.27)
RVP	Farsi et al. [43]	EP	2017	Iran	10 h.	205	3	61	Cardiologist echo.	100 (52–100)	100 (98–100)	∞[a]	0[a]
Aortic valve sclerosis	Evangelista et al. [34]	GP	2013	Spain	NR	393	23	71	Cardiologist echo.	81.6 (NR)	98.2 (NR)	45.3[a]	0.187[a]
Aortic stenosis	Evangelista et al. [35]	GP	2016	Spain	NR	1312	5	67	Cardiologist echo.	50.0 (36.1–64.0)	98.1 (97.0–99.1)	26.3[a]	0.510[a]
Aortic insufficiency	Evangelista et al. [34]	GP	2013	Spain	NR	393	27	71	Cardiologist echo.	86.1 (NR)	95.7 (NR)	76.9[a]	0.145[a]
	Evangelista et al. [35]	GP	2016	Spain	NR	1312	4	67	Cardiologist echo.	58.3 (43.3–73.3)	99.0 (98.3–99.6)	58.3[a]	0.421[a]
Dilated ascending aorta	Evangelista et al. [34]	GP	2013	Spain	NR	393	15	71	Cardiologist echo.	89.1 (NR)	100 (NR)	∞[a]	0.109[a]
	Evangelista et al. [35]	GP	2016	Spain	NR	1312	9	67	Cardiologist echo.	54.1 (37.1–70.2)	99.1 (98.4–99.6)	60.1[a]	0.463[a]
Mitral insufficiency	Evangelista et al. [34]	GP	2013	Spain	NR	393	48	71	Cardiologist echo.	89.1 (NR)	87.2 (NR)	6.96[a]	0.125[a]
	Evangelista et al. [35]	GP	2016	Spain	NR	1312	6	67	Cardiologist echo.	72.7 (61.2–84.2)	97.7 (96.8–98.6)	31.6[a]	0.279[a]

Table 2 (continued)

Test	Author	Op.	Year	Country or MA (studies)	Train.	*n*	Prev (%)	Age (years)	Criterion standard	Sn. (%) (95% CI)	Sp. (%) (95% CI)	LR+ (95% CI)	LR− (95% CI)
Mitral stenosis	Evangelista et al. [35]	GP	2016	Spain	NR	1312	1	67	Cardiologist echo.	62.8 (22.7–100)	98.1 (97.3–98.9)	33.1[a]	0.379[a]
Tricuspid insufficiency	Evangelista et al. [35]	GP	2016	Spain	NR	1312	4	67	Cardiologist echo.	41.4 (21.7–61.0)	98.9 (98.3–99.5)	37.6[a]	0.694[a]
Hypertrophic cardiomyopathy	Evangelista et al. [35]	GP	2016	Spain	NR	1312	1	67	Cardiologist echo.	44.4 (6.4–82.5)	99.8 (99.6–100)	222[a]	0.557[a]
Diastolic heart failure	Unlüer et al. [47]	EP	2012	Turkey	6 h.	69	74	63	Cardiologist echo.	89 (77–95)	80 (51–95)	4.5 (1.6–12)	0.14 (0.06–0.21)
	Ehrman et al. [48]	EP	2015	USA	3 h.	62	52	56	Cardiologist echo.	92 (60–100)	69 (50–83)	2.9	0.12
Restrictive mitral pattern	Nazerian et al. [50]	EP	2010	Italy	4 h.	125	35	78	Final diagnosis of AHF	82 (73–87)	90 (84–94)	8.27 (4.57–15.42)	0.21 (0.14–0.32)
Wall motion abnormality	Farsi et al. [43]	EP	2017	Iran	10 t.	205	33	61	Cardiologist echo.	97 (89–99)	87% (80–92)	8 (5–12)	0.03 (0.01–0.13)
	Croft et al. [52]	EP	2019	USA	NR	75	62	65	Cardiologist echo. or ventriculogram	88 (75–96)	92 (75–99)	11.5 (3.1–43.7)	0.13 (0.05–0.29)
Speckle tracking	Reardon et al. [53]	EP	2018	USA	NR	75	16	52	Cardiologist echo. or final diagnosis ACS	29 (17–46)	88 (72–96)	2.4[a]	0.81[a]
Pericardial effusion	Mandavia et al. [54]	EP	2001	USA	5 h.	515	20	NR	Cardiologist echo.	96.0 (90.4–98.9)	98.0 (95.8 to 99.1)	48.0[a]	0.0408[a]
	Farsi et al. [43]	EP	2017	Iran	10 h.	205	10	61	Cardiologist echo.	86 (63–96)	96 (91–98)	20 (10–40)	0.15 (0.05–0.40)
	Shah et al. [42]	EP	2016	Haiti	30 h.	117	8	36	Cardiologist echo.	88.9 (50.7–99.4)	99.1 (94.2–100)	98.8[a]	0.112[a]
	Bustam et al. [39]	EP	2014	Malaysia	3 h.	100	5	NR	Cardiologist echo.	60 (15[a]–95[a])	100 (96[a]–100[a])	∞[a]	0.40[a]

MA, meta-analysis (shown in italics with number of studies in brackets); Op., operators; Train., time spent in didactic intervention; *n*, size of population; Prev., prevalence; Age, median or mean age in years; Sn., sensitivity; Sp., specificity; CI, confidence interval; LR+, positive likelihood ratio; LR−, negative likelihood ratio; NR, not reported; echo., echocardiography; MAPSE, mitral annular plane systolic excursion; GP, general practitioner; LVH, left-ventricular hypertrophy; LVEF, left-ventricular ejection fraction; EP, emergency physician; LV, left ventricle; LA, left atrial; RVD, right-ventricular dilatation; RVP, right-ventricular pressure

[a] Calculated by the authors

Table 3 Summary of test accuracy findings in lung ultrasound

Test	Author	Op.	Year	Country (no. of studies in MA)	Train.	*n*	Prev (%)	Age	Criterion standard	Sn. in % (95% CI)	Sp. in % (95% CI)	LR+ (95% CI)	LR− (95% CI)
Diffuse interstitial syndrome in heart failure	*Martindale et al. [55]*	*EP*	*2016*	*MA (8)*	*NR*	*1914*	*48*	*NR*	*Final diagnosis*	*85.3 (82.8–87.5)*	*92.7 (90.9–94.3)*	*7.4 (4.2–12.8)*	*0.16 (0.05–0.51)*
	McGivery et al. [56]	*EP*	*2018*	*MA (5)[c]*	*NR*	*1387*	*NR*	*NR*	*Final diagnosis*	*88.6 (79.6–94.0)*	*83.2 (63.2–93.5)*	*5.27[a]*	*0.14[a]*
	Lian et al. [57]	*EP[d]*	*2018*	*MA (15)*	*NR*	*3309*	*NR*	*NR*	*Final diagnosis*	*85 (84–87)*	*91 (89–92)*	*8.94 (5.64–14.18)*	*0.14 (0.08–0.26)*
	Koh et al. [75]	EP	2018	Singapore	20 h.	231	36	68	Final diagnosis	71.4 (60.5–80.8)	80.9 (72.5–87.6)	3.73 (2.50–5.57)	0.35 (0.25–0.50)
	Maw et al. [58]	*EP[d]*	*2019*	*MA (6)*	*NR*	*1827*	*20–62*	*NR*	*Final diagnosis or echoc./BNP*	*88 (75–95)*	*90 (88–92)*	*8.63 (6.93–10.74)*	*0.14 (0.06–0.29)*
Pneumonia (adults)	*Staub et al. [59]*	*EP[d]*	*2019*	*MA (14)*	*NR*	*2778*	*24–88*	*NR*	*Final diagnosis*	*NR (75–90)[b]*	*NR (80–90)[b]*	*NR*	*NR*
	Pivetta et al. [60]	EP	2019	Italy	40 *x*	518	43	79	Final diagnosis	93.5 (87.7–97.2)	95.5 (90.5–98.3)	20.9 (9.54–45.7)	0.07 (0.03–0.13)
	Bekgoz et al. [76]	EP	2019	Turkey	2 h.	383	22	66	Final diagnosis	87 (79–93)	97 (94–98)	29[a]	0.13[a]
	Ye et al. [63]	*EP*	*2015*	*MA (5)*	*NR*	*742*	–	*NR*	*Final diagnosis*	*95 (93–97)*	*90 (86–94)*	*9.5[a]*	*0.056[a]*
	Orso et al. [62]	*EP*	*2018*	*MA (17)*	*NR*	*5108*	*NR*	*67*	*Final diagnosis or CXR and/or CCT*	*92 (87–96)*	*93 (86–97)*	*13[a]*	*0,086[a]*
	Staub et al. [59]	*EP[d]*	*2019*	*MA (14)*	*NR*	*1896*	*30–85*	*NR*	*Final diagnosis or CXR and/or CCT*	*NR (85–95)[b]*	*NR (75–90)[b]*	*NR*	*NR*
	Amatya et al. [64]	EP	2018	Nepal	1 h.	62	71	59	CCT	91 (78–97)[a]	61 (36–83)[a]	2.34 (1.30–4.20)[a]	0.15 (0.05–0.41)[a]
	Koh et al. [75]	EP	2018	Singapore	20 h.	231	21	68	Final diagnosis	65.3 (50.4–78.3)	82.0 (74.9–87.8)	3.63 (2.44–5.40)	0.42 (0.29–0.63)
	Bekgoz et al. [76]	EP	2019	Turkey	2 h.	383	24	66	Final diagnosis	82 (78–89)	98 (97–99)	41[a]	0.18[a]
Pneumonia (children)	Copetti and Cattarossi [65]	EP	2008	Italy	NR	79	76	5	CXR, CT or final diagnosis	100[a]	100[a]	∞[a]	0[a]
	Shah et al. [66]	EP	2013	USA	1 h.	200	18	3	CXR	86 (71–94)	89 (83–93)	7.8 (5.0–12.4)	0.2 (0.1–0.4)
Pneumothorax	*Ebrahimi et al. [70]*	*EP*	*2014*	*MA (14)[c]*	–	*1803*	*NR*	*NR*	*CCT*	*88 (82–94)*	*99 (98–100)*	*88[a]*	*0.12[a]*
	Staub et al. [71]	*EP[d]*	*2018*	*MA (13)*	–	*2378*	*14*	*NR*	*CXR, CCT or chest tube (with rush of air)*	*81 (71–88)*	*98 (97–99)*	*67.9 (26.3–148)*	*0.18 (0.11–0.29)*
	Riccardi et al. [72]	EP	2019	Italy	–	190	9	59	CXR and/or CCT	94	100	∞[a]	0.06[a]
	Bekgoz et al. [76]	EP	2019	Turkey	2 h.	383	2	66	Final diagnosis	85	100	∞[a]	0.15[a]
COPD/Asthma	Koh et al. [75]	EP	2018	Singapore	20 h.	231	27	68	Final diagnosis	64.5 (51.3–76.3)	89.8 (83.4–94.3)	6.31 (3.72–10.72)	0.40 (0.28–0.56)
	Bekgoz et al. [76]	EP	2019	Turkey	2 h.	383	28	66	Final diagnosis	96 (90–97)	75 (70–80)	3.8[a]	0.05[a]

MA, meta-analysis (shown in italics with number of studies in brackets); Op., operators; Train., time spent in didactic intervention; h., hours; *x*, number of examinations; *n*, size of population; Prev., prevalence; Age, median or mean age in years; Sn., sensitivity; Sp., specificity; CI, confidence interval; LR+, positive likelihood ratio; LR− negative likelihood ratio; EP, emergency physician; NR, not reported; echoc., echocardiography; BNP, brain-type natriuretic peptide; CXR, chest X-ray; CCT, chest computed tomography

[a] Calculated by the authors

[b] The approximate overall 95% confidence interval based on the area under the curve

[c] EP sub-group analyzed separately

[d] The majority of studies included involved EPs

Table 4 Summary of test accuracy findings in vascular ultrasound

Test	Author	Op.	Year	Country (no. of studies in MA)	Train.	*n*	Prev (%)	Age	Criterion standard	Sn. in % (95% CI)	Sp. in % (95% CI)	LR+ (95% CI)	LR− (95% CI)
AAA (> 3 cm)—screening in general practice	Bravo-Merino et al. [90]	GP	2019	Spain	NR	76	17[b]/4.6[c]	70	Vascular surgical services ultrasound	100[b]/93.3 (75.4–99.9)[c]	100[b]/98.5 (94.3–100)[c]	∞[b]/62.2[c]	0[b]/0.07[c]
	Blois et al. [88]	GP	2012	Canada	NR	45	4.4	73	Radiologist	100 (15.8–100)[a]	100 (91.8–100)[a]	∞[a]	0[a]
	Bailey et al. [89]	GP	2001	USA	2 h.	79	5.1	NR	Radiologist	100 (39.8–100)[a]	100 (95.2–100)[a]	∞[a]	0[a]
AAA on clinical indication (cm)													
> 3	*Rubano et al. [94]*	*EP*	*2013*	*MA (7)*	*NR*	*655*	*23*	*> 50*	*CT, MRI, radiologist US, aortography, surgical findings, autopsy*	*99 (96–100)*	*98 (97–99)*	*NR (10.8–∞)*	*NR (0–0.025)*
> 5	Lindgaard and Risgaard [93]	GP	2017	Denmark	2 d.	29	3	NR	Radiologist US	100 (2.5–100)[a]	100 (87.7–100)[a]	∞[a]	0[a]
DVT Mixed techniques (2-point, 3-point and duplex US)	*Pomero et al. [97]*	*EP*	*2013*	*MA (16)*	*10 m.–6 h.*	*2379*	*23*	*NR*	*Colour-flow duplex US by radiology or angiography*	*96.1 (90.6–98.5)*	*96.8 (94.6–98.1)*	*30.0 (17.2–52.2)*	*0.04 (0.02–0.10)*
DVT 2-point compression (CFV and PV)	Lee et al. *[98]*	*EP*	*2019*	*MA (9)*	*NR*	*1337*	*20*[a]	*49–73*	*Radiologist US*	*91 (68–98)*	*98 (96–99)*	*46*[a]	*0.09*[a]
	Torres-Macho et al. [99]	EP	2012	Spania	10 h.	76	35	NR	Radiologist US	92 (82–100)	98 (94–100)	46[a]	0.08[a]
	Mumoli et al. [96]	GP	2017	Italy	50 h.	1107	18	64	Vascular ultrasound physician experts	90.0 (88.2–91.8)	97.1 (96.2–98.1)	31.0[a]	0.10[a]
	Nygren et al. [101]	EP	2018	Sweden	45 m.	65	17	70	Radiologist US	100 (71.5–100)	90.7 (79.7–96.9)	10.8 (4.69–24.9)	0
DVT 3-point compression (CFV, SFV and PV)	*Lee et al. [98]*	*EP*	*2019*	*MA (8)*	*NR*	*1035*	*29*[a]	*47–68*	*Radiologist US and/or contrast venography*	*90 (83–95)*	*95 (83–99)*	*18*[a]	*0.11*[a]
	Crowhurst and Dunn [100]	EP	2013	Australia	2 h	178	14	57	Radiologist duplex US	77.8 (54.8–91.0)	91.4 (84.9–95.3)	9.04[a]	0.24[a]

MA, meta-analysis (shown in italics with number of studies in brackets); Op., operators; Train., time spent in didactic intervention; m., minutes; h., hours; d., days; *x*, examinations; *n*, size of population; Prev., prevalence; Age, median- or mean age; Sn., sensitivity; Sp., specificity; CI, confidence interval; LR+, positive likelihood ratio; LR−, negative likelihood ratio; GP, general practitioner; EP, emergency physician; NR, not reported; AAA, abdominal aortic aneurysm; DVT, deep vein thrombosis; CFV, common femoral vein; PV, popliteal vein; SFV, superficial femoral vein; CT, computed tomography; MRI, magnetic resonance imaging; US, ultrasound

[a] Only including the 20% that had the criterion standard applied

[b] By posterior probability distribution

[c] Calculated by the authors from available data

Table 5 Summary of test accuracy findings in abdominal ultrasound

Test	Author	Op.	Year	Country (no. of studies in MA)	Train.	*n*	Prev (%)	Age	Criterion standard	Sn. in % (95% CI)	Sp. in % (95% CI)	LR+ (95% CI)	LR− (95% CI)
Hydronephrosis/ nephrolithiasis	*Wong et al. [113]*	*EP*	*2018*	*MA (9)*	*NR*	*1773*	*35–84*	*NR*	*CT, visualisation of stone or surgical findings*	*70.2 (67.1–73.2)*	*75.4 (72.5–78.2)*	*2.85*	*0.39*
	Javaudin et al. [114]	EP	2017	France	16 h.	50	38	47	Radiologist US	100 (82–100)	71 (52–86)	3.4 (2.0–6.0)	0
Pediatric hydronephrosis in UTI	Guedj et al. [115]	EP	2015	France	2 h.	382	5	9 m.	Radiologist US	76.5 (58.1–94.6)	97.2 (95.2–99.2)	27.3	0.25
Scrotal pathology	Blaivas et al. [118]	EP	2001	USA	NR	36	58	45	Radiologist colour doppler US	95 (78–99)	94 (72–99)	16[a]	0.053[a]
Cholelithiasis	Esquerrà et al. [121]	GP	2012	Spain	212 h.	115	56	NR	Radiologist US	88.9 (83.2–94.6)	100 (NR)	∞[a]	0.111
	Lindgaard and Risgaard [93]	GP	2017	Denmark	2 d.	62	42	NR	Radiologist US	92 (75–99)[a]	92 (78–98)[a]	11[a] (3.7–33)[a]	0.08[a] (0.02–0.32)[a]
	Scruggs et al. [125]	EP	2008	USA	–	575	60	NR	Radiologist US	88 (84–91)	87 (82–91)	6.8[a]	0.13[a]
	Ross et al. [124]	*EP*	*2011*	*MA (8)*	*NR*	*710*	*46–80*	*NR*	*Radiologist US, CT, MRI or surgical findings*	*89.8 (86.4–92.5)*	*88 (83.7–91.4)*	*7.5 (NR)*	*0.12 (NR)*
	Hilsden et al. [126]	EP	2018	Canada	Cert.	283	16	NR	Need for cholecystectomy	55 (40–70)	92 (88–95)	5.6[a]	0.49[a]
Cholelithiasis OR Cholecystitis	Schlager et al. [122]	EP	1994	Canada	NR	65	54	NR	Radiologist US or surgical findings	86 (70[a]–95[a])	97 (83–100)[a]	26[a] (4–177)[a]	0.15[a] (0.07–0.33)[a]
Cholecystitis	Rosen et al. [127]	EP	2001	USA	NR	193	46	49	Clinical follow-up	92 (73–100)	78 (61–93)	4.2[a]	0.36[a]
	Summers et al. [128]	EP	2010	USA	NR	113	14	36	Surgical reports or clinical follow-up	87 (66–97)	82 (74–88)	4.7 (3.2–6.9)	0.16 (0.06–0.46)
	Shekarchi et al. [129]	EP	2018	Iran	4 h.	342	14	54	Radiologist US	89.58 (76.55–96.10)	96.59 (93.63–98.29)	4.30 (2.42–7.62)	0.017 (0.007–0.041)
	Tourghabe et al. [130]	EP	2018	Iran	NR	51	100	42	Surgical and pathology findings	37.84 (22.94–55.2)	100.0 (73.24–100.0)	∞	0.62 (0.48–0.80)
Appendicitis (pediatric)	*Benabbas et al. [134]*	*EP*	*2017*	*MA (4)*	–	*461*	*31–54*	*9–12*	*Final pathology*	*86 (79–90)*	*91 (87–94)*	*9.24 (6.42–13.28)*	*0.17 (0.09–0.30)*
	Nicole et al. [135]	EP	2018	Canada	2 d.	121	44	10	Pathology or clinical follow-up	53 (40–66)	82 (71–89)	2.94[a]	0.57[a]
Appendicitis (all ages)	*Lee and Yun [136]*	*EP*	*2019*	*MA (17)*	–	*2385*	*42[a]*	*6–37*	*Surgical or pathological findings*	*84 (72–92)*	*91 (85–95)*	*7.0 (3.2–15.3)*	*0.22 (0.12–0.42)*

Table 5 (continued)

Test	Author	Op.	Year	Country (no. of studies in MA)	Train.	*n*	Prev (%)	Age	Criterion standard	Sn. in % (95% CI)	Sp. in % (95% CI)	LR+ (95% CI)	LR− (95% CI)
Appendicitis (adults)	*Fields et al. [137]*	*EP*	*2017*	*MA (11)*[b]	*–*	*1621*	*NR*	*NR*	*CT, surgery, MRI or autopsy*	*80 (76–83)*	*92 (90–94)*	*10.2 (8.2–12.7)*	*0.22 (0.19–0.26)*
	Shahbazipar et al. [138]	EP	2018	Iran	8 h.	121	38	34	Pathology or clinical follow-up	63 (48–77)	99 (93–100)	63[a]	0.37[a]
	Sharif et al. [139]	EP	2018	Canada	NR	90	20	NR	Pathology, laparoscopy, CT and/or radiologist US	69.2 (48.1–84.9)	90.6 (80.0–96.1)	7.4 (3.3–16.5)	0.3 (0.2–0.6)
	Corson-Knowles and Russell [140]	EP	2018	USA	20 m	76	37	27[a]	Pathology results or clinical follow-up	42.8 (25.0–62.5)	97.9 (87.5–99.8)	20.6 (2.8–149.9)	0.58 (0.42–0.80)
Intussusception (pediatric)	Riera et al. [141]	EP	2012	USA	1 h.	82	16	24 m.	Radiologist US	85 (54–97)	97 (89–99)	29 (7.3–117)	0.16 (0.04–0.57)
	Lam et al. [142]	EP	2014	USA	1 h.	44	23	31	Radiologist study	100 (66–100)	97 (82–100)	32 (4.65–220)	0
Small bowel obstruction	Unlüer et al. [146]	EP	201	Turkey	6 h.	174	49	56	Surgical findings, CT or clinical follow-up	97.7 (94.5–100)	92.7 (87.0–98.3)	13.4 (6.2–28.9)	0.025[a]
	Jang et al. [147]	EP	2011	USA	10 m.	76	43	NR	Abdominal CT	91 (75–98)	84 (69–93)	5.6 (2.8–11.1)	0.1 (0.04–0.3)
	Frasure et al. [148]	EP	2018	USA	NR	47	68	63	Abdominal CT	93.8 (79.2–99.2)	93.3 (68.1–99.8)	14.1 (2.11–93.6)	0.07 (0.02–0.26)
	Becker et al. [145]	EP	2019	USA	30 m.	217	43	55	Abdominal CT	88 (80–94)	54 (45–63)	1.92 (1.56–2.35)	0.22 (0.12–0.39)
Ascites	Lindgaard and Riisgaard [93]	GP	2017	Denmark	2 d.	34	9	NR	Radiologist US	100 (29–100)[a]	100 (89–100)[a]	∞	0
Constipation in children	Doniger et al. [149]	EP	2018	USA	1.5 h.	50	64	10±4	Rome III questionnaire	86 (67–95)	71 (53–85)	3.0[a]	0.20[a]

MA, meta-analysis (shown in italics with number of studies in brackets); Op., operators; Train., time spent in didactic intervention; m., minutes; h., hours; d., days; *n*, size of population; Prev., prevalence; Age, median- or mean age; Sn., sensitivity; Sp., specificity; CI, confidence interval; LR+, positive likelihood ratio; LR−, negative likelihood ratio; GP, general practitioner; EP, emergency physician; NR, not reported; CT, computed tomography; MRI, magnetic resonance imaging; US, ultrasound

[a] Calculated by the authors from available data

[b] EP sub-group analyzed separately

Table 6 Summary of test accuracy findings in ocular ultrasound

Test	Author	Op.	Year	Country (no. of studies in MA)	Train.	*n*	Prev (%)	Age	Criterion standard	Sn. in % (95% CI)	Sp. in % (95% CI)	LR+ (95% CI)	LR− (95% CI)
Retinal detachment	*Gottlieb et al. [168]*	*EP*	*2019*	*MA (5)*[b]	*0.5–2 h.*	*455*[a]	*12–38*	*46–60*	*Orbital CT (1) or ophthalmology evaluation (6)*	*93.9 (78.7–98.5)*	*92.4 (85.6–96.1)*	*12.4*[a]	*0.0660*[a]
	Jacobsen et al. [169]	EP	2016	USA	0.5 h.	109	31	49	Ophthalmology evaluation	91 (76–98)	96 (89–99)	23[a]	0.094[a]
	Lahham et al. [170]	EP	2019	USA	1 h.	225	21	51	Ophthalmology evaluation	96.9 (80.6–99.6)	88.1 (81.8–92.4)	8.14[a]	0.0352[a]
	Ojaghihaghighi et al. [171]	EP	2019	Iran	16 h.	351	8	34	Ophthalmology evaluation	88.9 (70.8–97.6)	100.0 (98.9–100.0)	∞	0.11 (0.038–0.32)
Vitreous haemorrhage	Lahham et al. [170]	EP	2019	USA	1 h.	225	24	51	Ophthalmology evaluation	81.9 (63.0–92.4)	82.3 (75.4–87.5)	4.63[a]	0.220
	Ojaghihaghighi et al. [171]	EP	2019	Iran	16 h.	347	13	34	Ophthalmology evaluation	97.8 (88.2–99.9)	98.7 (96.7–99.6)	74.8 (28.2–198.0)	0.023 (0.032–0.16)
Vitreous detachment	Lahham et al. [170]	EP	2019	USA	1 h.	225	15	51	Ophthalmology evaluation	42.5 (24.7–62.4)	96.0 (91.2–98.2)	10.6[a]	0.599[a]
Lens dislocation	Ojaghi Haghighi et al. [172]	EP	2014	Iran	NR	130	10	35	Orbital CT	84.6 (53.7–97.3)	98.3 (93.3–99.7)	49.5 (12.3–199.4)	0.15 (0.04–0.56)
	Ojaghihaghighi et al. [171]	EP	2019	Iran	16 h.	348	9	34	Orbital CT	96.8 (83.3–99.9)	99.4 (97.8–99.9)	154.8 (38.8–617.0)	0.032 (0.005–0.22)
						346	9		Ophthalmology evaluation	96.6 (82.2–99.9)	98.8 (96.9–99.7)	77.7 (29.3–206.0)	0.035 (0.0051–0.24)
Globe foreign body	Ojaghihaghighi et al. [171]	EP	2019	Iran	16 h.	350	5	34	Orbital CT	100.0 (79.4–100.0)	99.7 (98.3–100.0)	335.0 (47.3–2,371.0)	0
Globe rupture (except clinically obvious)	Ojaghihaghighi et al. [171]	EP	2019	Iran	16 h.	350	1	34	Orbital CT	100.0 (39.7–100.0)	99.7 (98.4–100.0)	347.0 (49.0–2,456.0)	0
Retrobulbar haematoma	Ojaghihaghighi et al. [171]	EP	2019	Iran	16 h.	350	9	34	Orbital CT	95.7 (78.1–99.9)	99.7 (98.3–100.0)	313.7 (44.2–2225.0)	0.044 (0.0064–0.30)

MA, meta-analysis (shown in italics with number of studies in brackets); Op., operators; Train., time spent in didactic intervention; h., hours; *n*, size of population; Prev., prevalence; Age, median- or mean age; Sn., sensitivity; Sp., specificity; CI, confidence interval; LR+, positive likelihood ratio; LR−, negative likelihood ratio; EP, emergency physician; NR, not reported; CT, computed tomography

[a] Calculated by the authors from available data

[b] EP sub-group analyzed separately

Table 7 Summary of test accuracy findings in soft-tissue ultrasound

Test	Author	Op.	Year	Country (no. of studies in MA)	Train.	*n*	Prev (%)	Age	Criterion standard	Sn. in % (95% CI)	Sp. in % (95% CI)	LR+ (95% CI)	LR− (95% CI)
Abscess	*Barbic et al. [173]*	*EP*	*2017*	*MA (8)*	*15 m.–1 d.*	*747*	*NR*	*All*	*Positive I&D and/or follow-up*	*96.2 (91.1–98.4)*	*82.9 (60.4–93.9)*	*5.63 (2.2–14.6)*	*0.05 (0.01–0.11)*
	Subramaniam et al. [174]	*EP*	*2016*	*MA (6)*	*30 m.–2 d.*	*413[a]*	*NR*	*All*	*Positive I&D and/or follow-up*	*97 (94–98)*	*83 (75–88)*	*5.5 (3.7–8.2)*	*0.04 (0.02–0.08)*
	Gaspari et al. [175]	EP	2012	USA	NR	65	46	42	*Positive I&D and/or follow-up*	96.7 (87.9–99.4)	85.7 (77.4–88.0)	6.76[a]	*0.0385[a]*
	Mower et al. [177]	EP	2019	USA	NR	1216	68	36	Positive I&D immediately or 1 week	94.0 (92.1–95.4)	94.1 (91.3–96.2)	15.9 (10.7–23.6)	0.06 (0.05–0.08)
Peritonsillar abscess	Costantino et al. [182]	EP	2012	USA	NR	14	57	26	Positive I&D and follow-up	100 (63–100)[a]	100 (54–100)[a]	∞[a]	0[a]
Dental abscess	Adhikari et al. [183]	EP	2012	USA	NR	19	63	40	Positive I&D	92 (62–100)[a]	100 (59–100)[a]	∞[a]	0.08 (0.01–0.54)
Foreign body	Friedman et al. [186]	EP	2005	USA	NR	131	9	10	Identification of FB	66.7 (34.8–90.1)	96.6 (91.6–99.1)	19.8[a] (6.99–56.3)[a]	0.34[a] (0.15–0.77)[a]

MA, meta-analysis (shown in italics with number of studies in brackets); Op., operators; Train., time spent in didactic intervention; m., minutes; d., days; *n*, size of population; Prev., prevalence; Age, median- or mean age; Sn., sensitivity; Sp., specificity; CI, confidence interval; LR+, positive likelihood ratio; LR−, negative likelihood ratio; EP, emergency physician; NR, not reported; I&D, incision and drainage

[a] Calculated by the authors from available data

Table 8 Summary of test accuracy findings in musculoskeletal ultrasound

Test	Author	Op.	Year	Country (no. of studies in MA)	Train.	*n*	Prev (%)	Age	Criterion standard	Sn. in % (95% CI)	Sp. in % (95% CI)	LR+ (95% CI)	LR− (95% CI)
Ulnar ligamentous strain injuries	Lee and Yun [188]	EP	2018	South Korea	1 week	65	NR	31	MRI	97.2 (92.0–99.4)	96.8 (93.5–98.7)	30.4[a]	0.03[a]
	Oguz et al. [187]	EP	2017	Turkey	NR	80	19	46	MRI	66.7 (41.7–84.8)	100 (94.4–100)	∞[a]	0.333[a]
Ankle anterior talofibular ligament strain injury	Gün et al. [189]	EP	2013	Turkey	6 h.	65	49	34	MRI	93.8 (79.2–99.2)	100 (89.4–100)	∞	0.06
	Lee and Yun [190]	EP	2017	South Korea	1 week	85	77	27	MRI	98.5 (91.7–100)	95.0 (75.1–99.9)	19.7[a]	0.0158[a]
Ankle calcaneofibular ligament injury	Lee and Yun [190]	EP	2017	South Korea	1 week	85	21	27	MRI	96.4 (81.7–99.9)	100 (81.5, 100)	∞[a]	0.0360[a]
Achilles tendon rupture	Lee and Yun [190]	EP	2017	South Korea	1 week	85	8	27	MRI	100 (59.0–100)	100 (95.4–100)	∞[a]	0[a]
Hip effusion (paediatric)	Cruz et al. [194]	EP	2018	USA	NR		926	6	Final diagnosis	85 (79–89)	98 (96–99)	43[a]	0.15[a]
	Vieira and Levy [193]	EP	2010	USA	30 min	55	43	8	Radiologist performed US	80 (51–95)	98 (85–99)	32[a] (4.5–225)[a]	0.21[a] (0.07–0.57)[a]
Extremity tendon laceration	Wu et al. [191]	EP	2012	USA	2 h.	34	38	> 16	Wound exploration or MRI	100 (75–100)[a]	95 (76–100)	20[a]	0[a]
	Mohammadrezai et al. [192]	EP	2017	Iran	6 h.	60	30	30	Wound exploration	94.4 (72.7–99.8)	100.0 (91.5–100.0)	∞[a]	0.06 (0.01–0.37)
Shoulder dislocation	*Gottlieb* et al. [196]	*EP*	*2019*	*MA (7)*	–	*739*	*12–60*	*35*	X-ray	*99.1 (84.9–100)*	*99.9 (88.9–100)*	*796.2 (8.0–79,086)*	*0.01 (0–0.17)*
ACL or PCL ruptures	Lee and Yun [197]	EP	2019	South Korea	1 week	62	73	29	MRI	92.2 (81.1–97.8)	95.9 (88.5–99.1)	22.5[a]	0.0813[a]
Skull fractures (paediatric)	Weinberg et al. [198]	EP	2010	USA	1 h.	21	10	NR	CT	100 (20–100)	100 (79–100)	∞	0
	Riera and Chen [199]	EP	2012	USA	NR	46	24	2	CT	82 (48–97)	94 (79–99)	14[a]	0.085[a]
	Parri et al. [200]	EP	2013	Italia	1 h.	55	64	3.7	CT	100 (88.2–100)	95.0 (75.0–99.9)	20[a]	0[a]
	Rabiner et al. [201]	EP	2013	USA	30 m.	69	12	6.4	CT	88 (53–98)	97 (89–99)	27 (7–107)	0.13 (0.02–0.81)
	Choi et al. [202]	EP	2018	South Korea	1 h.	87	15	21 months	CT	76.9 (46.0–93.8)	100 (93.9–100)	∞[a]	0.231[a]
	Parri et al. [203]	EP	2018	Italia	NR	115	84	8 months	CT	90.9 (82.9–96.0)	85.2 (66.3–95.8)	6.14[a] (2.48–15.2)[a]	0.11[a] (0.05–0.21)[a]

Table 8 (continued)

Test	Author	Op.	Year	Country (no. of studies in MA)	Train.	n	Prev (%)	Age	Criterion standard	Sn. in % (95% CI)	Sp. in % (95% CI)	LR+ (95% CI)	LR− (95% CI)
Clavicle	Cross et al. [204]	EP	2010	USA	NR	100	43	11	X-ray	95 (83–99)	96 (87–99)	27 (7–106)	0.05 (0.01–0.19)
	Weinberg et al. [198]	EP	2010	USA	1 h.	15	60	NR	X-ray	89 (51–99)	83 (36–99)	5.3 (0.87–32.4)	0.13 (0.01–0.90)
	Chien et al. [205]	EP	2011	USA	15 m.	58	67	7	X-ray	89.7 (75.8–97.1)	89.5 (66.9–98.7)	8.53	0.11
Elbow fractures (paediatric)	*Lee and Yun [206]*	*EP*	*2019*	*MA (5)*[b]	*NR*	*445*	*44*	*6–9*	X-ray	*95 (87–100)*	*94 (88–100)*	*16*[a]	*0.053*
Forearm fractures (paediatric)	*Chartier et al. [208]*	*EP*[c]	*2017*	*MA (10)*	*NR*	*NR*	*NR*	*NR*	X-ray	*93.1 (87.2–96.4)*	*92.9 (86.6–96.4)*	*14.1 (6.71–25)*	*0.08 (0.04–0.15)*
	Hedelin et al. [209]	EP	2017	Sweden	1.5 h.	116	65	11	X-ray	97.4 (90.9–99.7)	84 (67.2–94.7)	6.23[a] (2.78–13.96)[a]	0.03[a] (0.01–0.12)[a]
	Rowlands et al. [210]	EP	2017	Australia	3.5 h.	419	56	9	X-ray	91.5 (87.1–94.7)[a]	87.5 (81.9–92.0)[a]	7.36[a] (5.01–10.8)[a]	0.10[a] (0.06–0.15)[a]
Distal forearm fractures (all ages)	*Douma-den Hamer et al. [211]*	*EP*[c]	*2016*	*MA (16)*	*NR*	*1204*	*53*	*NR*	X-ray	*97 (93–99)*	*95 (89–98)*	*20 (8.5–47.2)*	*0.03 (0.01–0.08)*
	Sivrikaya et al. [212]	EP	2016	Turkey		93		47	CT/X-ray and orthopaedic evaluation	97.4 (90.2e99.5)	92.6 (85.5–96.5)	13.1 (6.7–25.6)	0.02 (0–0.10)
Wrist fracture (any)	Oguz et al. [187]	EP	2017	Turkey	NR	80	80	46	X-ray and/or CT	95.31 (87.10–98.39)	93.75 (71.67–98.89)	15.25[a] (2.28–101)[a]	0.05[a] (0.02–0.15)[a]
Metacarpal or phalangeal fractures	Tayal et al. [213]	EP	2007	USA	NR	78	40	34	X-ray or surgical findings	90 (74–97)	98 (95–100)	42.5 (NR)	0.1 (NR)
	Neri et al. [214]	EP[d]	2014	Italy	2 h.	153	39	12	X-ray	91.5 (84.4–98.7)	96.8 (93.2–100)	28.7[a] (9.39–87.5)[a]	0.09[a] (0.04–0.20)[a]
Metacarpal fractures	Kozaci et al. [215]	EP	2015	Turkey	NR	66	55	24	X-ray (reported by EPs)	92 (NR)	87 (NR)	7.1[a]	0.091[a]
	Kocaoğlu et al. [219]	EP	2016	Turkey	0	96	40	30	X-ray (reported by EP)	92.5 (78.5–98.0)	98.3 (89.5–99.9)	54.4[a]	0.08[a]
Fifth metacarpal fracture	Aksay et al. [216]	EP	2015	Turkey	1 h.	81	48	28	X-ray (reported by OS) or CT	97.4 (84.9–99.9)	92.9 (79.4–98.1)	14 (4.58–41)	0.03 (0.00–0.19)
Proximal or middle phalanx fracture	Aksay et al. [217]	EP	2016	Turkey	NR	119	24	27	X-ray (reported by OS)	79.3 (59.7–91.2)	90 (81.4–95)	7.93 (4.15–15)	0.23 (0.11–0.47)
Distal phalanx fracture	Gungor et al. [218]	EP	2016	Turkey	3 h.	45	29	32	X-ray reported by EP	100 (79–100)	98 (91–100)	59 (8–412)	0

Table 8 (continued)

Test	Author	Op.	Year	Country (no. of studies in MA)	Train.	*n*	Prev (%)	Age	Criterion standard	Sn. in % (95% CI)	Sp. in % (95% CI)	LR+ (95% CI)	LR− (95% CI)
Nail bed injury	Gungor et al. [218]	EP	2016	Turkey	3 h.	45	73	32	Visual inspection	93 (80–99)	100 (74–100)	∞	0.06 (0.02–0.23)
Tibia and/or fibula (anywhere)	Kozaci et al. [220]	EP	2017	Turkey	2 h.	62	34	5–55	X-ray reported by EP	100 (84–100)[a]	93 (80–98)[a]	13.7[a] (4.60–40.6)[a]	0[a]
Medial or lateral malleolus fracture	*Chartier et al. [208]*	*EP[c]*	*2017*	*MA (4)*	*NR*	*609[a]*	*7–23*	*Adults*	*X-ray and/or CT*	*89.5 (77.0–95.6)*	*94.2 (86.1–97.7)*	*16.4 (6.57–33.5)*	*0.12 (0.05–0.24)*
Lateral malleolus	Ozturk et al. [223]	EP	2018	Turkey	2 h.	120	35	41	X-ray and/or CT evaluated by OS	100 (90–100)	93 (85–98)	8.4 (3.6–19.3)	0
Malleolar fracture OR fifth metatarsal fracture	Tollefson et al. [222]	EP	2016	USA	1 h.	50	36	35	X-ray reported by radiologist	100 (78–100)	100 (87–100)	∞[a]	0[a]
Navicular fracture	Atilla et al. [221]	EP	2014	Turkey	4 h.	34	15	37	X-ray and/or CT evaluated by OS	40 (7–83)	93 (76–99)	5.7[a]	0.65[a]
Fifth metatarsal fracture	Atilla et al. [221]	EP	2014	Turkey	4 h.	97	30	37	X-ray and/or CT evaluated by OS	100 (85–100)	96 (87–99)	25[a]	0[a]
	Yesilaras et al [224]	EP	2014	Turkey	0	84	41	36	X-ray reported by OS	97.1 (82.9–99.8)	100 (91.1–100)	∞	0.03 (0.01–0.21)
	Kozaci et al. [225]	EP	2017	Turkey	2 h.	72	39	5–55	X-ray reported by EP	93 (77–99)[a]	89 (75–96)[a]	8.17[a] (3.56–18.7)[a]	0.08[a] (0.02–0.31)[a]

MA, meta-analysis (shown in italics with number of studies in brackets); Op., operators; Train., time spent in didactic intervention; m., minutes; h., hours; *n*, size of population; Prev., prevalence; Age, median- or mean age; Sn., sensitivity; Sp., specificity; CI, confidence interval; LR+, positive likelihood ratio; LR−, negative likelihood ratio; EP, emergency physician; NR, not reported; CT, computed tomography; MRI, magnetic resonance imaging; US, ultrasound; OS, orthopaedic surgeon

[a] Calculated by the authors from available data

[b] EP sub-group analyzed separately

[c] The majority of studies included involved EPs

other clinical parameters for ADHF ever studied [55]. One meta-analysis only included studies where also chest X-ray (CXR) had been compared with LUS towards the same gold standard, and found that CXR had the same specificity (90%) but lower sensitivity than LUS (73% vs 88%) [58]. A recent randomised-controlled study by Pivetta et al. [60], not analyzed in these meta-analyses, allocated patients after the initial suspicion of ADHF into groups receiving CXR and pro-brain natriuretic peptide (pro-BNP) or LUS, and found not only that LUS had both superior specificity and sensitivity compared to the criterion standard of final chart diagnosis, but also a shorter time to the diagnosis (5 min vs 104.5 min). Finally, one Australian study analyzed inter-rater agreement between experienced and novice EP lung sonographers which was found to be good, with a Cohen's kappa coefficient of 0.70 [61].

Three meta-analyses were identified that assessed the accuracy of LUS in diagnosing pneumonia in unselected adult populations [59, 62, 63]. Orso et al. found 17 studies in ED populations where focal subpleural consolidations, focal B lines, or a combination of these were considered a positive finding, using X-ray and/or CT as the criterion standard, and found a pooled sensitivity of 92% and a specificity of 93%, similar to the findings in the meta-analysis by Staub et al. [59]. Ye et al. [63] only included studies where LUS was directly compared to CXR using the final diagnosis as the criterion standard, and found that LUS had a sensitivity of 95% against 77% for CXR, while the specificity was the same, 90%. A recent study not included in these meta-analyses found a similar superiority to CXR in a Nepalese ED population [64].

An Italian study on PoCUS for pneumonia in a paediatric population by one expert EP ($n=79$) agreed with the final diagnosis of pneumonia in all cases and had no false-positive findings [65]. A later study in 200 children with suspected pneumonia (prevalence = 18%) showed sensitivity and specificity of 86% and 89%, respectively, when compared to CXR as the gold standard [66]. Ultrasound has been shown to be more sensitive than CXR in a study of a paediatric ED population, but less specific [67], and another study showed a 39% reduction in use of CXR for the final diagnosis of pneumonia in children in a randomised trial, with no cases of missed diagnoses or complications [68]. PoCUS by paediatric EPs instead of CXR was in one study associated with less time spent and decreased overall costs [69].

The absence of pleural sliding and B lines is a sign of pneumothorax, and finding the point where the pleural layers separates from each other, the lung point, is pathognomonic. A recent meta-analysis showed a very high accuracy of PoCUS when performed by EPs, with 88% sensitivity and 99% specificity, and it was superior to CXR which had 46% sensitivity and 100% specificity [70]. The findings were similar in another recent meta-analysis, albeit with a somewhat heterogeneous operator group [71], as well as in a recent original prospective observational study [72].

Two studies from 2017 used the total cases of positive findings of rib fractures found by either LUS or CXR as the criterion standard (assuming that there were no false-positive findings) and found a sensitivity of 81–98% in LUS compared to 41–53% for CXR [73, 74]. A third study found a similar concordance between LUS and CXR and/or CCT [72].

Two studies evaluated the accuracy of PoCUS through present lung sliding and predominant A lines as a marker for asthma or chronic obstructive pulmonary disease (COPD) in the setting of dyspnoea, and found an LR+ of 3.8–6.3 and an LR− of 0.05–0.40 [75, 76]. Such LUS findings can also be seen in patients without pulmonary pathology, which may explain the poorer test characteristics seen in the undifferentiated ED populations compared to what has been seen in intensive-care unit populations [59].

Finally, we identified 11 articles which studied the impact of different PoCUS protocols on the overall diagnosis of patients presenting with undifferentiated respiratory or chest symptoms. An Italian ED-based study showed that LUS in the setting of pleuritic pain without dyspnoea had 97% sensitivity and 96% specificity for detecting lesions that did not show up on CXR, using other imaging modalities and final diagnosis as their criterion standard [77]. Another Italian study found that LUS in dyspnoeic patients changed the diagnosis in 44% of cases and altered management in 58% [78]. Danish EPs evaluating dyspnoeic patients with PoCUS of heart, lung, and deep veins found life-threatening diagnoses that were missed in the primary assessment in 14% of patients, reporting a total of 100% sensitivity and 93% specificity for the diagnosis of such conditions [79]. The same group randomised 320 dyspnoeic patients (and $SpO2 < 95\%$) into a PoCUS group or management as usual, and found as their primary endpoint a significant 24% higher accuracy in diagnosis at 4 h (88% vs 64%), using masked audit as the gold standard [80]. Similarly, two studies found a significant reduction in time needed for diagnosis using integrated ultrasound on dyspnoeic patients [81, 82]. It has also been shown that the addition of heart and lung PoCUS allowed the EPs to reduce the number of diagnoses on their differential diagnosis list from 5 to 3 ($p < 0.001$) [83], and also three other studies showed statistical significance in PoCUS overall diagnostic accuracy in patients with dyspnoea [84–86]. One USA study could not show significant diagnostic or management changes when a PoCUS protocol was applied to dyspnoeic patients in ED significantly, but it improved EPs' confidence levels [87].

Vessels

Main test characteristic findings can be found in Table 4.

Screening for abdominal aortic aneurysms (AAA) by GPs would require a very high accuracy to avoid false positive in a relatively low pre-test probability population, even if one selects the population who is at risk, men who have smoked in the ages between 65 and 75. We identified three small studies of GPs' screening for AAA in such populations against a gold standard [88–90]. All found 100% accuracy for AAA greater than 3 cm and concluded screening by GPs were feasible. One larger feasibility study only confirmed positive cases [91]. Hoffmann et al. [92] also found screening by EPs in the emergency department feasible, but requiring substantial resources for a low success rate.

In a Danish study, inexperienced GPs achieved 100% accuracy for AAA > 5 cm compared to radiologists when the scan was performed on clinical indication [93]. Similarly, one meta-analysis showed that EPs have very high accuracy for detecting AAA > 3 cm compared to formal radiologist performed ultrasound when performed on indication [94].

One Japanese retrospective study investigated the impact of GPs screening of carotid intima media thickness in patients at risk of coronary artery disease (CAD) on later interventions, and found an increase in the prevalence of CAD in patients referred to a local specialist centre and higher probability of coronary angiograms and revascularization [95].

One multi-centre study assessed Italian GPs' accuracy of a two-point compression technique for the identification of lower extremity deep vein thrombosis (DVT) and found 90% sensitivity and 97% specificity compared to radiologist ultrasound [96]. A meta-analysis on EPs use of PoCUS for detection of DVT found even higher accuracy with a sensitivity of 96% and a specificity of 97% [97]. A newer meta-analysis from 2019 shows a pooled sensitivity of 91% and a specificity of 98% for the two-point compression technique (assessing the common femoral vein and the popliteal vein) and similarly 90% and 95% for the three-point compression technique (including the superficial femoral vein) [98]. Three other studies not analyzed in above meta-analyses show similar test accuracies [99–101]. One study showed a > 4-fold reduction in ED length of stay for the group with EP-performed DVT studies vs the radiology department patients [102].

Ultrasound-guided peripheral venous catheter (PVC) insertion has been shown in some studies to reduce time and attempts [103–105], while others show similar or even worse success rate [106–108]. One study found that ultrasound-guided PVC insertion was associated with a higher rate of extravasation, 3.6% vs 0.3% [109]. Another study showed a 73% success of cannulation of the brachial or the basilic vein after two failed attempts without ultrasound, but also showed an 8% rate of extravasation at 1 h [110]. One group evaluated EPs use of PoCUS before peripheral venous cannulation of children less than 7 years before cannulation as usual, and found visible veins on ultrasound a strong predictor for successful cannulation [111]. It has also been found that EPs could insert a standard 2.5-in., 18-gauge peripheral venous catheter in the internal jugular vein with a success rate of 97.1% after two failed attempts by management as usual by nursing staff [112].

Abdomen

The main findings on diagnostic test accuracy of abdominal PoCUS are listed in Table 5.

One meta-analysis of EPs' findings of hydronephrosis as a surrogate for nephrolithiasis in patients presenting with renal colic found only moderate sensitivity and specificity [113]. Moderate-to-severe hydronephrosis is highly specific for the presence of a stone at 94%, but only with a sensitivity of 29%. One study not included in this meta-analysis found 100% sensitivity, but moderate specificity [114]. A French study found that EPs correctly identified hydronephrosis in children with urinary tract infections (prevalence = 5%) with a sensitivity of 76.5% and a specificity of 97.2% [115]. Finally, one large (n = 2759) study, randomising patients into diagnosis through EP PoCUS, radiologist ultrasound or computed tomography (CT), found no difference in high-risk diagnoses that could be due to missed or delayed diagnosis after 30 days, and showed overall lower cumulative radiation exposure at 6 months for both ultrasound groups compared to the CT group [116]. They also showed a slight, but significant, reduction in ED length of stay, while another study found halving of the length of stay [117].

Only one small, retrospective study reviewed EPs diagnostic accuracy of scrotal PoCUS, and found that the EPs correctly diagnosed epididymitis, orchitis, and testicular torsion in 35 of 36 cases [118]. No cases of testicular torsion were missed.

Two Norwegian studies demonstrated clinical usefulness for the use of GP operated PoCUS to demonstrate cholelithiasis already in the 80s [119, 120], and also a more recent study shows high agreement between GP and radiologist performed ultrasound [121]. In the ED setting, a high accuracy was shown already in a 1994 study [122] and Blaivas et al. [123] showed a significant reduction in the length of stay in the emergency department when EPs used PoCUS for diagnosis of biliary disease. One meta-analysis found an LR+ of 7.5 and LR− of 0.12 on EP-performed PoCUS for cholelithiasis [124], similar to a large, retrospective study not included in the meta-analysis [125]. A similar high specificity was found in a more recent study, and a sensitivity of 55% when using eventual need for cholecystectomy as their gold standard [126]. When it comes to cholecystitis, the LR+ ranged from 4.2 to 4.7 and the LR− from 0.05 to 0.39 in three studies of varying design [127–129]. Summers et al. [128] found that there were close agreement with radiology department ultrasound when compared to the criterion standard of surgical reports and follow-up, and suggested that patients with negative EP scans are unlikely to require surgery. Another study could not conclude the same, as they, in contrast to the other studies, only found 38% sensitivity using surgical findings as the criterion standard [130]. The positive likelihood ratio was high nevertheless, as specificity in their study was 100%. A Turkish study found that diagnosis and management were more likely to be affected if the clinician had moderate, rather than low or high, suspicion about the diagnosis prior to the study [131]. One study performed PoCUS on patients presenting with non-traumatic epigastric pain, and found a cholelithiasis prevalence of 39% in this population, even though the treating EP did not initially consider the need for biliary ultrasound in 85% of these cases [132]. A USA study found that the presence of a dilated common bile duct on EP-performed PoCUS, in the absence of laboratory findings or signs of cholecystitis on ultrasound, was unlikely to be a good indicator for complicated biliary pathology (sensitivity 23.7% and specificity 77.9%) [133].

Appendicitis has several hall-mark findings such as oedematous wall and overall thickness. One meta-analysis found an LR+ of 9.24 on EP-performed ultrasound for appendicitis in children [134], reproduced in one study published since [135]. Lee and Yun [136] found LR+ of 7.0 in a 2019 meta-analysis of PoCUS on all ages, while Fields et al. [137] found LR+ of 10.2 in their sub-group analysis of EP-performed PoCUS for appendicitis in a 2017 meta-analysis. The LR−, however, ranged from 0.17 to 0.22, and one can conclude that EP-performed PoCUS is useful to rule in appendicitis, but not sufficient on its own to rule it out. This can also be concluded from the latest three studies not included in the above-mentioned meta-analyses [138–140].

Concentric rings on ultrasound of the small bowel indicate intussusception in children in whom one suspects this condition [141]. We identified one prospective observational study and one retrospective analysis of EP-performed PoCUS for intussusception after only short periods of training, both showing high specificities of 94–97%, but varying sensitivities of 85–100% [141, 142]. One retrospective study was limited by its design giving an absence of true negative findings, but showed sensitivity of 79% in novices and 90% in a certified paediatric EP [143], while a South Korean group found that PoCUS significantly reduced the door-to-reduction time and overall stay in their ED [144].

Small bowel obstruction can be seen using ultrasound by identifying features such as small bowel dilation, abnormal peristalsis, small bowel wall oedema, and intraperitoneal free fluid [145]. Four studies in the ED showed sensitivities from 88 to 98% [145–148], with two studies showing a higher sensitivity, but lower specificity for EPs than for radiologist ultrasound when compared to CT [146, 147]. One of the studies showed lower specificity than the other three studies (54% vs 84–94%), citing a shorter didactic session and experience requirements as a possible explanation [145].

One small study found that GPs had 100% agreement with radiologists on the use of PoCUS for finding ascites on indication [93].

A small study ($n = 50$) compared ultrasound measured transverse diameter of the rectum against Roma III criteria for constipation in children, and found high sensitivity of 86%, but a somewhat low specificity of 71% [149]. However, ultrasound was not less sensitive than abdominal X-ray (87%) and trended towards being more specific (71% vs 40%). A rectal diameter of 3.8 cm or greater correlated well with constipation.

Two studies were identified using several of the above-mentioned techniques to help diagnose patients presenting with abdominal pain and found an overall improvement in diagnostic accuracy compared to work-up as usual [150, 151].

Obstetric ultrasound

Inexperienced Danish GPs had 28 of 30 measurements of gestational age (GA) within 3 days of the obstetrician performed estimate, while the final 2 were within 7 days [93]. Johansen et al. [152] found that GP's measurements of GA in an 11 year period ($n = 356$) showed the same agreement with actual date of birth as did those of the local obstetric service ($n = 14{,}550$). The same agreement was found in six other GP studies between 1985 and 2001 [153–158].

Also EP measured crown-rump length (CRL), used in first trimester estimation of GA, showed in two studies correlation coefficients of 0.95–0.98 when compared with obstetric ultrasound [159, 160]. Another study found that EPs were accurate stratifying GA into before and after 24 weeks, and thus foetal potential viability if one decides to go ahead with an emergent caesarean section in patients unable to give an accurate history due to lowered consciousness [161].

One meta-analysis assessed EPs' accuracy in diagnosing ectopic pregnancy by PoCUS, defining a positive finding as an empty uterus in a patient with a confirmed pregnancy [162]. Using this "safe" definition, the pooled sensitivity was high at 99.3%, while the specificity ranged from 42 to 89%, pooled specificity estimate not being possible to calculate due to study heterogeneity.

Another meta-analysis included six studies aimed to show whether EP-performed pelvic ultrasound on women with symptomatic early pregnancy in the ED caused a reduction in the length of stay (LOS) in the ED, and confirmed this, with a mean reduction in LOS of 74 min (95% CI 49–99) [163].

Among those visiting ED due to bleeding in the first trimester, one study showed 42% had the expectation of getting confirmation of foetal viability by ultrasound and blood work [164]. In addition to identifying an intrauterine pregnancy, confirming foetal heart activity is decisive in diagnosing a threatened or missed abortion. We identified four studies where GPs had 100% accuracy (total $n=295$) [93, 152, 153, 165] and one study of EPs showing a sensitivity of 89% and a specificity of 100% by use of transabdominal transducer [166]. In this study, mean GA was 9.5 weeks, and only the heart activity of the very earliest pregnancies was missed when compared to a radiologist using transvaginal transducer.

Two studies (total $n=387$) showed that both GPs and EPs had 100% accuracy in detecting foetal position in the third trimester [152, 167].

The eye

Studies on ocular PoCUS are listed in Table 6. Retinal detachment may be seen on ultrasound as a hyperechoic line separating from the choroid while being tethered to the optic disc. One recent meta-analysis determined the test characteristics of ocular PoCUS for this condition [168]. A sub-group analysis of five studies where the provider was an EP working in the ED found a sensitivity of 94% and a specificity of 91%. One retrospective study excluded from this meta-analysis, due to its retrospective design, showed similar numbers [169], as did two more recent prospective studies [170, 171] (see Table 6).

One study was identified estimated test accuracies for the important differential diagnoses of vitreous haemorrhage and detachment, and found high total accuracy for haemorrhage and high specificity for vitreous detachment [170]. Another study evaluated 232 patients (351 eyes) after trauma (excluding obvious globe rupture), and found high accuracy for the detection of vitreous haemorrhage, lens dislocation, globe foreign body, globe rupture, and retrobulbar haematoma [171]. The same group also found high accuracy for the detection of traumatic lens dislocation in a different study 5 years previously [172].

Soft tissue

Linear, high-frequency ultrasound can give detailed images of structures in the soft tissue, and findings from studies are summarized in Table 7. A 2017 meta-analysis included eight studies on adult and paediatric ED populations determining the accuracy of EPs using PoCUS to detect the presence of an abscess in patients presenting with signs of skin and soft-tissue infection, and found a pooled sensitivity of 96% and a specificity of 83% [173]. The pooled sensitivity of the paediatric sub-group was slightly lower at 94%, but had the same specificity. The decision of whether to lance or not was changed in 14–56% of the cases. Pre-study teaching varied from 15 min to 1 day. A 2016 meta-analysis including six studies showed the same test accuracy [174]. Another study compared EP PoCUS and CT for abscesses head-to-head and found significantly better sensitivity for PoCUS (97% vs 77%), and similar specificity (86% vs 91% with overlapping 95% confidence intervals) [175]. In a primary care outpatient setting, it has been showed that the size of abscesses was estimated incorrectly by clinical examination in 52% of cases and ultrasound changed management in 55% of cases [176]. One study compared the test accuracy of clinical examination with and without PoCUS on finding soft-tissue abscesses [177]. They found very high accuracy and no significant difference between the groups in the population for which the EP indicated that she was clinically certain about the diagnosis ($n=1111$). However, in the uncertain cases ($n=105$), ultrasound changed management in a quarter, appropriately so in 85% of these. Also in a paediatric ED population, it was found that ultrasound did not change the ED treatment failure rate, even though ultrasound changed management from surgical to medical or vice versa in 25% of cases [178]. This is in contrary to another study in a paediatric population who did see a significant reduction in failure rate, with three times higher failure rates in the non-PoCUS vs PoCUS groups (14% vs 4%) [179]. The same group found similar rates in adults ($n=125$), with 17% vs 3.7%, but the 95% confidence intervals showed 0–19.4% difference between the groups, leaving it barely statistically significant [180]. A US study showed that the ED length of stay was significantly reduced, by a mean of 73 min, when patients received EP PoCUS rather than radiology ultrasound [181]. They also found significant differences in the two groups on incision and drainage rate which was twice as high in the PoCUS group and rate of ED intravenous antibiotics, which was 60%.

Two small studies on the use of PoCUS for the detection of peritonsillar abscess [182] and dental abscess [183] showed near 100% test accuracy, but had wide confidence intervals due to small populations.

Two studies ($n=27$ and $n=75$) evaluated EP PoCUS diagnostic accuracy on paediatric soft-tissue neck masses and found a Cohen's kappa coefficient when compared to the final diagnosis of 0.69 (95% CI 0.44–0.94) and 0.71 (0.60–0.83), respectively [184, 185].

One clinical study on the use of PoCUS for identification of soft-tissue foreign bodies showed that ultrasound identified two-thirds of all foreign bodies with a specificity of 97% [186]. There were no significant differences in performance characteristics of X-ray which showed sensitivity of 58% and a specificity of 90%.

Musculoskeletal ultrasound

The retrieved studies on musculoskeletal ultrasound were on the ability to detect acute tendon trauma, joint fluid, shoulder dislocation, and bone fractures, and the test accuracy findings are summarized in Table 8.

Two studies studied the accuracy of EP-performed PoCUS on suspected ligamentous injuries in the ulnar part of the wrist and showed high specificity, but mixed sensitivity [187, 188], using magnetic resonance imaging (MRI) as the criterion standard. Two studies evaluating the same in the ankle showed high test accuracies against the same Ref. [189, 190]. A US study showed a higher specificity for ligamentous laceration on extremity penetrating trauma than clinical examination without ultrasound when compared to surgical exploration or MRI [191], and this study and an Iranian study [192] showed 94–100% sensitivity and specificity.

Two studies showed high specificity (both 98%) for paediatric hip effusions, but a somewhat reduced sensitivity of 80–85%, compared to a chart review or radiologist performed ultrasound [193, 194]. One study showed that 50% of planned joint aspirations were avoided after PoCUS of swollen joints [195].

One meta-analysis on the use of PoCUS on patients with shoulder dislocations included seven studies ($n=739$), and showed 99.1% sensitivity and 99.8% specificity when compared to X-ray [196]. The accuracy was similar for associated fractures, but one could not determine the clinical significance due to wide confidence intervals.

A South Korean study found high accuracy for the detection of anterior and posterior cruciate ligament tears by PoCUS [197].

Finding or excluding a bony fracture could be a useful utility of ultrasound in a GP setting given a high enough accuracy, as X-ray is usually not immediately available and may require significant travelling for the patient. We identified three meta-analyses and 25 primary studies evaluating the test accuracy of EP-performed ultrasound on different fractures, all summarized in Table 8. The main finding is that there is generally a very high sensitivity and specificity for detecting the cortical disruption representing the fracture ultrasound, but less for fractures near joints.

Six diagnostic accuracy studies on the use of EP-performed PoCUS to detect paediatric skull fractures found sensitivities ranging from 77 to 100 and specificities from 85 to 100 [198–203].

Clavicular fractures were studied in three studies, all showing high accuracy [198, 204, 205], with false-negative cases being clinically non-significant green-stick fractures.

One meta-analysis of ultrasound for elbow fractures included a sub-group analysis of five studies where the operators were EPs, and showed a specificity of 95% and a sensitivity of 94% [206]. Elbow fractures can be identified on ultrasound by cortical disruption and/or posterior fat pad sign. The latter is rare in radial head subluxation without fractures according to a US study, indicating that PoCUS may be an adequate rule out test before reduction of the subluxation [207].

One meta-analysis assessed the test characteristics of ultrasound to detect paediatric forearm fractures [208] and found sensitivity and specificity of 93, and also two studies published since showed high accuracy [209, 210]. Another meta-analysis, also including studies with adults, showed even higher accuracy with a pooled sensitivity of 97% and a specificity of 95% [211], and also showed no significant accuracy differences between inexperienced and experienced physicians. A Turkish study published after this meta-analysis has shown similar test accuracy in adults [212].

Studies on metacarpal and phalangeal fractures showed sensitivities ranging from 79 to 100% and specificities from 87 to 98%, with the poorest accuracy for periarticular fractures and for the third and fourth metacarpal bones which are only available to scan from two surfaces [213–219]. The study of the distal phalanx fractures also assessed the accuracy of PoCUS to detect nail bed injuries before lifting the nail and visually inspecting, and found a 93% sensitivity and 100% specificity for this [218].

One study aimed to determine the combined accuracy for any tibia or fibula fracture, and found 100% sensitivity and 93% specificity against X-ray, and also found that all false positives were true positives when compared to CT, indicating a higher accuracy than X-ray [220].

One study showed poor sensitivity for navicular bone fracture [221].

One meta-analysis from 2017 [208] and two more recent studies [222, 223] all showed high accuracy in detection of fractures in the ankle malleoli. Three studies determined the accuracy of PoCUS specifically for fifth metatarsal fracture, and found total accuracies in the 90s [221, 224, 225].

Discussion

Strengths and limitations

This review is based on a search strategy that was designed to be comprehensive and sensitive enough to identify all relevant meta-analyses and primary research papers available, and included studies written in English, Spanish, Norwegian, and Swedish. In addition, reference lists of included studies were manually searched to identify further studies to include. However, the search only included searches through PubMed/MEDLINE, not EMBASE or similar proprietary databases. The main screening was only performed by one of the authors, which could be a source of bias.

One comprehensive systematic review only including clinical studies on the training and use of PoCUS by GPs already exists [12]. Given the scarcity of data, it was difficult to draw conclusions other than PoCUS has a potential of being a valuable tool for the general practitioner. A strength of our review is the wealth of data on GP relevant indications which we draw on from our EP colleagues. However, this may be one of the main weaknesses as well, as even though there is a considerable overlap in knowledge and skill bases, generalist approach, and even populations, there are also considerable differences. GPs tend to work more independently with less possibility of daily peer interaction, and have a broader scope of practice, not only including working with patients with conditions which require immediate action. In areas where patients can self-refer to emergency departments staffed by EPs, the pre-test probability of any given diagnosis will be different, with a skew towards more life-threatening conditions in EDs compared to those presenting to primary care run services. However, in other regions, where GPs may, indeed, be the first responder to any emergency, this may not be the case.

Nevertheless, much of a GP's evidence-based practice, is, and will likely always be, based on work done in other fields. In fact, there are most likely relevant studies on the use of ultrasound done by, e.g., physiotherapist, sports medicine physicians, paediatricians, internal medicine specialist, surgeons, etc., which also could be relevant for GPs.

The studies identified were heterogenous and ranged from small pilot studies, through prospective and retrospective convenience sample observational studies, some randomised control trials and on to large, rigorous meta-analyses. In terms of operators, they include in some cases one expert GP or EP sonographer, while, in other cases, the operators were many, of different levels of experience, including novices, all only receiving short, specific didactic interventions. There were no attempts at formally assessing the quality of the primary studies by available quality assessment tools, but most of the meta-analyses will have had such assessment done by their respective authors.

Being a very heterogenous group of physicians, it is hard to establish an absolute list of possible indications for which any given GP may find PoCUS of clinical relevance. We think that we have created an overview where most GPs can find some areas of interest, but also acknowledge that others may criticise the exclusion of indications listed in Appendix 1.

Conclusions

This systematic review shows that ultrasound, at the point of care, is increasingly being utilised by GPs and EPs across the world. It also shows that generalists can, given a certain level of pre-test probability, safely use ultrasound in a wide range of clinical settings to aid diagnosis. For many conditions, the sensitivity is high and can help the physician rule out a condition, while for others, the specificity is high, helping to rule in a diagnosis. For some conditions, the total test accuracy is high, and it may, in fact, be a valuable screening tool. For some conditions, such as identifying foreign bodies and in shoulder dislocations, PoCUS seems to have similar accuracy as X-ray, while for others, such as rib fractures, tibia and fibula fractures, pneumothorax, pneumonia, and in patients presenting with pleuritic pain of any cause, it seems to outperform conventional X-ray. PoCUS has also shown to decrease the length of time to diagnosis and discharge in some settings, decrease failure rates of treatment, and to aid in difficult intravenous access.

GPs are by no means a homogenous group of physicians, neither are EPs. It is likely that if many EPs can learn to safely use clinical ultrasound, so can many interested GPs, as both groups are trained and used to applying a wide range of methods to assess a wide range of patients and conditions. It is likely that the patient population will vary from GP to GP as well, as we all work in different regions with populations of different disease prevalence profiles and health service seeking behaviors. It is important for both GPs and EPs to be aware of one's population's characteristics and pre-test probabilities for any given condition with regards to all aspects of clinical work, including history taking, examination, and diagnostic studies. Given the varying prevalence in each clinician's population, we, therefore, encourage the use of the likelihood ratios using Fagan's nomogram [226], which as a pre-requisite for usage only requires an estimate of pre-test likelihood rather than having the exact same prevalence as in the respective studies from which the data were obtained.

This systematic review will potentially be a valuable reference for physicians searching for evidence for the use of PoCUS in their given primary care setting. Even though most of the studies involved ultrasound performed by EPs, we believe what has been found is relevant also in a GP setting, and is, to date, the best evidence available. We hope also that our review can be of value in showing the need for further research in a primary care setting, and we see a need for more rigorous study designs, with more studies with multi-centre, randomised and controlled designs.

Abbreviations

AAA: abdominal aortic aneurysm; ADHF: acute decompensated heart failure; CAD: coronary artery disease; COPD: chronic obstructive pulmonary disease; CRL: crown-rump length; CT: computed tomography; CXR: chest X-ray; DVT: deep vein thrombosis; ED: emergency department; EP: emergency physician; GA: gestational age; GP: general practitioner/family physician; LOS: length of stay; LR+: positive likelihood ratio; LR−: negative likelihood ratio; LUS: lung ultrasound; LVEF: left-ventricular ejection fraction; LVH: left-ventricular hypertrophy; MAPSE: mitral annular plane systolic excursion; MeSH: medical subject headings; MRI: magnetic resonance imaging; OOH: out-of-hours; PoCUS: point-of-care ultrasound; pro-BNP: pro-brain natriuretic peptide; PVC: peripheral venous catheter.

Acknowledgements

Not applicable.

Authors' contributions
BS is the corresponding author. Both BS and SH collaboratively conceived, designed the study, and wrote the manuscript. BS performed the search and screened the articles. Both authors read and approved the final manuscript.

Authors' information
Bjarte Sorensen: BSc(Med) MB BS, Specialist in General Practice (Norwegian certification), Fellow of the Royal Australian College of General Practitioners (FRACGP), Hjelmeland General Practice Surgery, Prestagarden 13, 4130 Hjelmeland, Norway.

Steinar Hunskaar: MD PhD, Specialist in General Practice (Norwegian certification), Professor at the Department of Global Public Health and Primary Care, University of Bergen, Bergen, Norway and Vice Dean of Education at the Faculty of Medicine, University of Bergen. Senior Researcher at the National Centre for Emergency Primary Health Care, NORCE Norwegian Research Centre AS, Bergen, Norway.

Author details
[1] Hjelmeland General Practice Surgery, Prestagarden 13, 4130 Hjelmeland, Norway. [2] Department of Global Public Health and Primary Care, University of Bergen, Bergen, Norway. [3] National Centre for Emergency Primary Health Care, NORCE Norwegian Research Centre AS, Bergen, Norway.

Appendix 1

See Table 9.

Table 9 Indications excluded due to less relevance for general practice

Organ	Indication
Heart	Echocardiography during resuscitation Paediatric echocardiography
Lungs	Thoracic aortic aneurysm Pulmonary embolism
Vessels	Type A dissection of the ascending aorta Ruptured abdominal aortic aneurysm
Abdomen and pelvis	Hepatic abscess Tubo-ovarian abscess Pneumonperitoneum Mesenteric ischemia
Central nervous system	Ventriculoperitoneal shunt malfunction Intracranial pressure through optic nerve sheath diametre Transcranial ultrasound for MCA perfusion
Trauma	Focused abdominal sonography in trauma (FAST)/extended FAST (eFAST) Hemothorax Pelvic fracture
Procedures	Regional nerve blocks Closed reduction of fractures under sedation Intubation Pericardiocentesis Neonatal intracranial bleeding Lumbar puncture Nasogastric tube placement verification Cystostomy
Others	Undifferentiated hypotension/dehydration Studies from prehospital emergency medical services Mass casualty trauma triage Gastric content

Appendix 2

Ultrasound and general practice (MeSH terms)

"ultrasonography"[MeSH Terms] AND ("primary health care"[MeSH Terms] OR "general practice"[MeSH Terms] OR "general practitioners"[MeSH Terms] OR "physicians, primary care"[MeSH Terms] OR "physicians, family"[MeSH Terms])

Ultrasound and emergency medicine (MeSH terms)

"ultrasonography"[MeSH Terms] AND ("emergency medical services"[MeSH Terms] OR "emergency treatment"[MeSH Terms] OR "emergency medicine"[MeSH Terms] OR "emergencies"[MeSH Terms])

Ultrasound and general practice (keywords)*

((((((ultrasonography) OR pocus) OR ultrasound)) OR echocardiography)) AND ((((((primary care physician)) OR (family practice)) OR (primary health care)) OR (family physician)) OR ((general practice) OR general practitioner))

automatically expanded by PubMed to

(((("diagnostic imaging"[Subheading] OR ("diagnostic"[All Fields] AND "imaging"[All Fields]) OR "diagnostic imaging"[All Fields] OR "ultrasonography"[All Fields] OR "ultrasonography"[MeSH Terms]) OR pocus[All Fields]) OR ("diagnostic imaging"[Subheading] OR ("diagnostic"[All Fields] AND "imaging"[All Fields]) OR "diagnostic imaging"[All Fields] OR "ultrasound"[All Fields] OR "ultrasonography"[MeSH Terms] OR "ultrasonography"[All Fields] OR "ultrasound"[All Fields] OR "ultrasonics"[MeSH Terms] OR "ultrasonics"[All Fields])) OR ("echocardiography"[MeSH Terms] OR "echocardiography"[All Fields])) AND ((((("physicians, primary care"[MeSH Terms] OR ("physicians"[All Fields] AND "primary"[All Fields] AND "care"[All Fields]) OR "primary care physicians"[All Fields] OR ("primary"[All Fields] AND "care"[All Fields] AND "physician"[All Fields]) OR "primary care physician"[All Fields]) OR ("family practice"[MeSH Terms] OR ("family"[All Fields] AND "practice"[All Fields]) OR "family practice"[All Fields])) OR ("primary health care"[MeSH Terms] OR ("primary"[All Fields] AND "health"[All Fields] AND "care"[All Fields]) OR "primary health care"[All Fields])) OR ("physicians, family"[MeSH Terms] OR ("physicians"[All Fields] AND "family"[All Fields]) OR "family physicians"[All Fields] OR ("family"[All Fields] AND "physician"[All Fields]) OR "family physician"[All Fields])) OR (("general practice"[MeSH Terms] OR ("general"[All Fields] AND "practice"[All Fields]) OR "general practice"[All Fields]) OR ("general practitioners"[MeSH Terms] OR ("general"[All Fields] AND "practitioners"[All Fields]) OR "general practitioners"[All Fields] OR ("general"[All Fields] AND "practitioner"[All Fields]) OR "general practitioner"[All Fields])))

Ultrasound and emergency medicine (keywords)*

((((((emergency medical services) OR emergency medicine) OR emergency treatment) OR emergency physician) OR prehospital medicine)) AND (((ultrasound)) OR (((ultrasonography) OR pocus) OR echocardiography))

automatically expanded by PubMed to

((((("emergency medical services"[MeSH Terms] OR ("emergency"[All Fields] AND "medical"[All Fields] AND "services"[All Fields]) OR "emergency medical services"[All Fields]) OR ("emergency medicine"[MeSH Terms] OR ("emergency"[All Fields] AND "medicine"[All Fields]) OR "emergency medicine"[All Fields])) OR ("emergency treatment"[MeSH Terms] OR ("emergency"[All Fields] AND "treatment"[All Fields]) OR "emergency treatment"[All Fields])) OR (("emergencies"[MeSH Terms] OR "emergencies"[All Fields] OR "emergency"[All Fields]) AND ("physicians"[MeSH Terms] OR "physicians"[All Fields] OR "physician"[All Fields]))) OR (prehospital[All Fields] AND ("medicine"[MeSH Terms] OR "medicine"[All Fields]))) AND (("diagnostic imaging"[Subheading] OR ("diagnostic"[All Fields] AND "imaging"[All Fields]) OR "diagnostic imaging"[All Fields] OR "ultrasound"[All Fields] OR "ultrasonography"[MeSH Terms] OR "ultrasonography"[All Fields] OR "ultrasound"[All Fields] OR "ultrasonics"[MeSH Terms] OR "ultrasonics"[All Fields]) OR ((("diagnostic imaging"[Subheading] OR ("diagnostic"[All Fields] AND "imaging"[All Fields]) OR "diagnostic imaging"[All Fields] OR "ultrasonography"[All Fields] OR "ultrasonography"[MeSH Terms]) OR pocus[All Fields]) OR ("echocardiography"[MeSH Terms] OR "echocardiography"[All Fields])))

* To exclude indexed articles (which presumably were found by searching with MeSH terms) the keyword searches was done with the following filter:

((publisher[sb] NOT pubstatusnihms NOT pubstatuspmcsd NOT pmcbook) OR inprocess[sb] OR pubmednotmedline[sb] OR ((pubstatusnihms OR pubstatuspmcsd) AND publisher[sb])) OR pubmednotmedline[sb]

((publisher[sb] NOT pubstatusnihms NOT pubstatuspmcsd NOT pmcbook) OR pubmednotmedline[sb] OR ((pubstatusnihms OR pubstatuspmcsd) AND publisher[sb]))
inprocess[sb]

References

1. Moore CL, Copel JA (2011) Point-of-care ultrasonography. N Engl J Med 364(8):749–757
2. Weile J, Brix J, Moellekaer AB (2018) Is point-of-care ultrasound disruptive innovation? Formulating why POCUS is different from conventional comprehensive ultrasound. Crit Ultrasound J 10(1):25
3. Huibers L, Giesen P, Wensing M, Grol R (2009) Out-of-hours care in western countries: assessment of different organizational models. BMC Health Serv Res 9:105
4. Pandit T, Ray R, Sabesan S (2019) Review article: Managing medical emergencies in rural Australia: a systematic review of the training needs. Emerg Med Australas 31(1):20–28
5. Bosco C, Oandasan I (2016) Review of family medicine within rural and remote Canada: education, practice, and policy. The College of Family Physicians of Canada, Mississauga
6. Nieber T, Hansen EH, Bondevik GT (2007) Organization of Norwegian out-of-hours primary health care services. Tidsskr Nor Laegeforen 127:1335–1338
7. St John and the PRIME programme. https://www.stjohn.org.nz/What-we-do/Community-programmes/Partnered-programmes/PRIME/. Accessed 9 Sept 2019
8. Lopez DG, Hamdorf JM, Ward AM, Emery J (2006) Early trauma management skills in Australian general practitioners. ANZ J Surg 76(10):894–897
9. Huibers LAMJ, Moth G, Bondevik GT, Kersnik J, Huber CA, Christensen MB, Leutgeb R, Casado AM, Remmen R, Wensing M (2011) Diagnostic scope in out-of-hours primary care services in eight European countries: an observational study. BMC Fam Pract 12:30
10. Hall JWW, Holman H, Bornemann P, Barreto T, Henderson D, Bennett K, Chamberlain J, Maurer DM (2015) Point of care ultrasound in family medicine residency programs: a CERA study. Fam Med 47(9):706–711
11. Bornemann P, Barreto T (2018) Point-of-care ultrasonography in family medicine. Am Fam Physician 98(4):200–202
12. Andersen CA, Holden S, Vela J, Rathleff MS, Jensen MB (2019) Point-of-care ultrasound in general practice: a systematic review. Ann Fam Med 17(1):61–69
13. Myhr K, Sandvik H, Morken T, Hunskaar S (2017) Point-of-care ultrasonography in Norwegian out-of-hours primary health care. Scand J Prim Health Care 35(2):120–125
14. Mengel-Jørgensen T, Jensen MB (2016) Variation in the use of point-of-care ultrasound in general practice in various European countries. Results of a survey among experts. Eur J Gen Pract 22(4):274–277
15. Flynn CJ, Weppler A, Theodoro D, Haney E, Milne WK (2012) Emergency medicine ultrasonography in rural communities. Can J Rural Med 17(3):99–104
16. Léger P, Fleet R, Maltais-Giguère J, Plant J, Piette É, Légaré F, Poitras J (2015) A majority of rural emergency departments in the province of Quebec use point-of-care ultrasound: a cross-sectional survey. BMC Emerg Med 15:36
17. Leschyna M, Hatam E, Britton S, Myslik F, Thompson D, Sedran R, VanAarsen K, Detombe S (2019) Current state of point-of-care ultrasound usage in Canadian emergency departments. Cureus 11(3):e4246
18. Bobbia X, Zieleskiewicz L, Pradeilles C, Hudson C, Muller L, Claret PG, Leone M, de La Coussaye J-E, Winfocus France Group (2017) The clinical impact and prevalence of emergency point-of-care ultrasound: a prospective multicenter study. Anaesth Crit Care Pain Med 36(6):383–389
19. Bobbia X, Abou-Badra M, Hansel N, Pes P, Petrovic T, Claret PG, Lefrant JY, de La Coussaye JE, Winfocus France Group (2017) Changes in the availability of bedside ultrasound practice in emergency rooms and prehospital settings in France. Anaesth Crit Care Pain Med 37(3):201–205
20. Nielsen K, Lauridsen JRM, Laursen CB, Brabrand M (2015) Physicians using ultrasound in Danish emergency departments are mostly summoned specialists. Scand J Trauma Resusc Emerg Med 23:51
21. Shi D, Walline JH, Yu X, Xu J, Song PP, Zhu H (2018) Evaluating and assessing the prevalence of bedside ultrasound in emergency departments in China. J Thorac Dis 10(5):2685–2690
22. Ahn C, Kim C, Kang BS, Choi HJ, Cho JH (2015) Variation of availability and frequency of emergency physician-performed ultrasonography between adult and pediatric patients in the academic emergency department in Korea. Clin Exp Emerg Med 2(1):16–23
23. Henwood PC, Beversluis D, Genthon AA et al (2014) Characterizing the limited use of point-of-care ultrasound in Colombian emergency medicine residencies. Int J Emerg Med 7(1):7
24. American College of Emergency Physicians (2017) Ultrasound guidelines: emergency, point-of-care and clinical ultrasound guidelines in medicine. Ann Emerg Med 69(5):e27–e54
25. Moore CL, Molina AA, Lin H (2006) Ultrasonography in community emergency departments in the United States: access to ultrasonography performed by consultants and status of emergency physician-performed ultrasonography. Ann Emerg Med 47(2):147–153
26. Talley BE, Ginde AA, Raja AS, Sullivan AF, Espinola JA, Camargo CA Jr (2011) Variable access to immediate bedside ultrasound in the emergency department. West J Emerg Med 12(1):96–99
27. Herbst MK, Camargo CA Jr, Perez A, Moore CL (2015) Use of point-of-care ultrasound in Connecticut emergency departments. J Emerg Med 48(2):191–196.e2
28. Sanders JL, Noble VE, Raja AS, Sullivan AF, Camargo CA Jr (2015) Access to and use of point-of-care ultrasound in the emergency department. West J Emerg Med 16(5):747–752
29. Amini R, Wyman MT, Hernandez NC, Guisto JA, Adhikari S (2017) Use of emergency ultrasound in Arizona community emergency departments. J Ultrasound Med 36(5):913–921
30. Mengarelli M, Nepusz A, Kondrashova T (2018) A comparison of point-of-care ultrasonography use in rural versus urban emergency departments throughout Missouri. Mo Med 115(1):56–60
31. Bratland SZ (1985) Ultrasonic diagnosis in general practice. An evaluation study. Tidsskr Nor Laegeforen 105(28):1939–1940
32. Gillespie ND, Pringle S (1998) A pilot study of the role of echocardiography in primary care. Br J Gen Pract 48(429):1182
33. Mjølstad OC, Snare SR, Folkvord L, Helland F, Grimsmo A, Torp H, Haraldseth O, Haugen BO (2012) Assessment of left ventricular function by GPs using pocket-sized ultrasound. Fam Pract 29(5):534–540
34. Evangelista L, Juncadella E, Copetti S, Pareja A, Torrabadella J, Evangelista A (2013) Diagnostic usefulness of pocket echography performed in hypertensive patients by a general practitioner. Med Clin 141(1):1–7
35. Evangelista A, Galuppo V, Méndez J et al (2016) Hand-held cardiac ultrasound screening performed by family doctors with remote expert support interpretation. Heart 102(5):376–382
36. Moore CL, Rose GA, Tayal VS, Sullivan DM, Arrowood JA, Kline JA (2002) Determination of left ventricular function by emergency physician echocardiography of hypotensive patients. Acad Emerg Med 9(3):186–193
37. Randazzo MR, Snoey ER, Levitt MA, Binder K (2003) Accuracy of emergency physician assessment of left ventricular ejection fraction and central venous pressure using echocardiography. Acad Emerg Med 10(9):973–977
38. Secko MA, Lazar JM, Salciccioli LA, Stone MB (2011) Can junior emergency physicians use E-point septal separation to accurately estimate left ventricular function in acutely dyspneic patients? Acad Emerg Med 18(11):1223–1226
39. Bustam A, Noor Azhar M, Singh Veriah R, Arumugam K, Loch A (2014) Performance of emergency physicians in point-of-care echocardiography following limited training. Emerg Med J 31(5):369–373

40. McKaigney CJ, Krantz MJ, La Rocque CL, Hurst ND, Buchanan MS, Kendall JL (2014) E-point septal separation: a bedside tool for emergency physician assessment of left ventricular ejection fraction. Am J Emerg Med 32(6):493–497
41. Unlüer EE, Karagöz A, Akoğlu H, Bayata S (2014) Visual estimation of bedside echocardiographic ejection fraction by emergency physicians. West J Emerg Med 15(2):221–226
42. Shah SP, Shah SP, Fils-Aime R, Desir W, Joasil J, Venesy DM, Muruganandan KM (2016) Focused cardiopulmonary ultrasound for assessment of dyspnea in a resource-limited setting. Crit Ultrasound J 8(1):7
43. Farsi D, Hajsadeghi S, Hajighanbari MJ, Mofidi M, Hafezimoghadam P, Rezai M, Mahshidfar B, Abiri S, Abbasi S (2017) Focused cardiac ultrasound (FOCUS) by emergency medicine residents in patients with suspected cardiovascular diseases. J Ultrasound 20(2):133–138
44. Dehbozorgi A, Eslami Nejad S, Mousavi-Roknabadi RS, Sharifi M, Tafakori A, Jalli R (2019) Lung and cardiac ultrasound (LuCUS) protocol in diagnosing acute heart failure in patients with acute dyspnea. Am J Emerg Med. https://doi.org/10.1016/j.ajem.2019.02.040
45. Dinh VA, Ko HS, Rao R, Bansal RC, Smith DD, Kim TE, Nguyen HB (2012) Measuring cardiac index with a focused cardiac ultrasound examination in the ED. Am J Emerg Med 30(9):1845–1851
46. Betcher J, Majkrzak A, Cranford J, Kessler R, Theyyunni N, Huang R (2018) Feasibility study of advanced focused cardiac measurements within the emergency department. Crit Ultrasound J 10(1):10
47. Unlüer EE, Bayata S, Postaci N, Yeşil M, Yavaşi Ö, Kara PH, Vandenberk N, Akay S (2012) Limited bedside echocardiography by emergency physicians for diagnosis of diastolic heart failure. Emerg Med J 29(4):280–283
48. Ehrman RR, Russell FM, Ansari AH, Margeta B, Clary JM, Christian E, Cosby KS, Bailitz J (2015) Can emergency physicians diagnose and correctly classify diastolic dysfunction using bedside echocardiography? Am J Emerg Med 33(9):1178–1183
49. Del Rios M, Colla J, Kotini-Shah P, Briller J, Gerber B, Prendergast H (2018) Emergency physician use of tissue Doppler bedside echocardiography in detecting diastolic dysfunction: an exploratory study. Crit Ultrasound J 10(1):4
50. Nazerian P, Vanni S, Zanobetti M, Polidori G, Pepe G, Federico R, Cangioli E, Grifoni S (2010) Diagnostic accuracy of emergency Doppler echocardiography for identification of acute left ventricular heart failure in patients with acute dyspnea: comparison with Boston criteria and N-terminal prohormone brain natriuretic peptide. Acad Emerg Med 17(1):18–26
51. Saul T, Avitabile NC, Berkowitz R, Siadecki SD, Rose G, Toomarian M, Kaban NL, Governatori N, Suprun M (2016) The inter-rater reliability of echocardiographic diastolic function evaluation among emergency physician sonographers. J Emerg Med 51(4):411–417
52. Croft PE, Strout TD, Kring RM, Director L, Vasaiwala SC, Mackenzie DC (2019) WAMAMI: emergency physicians can accurately identify wall motion abnormalities in acute myocardial infarction. Am J Emerg Med. https://doi.org/10.1016/j.ajem.2019.03.037
53. Reardon L, Scheels WJ, Singer AJ, Reardon RF (2018) Feasibility and accuracy of speckle tracking echocardiography in emergency department patients. Am J Emerg Med 36(12):2254–2259
54. Mandavia DP, Hoffner RJ, Mahaney K, Henderson SO (2001) Bedside echocardiography by emergency physicians. Ann Emerg Med 38(4):377–382
55. Martindale JL, Wakai A, Collins SP, Levy PD, Diercks D, Hiestand BC, Fermann GJ, deSouza I, Sinert R (2016) Diagnosing acute heart failure in the emergency department: a systematic review and meta-analysis. Acad Emerg Med 23(3):223–242
56. McGivery K, Atkinson P, Lewis D, Taylor L, Harris T, Gadd K, Fraser J, Stoica G (2018) Emergency department ultrasound for the detection of B-lines in the early diagnosis of acute decompensated heart failure: a systematic review and meta-analysis. CJEM 20(3):343–352
57. Lian R, Zhang GC, Yan ST, Sun LC, Zhang SQ, Zhang GQ (2018) Role of ultrasound lung comets in the diagnosis of acute heart failure in emergency department: a systematic review and meta-analysis. Biomed Environ Sci 31(8):596–607
58. Maw AM, Hassanin A, Ho PM et al (2019) Diagnostic accuracy of point-of-care lung ultrasonography and chest radiography in adults with symptoms suggestive of acute decompensated heart failure: a systematic review and meta-analysis. JAMA Netw Open 2(3):e190703
59. Staub LJ, Mazzali Biscaro RR, Kaszubowski E, Maurici R (2019) Lung ultrasound for the emergency diagnosis of pneumonia, acute heart failure, and exacerbations of chronic obstructive pulmonary disease/asthma in adults: a systematic review and meta-analysis. J Emerg Med 56(1):53–69
60. Pivetta E, Goffi A, Nazerian P et al (2019) Lung ultrasound integrated with clinical assessment for the diagnosis of acute decompensated heart failure in the emergency department: a randomized controlled trial. Eur J Heart Fail. https://doi.org/10.1002/ejhf.1379
61. Baker K, Mitchell G, Stieler G (2013) Limited lung ultrasound protocol in elderly patients with breathlessness; agreement between bedside interpretation and stored images as acquired by experienced and inexperienced sonologists. Australas J Ultrasound Med 16(2):86–92
62. Orso D, Guglielmo N, Copetti R (2018) Lung ultrasound in diagnosing pneumonia in the emergency department: a systematic review and meta-analysis. Eur J Emerg Med 25(5):312–321
63. Ye X, Xiao H, Chen B, Zhang S (2015) Accuracy of lung ultrasonography versus chest radiography for the diagnosis of adult community-acquired pneumonia: review of the literature and meta-analysis. PLoS ONE 10(6):e0130066
64. Amatya Y, Rupp J, Russell FM, Saunders J, Bales B, House DR (2018) Diagnostic use of lung ultrasound compared to chest radiograph for suspected pneumonia in a resource-limited setting. Int J Emerg Med 11(1):8
65. Copetti R, Cattarossi L (2008) Ultrasound diagnosis of pneumonia in children. Radiol Med 113(2):190–198
66. Shah VP, Tunik MG, Tsung JW (2013) Prospective evaluation of point-of-care ultrasonography for the diagnosis of pneumonia in children and young adults. JAMA Pediatr 167(2):119–125
67. Yilmaz HL, Özkaya AK, Sarı Gökay S, Tolu Kendir Ö, Şenol H (2017) Point-of-care lung ultrasound in children with community acquired pneumonia. Am J Emerg Med 35(7):964–969
68. Jones BP, Tay ET, Elikashvili I, Sanders JE, Paul AZ, Nelson BP, Spina LA, Tsung JW (2016) Feasibility and safety of substituting lung ultrasonography for chest radiography when diagnosing pneumonia in children: a randomized controlled trial. Chest 150(1):131–138
69. Harel-Sterling M, Diallo M, Santhirakumaran S, Maxim T, Tessaro M (2019) Emergency department resource use in pediatric pneumonia: point-of-care lung ultrasonography versus chest radiography. J Ultrasound Med 38(2):407–414
70. Ebrahimi A, Yousefifard M, Mohammad Kazemi H, Rasouli HR, Asady H, Moghadas Jafari A, Hosseini M (2014) Diagnostic accuracy of chest ultrasonography versus chest radiography for identification of pneumothorax: a systematic review and meta-analysis. Tanaffos 13(4):29–40
71. Staub LJ, Biscaro RRM, Kaszubowski E, Maurici R (2018) Chest ultrasonography for the emergency diagnosis of traumatic pneumothorax and haemothorax: a systematic review and meta-analysis. Injury 49(3):457–466
72. Riccardi A, Spinola MB, Ghiglione V, Licenziato M, Lerza R (2019) PoCUS evaluating blunt thoracic trauma: a retrospective analysis of 18 months of emergency department activity. Eur J Orthop Surg Traumatol 29(1):31–35
73. Lalande É, Guimont C, Émond M, Parent MC, Topping C, Kuimi BLB, Boucher V, Le Sage N (2017) Feasibility of emergency department point-of-care ultrasound for rib fracture diagnosis in minor thoracic injury. CJEM 19(3):213–219
74. Pishbin E, Ahmadi K, Foogardi M, Salehi M, Seilanian Toosi F, Rahimi-Movaghar V (2017) Comparison of ultrasonography and radiography in diagnosis of rib fractures. Chin J Traumatol 20(4):226–228
75. Koh Y, Chua MT, Ho WH, Lee C, Chan GWH, Sen Kuan W (2018) Assessment of dyspneic patients in the emergency department using point-of-care lung and cardiac ultrasonography—a prospective observational study. J Thorac Dis 10(11):6221–6229
76. Bekgoz B, Kilicaslan I, Bildik F, Keles A, Demircan A, Hakoglu O, Coskun G, Demir HA (2019) BLUE protocol ultrasonography in emergency department patients presenting with acute dyspnea. Am J Emerg Med. https://doi.org/10.1016/j.ajem.2019.02.028
77. Volpicelli G, Cardinale L, Berchialla P, Mussa A, Bar F, Frascisco MF (2012) A comparison of different diagnostic tests in the bedside evaluation of pleuritic pain in the ED. Am J Emerg Med 30(2):317–324
78. Goffi A, Pivetta E, Lupia E, Porrino G, Civita M, Laurita E, Griot G, Casoli G, Cibinel G (2013) Has lung ultrasound an impact on the management of

patients with acute dyspnea in the emergency department? Crit Care 17(4):R180
79. Laursen CB, Sloth E, Lambrechtsen J, Lassen AT, Madsen PH, Henriksen DP, Davidsen JR, Rasmussen F (2013) Focused sonography of the heart, lungs, and deep veins identifies missed life-threatening conditions in admitted patients with acute respiratory symptoms. Chest 144(6):1868–1875
80. Laursen CB, Sloth E, Lassen AT, Christensen RD, Lambrechtsen J, Madsen PH, Henriksen DP, Davidsen JR, Rasmussen F (2014) Point-of-care ultrasonography in patients admitted with respiratory symptoms: a single-blind, randomised controlled trial. Lancet Respir Med 2(8):638–646
81. Zanobetti M, Scorpiniti M, Gigli C et al (2017) Point-of-care ultrasonography for evaluation of acute dyspnea in the ED. Chest 151(6):1295–1301
82. Seyedhosseini J, Bashizadeh-Fakhar G, Farzaneh S, Momeni M, Karimi-alavijeh E (2017) The impact of the BLUE protocol ultrasonography on the time taken to treat acute respiratory distress in the ED. Am J Emerg Med 35(12):1815–1818
83. Buhumaid RE, St-Cyr Bourque J, Shokoohi H, Ma IWY, Longacre M, Liteplo AS (2019) Integrating point-of-care ultrasound in the ED evaluation of patients presenting with chest pain and shortness of breath. Am J Emerg Med 37(2):298–303
84. Zanobetti M, Poggioni C, Pini R (2011) Can chest ultrasonography replace standard chest radiography for evaluation of acute dyspnea in the ED? Chest 139(5):1140–1147
85. Sforza A, Mancusi C, Carlino MV, Buonauro A, Barozzi M, Romano G, Serra S, de Simone G (2017) Diagnostic performance of multi-organ ultrasound with pocket-sized device in the management of acute dyspnea. Cardiovasc Ultrasound 15(1):16
86. Carlino MV, Paladino F, Sforza A, Serra C, Liccardi F, de Simone G, Mancusi C (2018) Assessment of left atrial size in addition to focused cardiopulmonary ultrasound improves diagnostic accuracy of acute heart failure in the emergency department. Echocardiography 35(6):785–791
87. Papanagnou D, Secko M, Gullett J, Stone M, Zehtabchi S (2017) Clinician-performed bedside ultrasound in improving diagnostic accuracy in patients presenting to the ED with acute dyspnea. West J Emerg Med 18(3):382–389
88. Blois B (2012) Office-based ultrasound screening for abdominal aortic aneurysm. Can Fam Physician 58(3):e172–e178
89. Bailey RP, Ault M, Greengold NL, Rosendahl T, Cossman D (2001) Ultrasonography performed by primary care residents for abdominal aortic aneurysm screening. J Gen Intern Med 16(12):845–849
90. Bravo-Merino L, González-Lozano N, Maroto-Salmón R, Meijide-Santos G, Suárez-Gil P, Fañanás-Mastral A (2019) Validity of the abdominal ecography in primary care for detection of aorta abdominal aneurism in male between 65 and 75 years. Aten Primaria 51(1):11–17
91. Sisó-Almirall A, Kostov B, Navarro González M et al (2017) Abdominal aortic aneurysm screening program using hand-held ultrasound in primary healthcare. PLoS ONE 12(4):e0176877
92. Hoffmann B, Um P, Bessman ES, Ding R, Kelen GD, McCarthy ML (2009) Routine screening for asymptomatic abdominal aortic aneurysm in high-risk patients is not recommended in emergency departments that are frequently crowded. Acad Emerg Med 16(11):1242–1250
93. Lindgaard K, Riisgaard L (2017) Validation of ultrasound examinations performed by general practitioners. Scand J Prim Health Care 35(3):256–261
94. Rubano E, Mehta N, Caputo W, Paladino L, Sinert R (2013) Systematic review: emergency department bedside ultrasonography for diagnosing suspected abdominal aortic aneurysm. Acad Emerg Med 20(2):128–138
95. Okahara A, Sadamatsu K, Matsuura T, Koga Y, Mine D, Yoshida K (2016) Coronary artery disease screening with carotid ultrasound examination by a primary care physician. Cardiol Res Pract 7(1):9–16
96. Mumoli N, Vitale J, Giorgi-Pierfranceschi M et al (2017) General practitioner-performed compression ultrasonography for diagnosis of deep vein thrombosis of the leg: a multicenter, prospective cohort study. Ann Fam Med 15(6):535–539
97. Pomero F, Dentali F, Borretta V, Bonzini M, Melchio R, Douketis JD, Fenoglio LM (2013) Accuracy of emergency physician-performed ultrasonography in the diagnosis of deep-vein thrombosis: a systematic review and meta-analysis. Thromb Haemost 109(1):137–145
98. Lee JH, Lee SH, Yun SJ (2019) Comparison of 2-point and 3-point point-of-care ultrasound techniques for deep vein thrombosis at the emergency department: a meta-analysis. Medicine 98(22):e15791
99. Torres-Macho J, Antón-Santos JM, García-Gutierrez I et al (2012) Initial accuracy of bedside ultrasound performed by emergency physicians for multiple indications after a short training period. Am J Emerg Med 30(9):1943–1949
100. Crowhurst TD, Dunn RJ (2013) Sensitivity and specificity of three-point compression ultrasonography performed by emergency physicians for proximal lower extremity deep venous thrombosis. Emerg Med Australas 25(6):588–596
101. Nygren D, Hård Af Segerstad C, Ellehuus Hilmersson C, Elf J, Ulf E, Lundager Forberg J (2018) Good outcomes when emergency physicians diagnosed deep vein thrombosis. Lakartidningen 115(3):92–95
102. Seyedhosseini J, Fadavi A, Vahidi E, Saeedi M, Momeni M (2018) Impact of point-of-care ultrasound on disposition time of patients presenting with lower extremity deep vein thrombosis, done by emergency physicians. Turk J Emerg Med 18(1):20–24
103. Costantino TG, Parikh AK, Satz WA, Fojtik JP (2005) Ultrasonography-guided peripheral intravenous access versus traditional approaches in patients with difficult intravenous access. Ann Emerg Med 46(5):456–461
104. Dargin JM, Rebholz CM, Lowenstein RA, Mitchell PM, Feldman JA (2010) Ultrasonography-guided peripheral intravenous catheter survival in ED patients with difficult access. Am J Emerg Med 28(1):1–7
105. Vinograd AM, Zorc JJ, Dean AJ, Abbadessa MKF, Chen AE (2018) First-attempt success, longevity, and complication rates of ultrasound-guided peripheral intravenous catheters in children. Pediatr Emerg Care 34(6):376–380
106. Stein J, George B, River G, Hebig A, McDermott D (2009) Ultrasonographically guided peripheral intravenous cannulation in emergency department patients with difficult intravenous access: a randomized trial. Ann Emerg Med 54(1):33–40
107. Oakley E, Wong A-M (2010) Ultrasound-assisted peripheral vascular access in a paediatric ED. Emerg Med Australas 22(2):166–170
108. Otani T, Morikawa Y, Hayakawa I et al (2018) Ultrasound-guided peripheral intravenous access placement for children in the emergency department. Eur J Pediatr 177(10):1443–1449
109. Rupp JD, Ferre RM, Boyd JS, Dearing E, McNaughton CD, Liu D, Jarrell KL, McWade CM, Self WH (2016) Extravasation risk using ultrasound-guided peripheral intravenous catheters for computed tomography contrast administration. Acad Emerg Med 23(8):918–921
110. Keyes LE, Frazee BW, Snoey ER, Simon BC, Christy D (1999) Ultrasound-guided brachial and basilic vein cannulation in emergency department patients with difficult intravenous access. Ann Emerg Med 34(6):711–714
111. Schnadower D, Lin S, Perera P, Smerling A, Dayan P (2007) A pilot study of ultrasound analysis before pediatric peripheral vein cannulation attempt. Acad Emerg Med 14(5):483–485
112. Zitek T, Busby E, Hudson H, McCourt JD, Baydoun J, Slattery DE (2018) Ultrasound-guided placement of single-lumen peripheral intravenous catheters in the internal jugular vein. West J Emerg Med 19(5):808–812
113. Wong C, Teitge B, Ross M, Young P, Robertson HL, Lang E (2018) The accuracy and prognostic value of point-of-care ultrasound for nephrolithiasis in the emergency department: a systematic review and meta-analysis. Acad Emerg Med 25(6):684–698
114. Javaudin F, Mounier F, Pes P, Arnaudet I, Vignaud F, Frampas E, Le Conte P, Winfocus-France study group (2017) Evaluation of a short formation on the performance of point-of-care renal ultrasound performed by physicians without previous ultrasound skills: prospective observational study. Crit Ultrasound J 9(1):23
115. Guedj R, Escoda S, Blakime P, Patteau G, Brunelle F, Cheron G (2015) The accuracy of renal point of care ultrasound to detect hydronephrosis in children with a urinary tract infection. Eur J Emerg Med 22(2):135–138
116. Smith-Bindman R, Aubin C, Bailitz J et al (2014) Ultrasonography versus computed tomography for suspected nephrolithiasis. N Engl J Med 371(12):1100–1110
117. Park YH, Jung RB, Lee YG, Hong CK, Ahn J-H, Shin TY, Kim YS, Ha YR (2016) Does the use of bedside ultrasonography reduce emergency department length of stay for patients with renal colic?: a pilot study. Clin Exp Emerg Med 3(4):197–203

118. Blaivas M, Sierzenski P, Lambert M (2001) Emergency evaluation of patients presenting with acute scrotum using bedside ultrasonography. Acad Emerg Med 8(1):90–93
119. Bratland SZ, Nordshus T (1985) Ultrasonography of the gallbladder in general practice. Tidsskr Nor Laegeforen 105(28):1946–1948
120. Eggebø TM, Sørvang S, Dalaker K (1990) Ultrasonic diagnosis of the upper abdomen performed in general practice. Tidsskr Nor Laegeforen 110(9):1096–1098
121. Esquerrà M, Roura Poch P, Masat Ticó T, Canal V, Maideu Mir J, Cruxent R (2012) Abdominal ultrasound: a diagnostic tool within the reach of general practitioners. Aten Primaria 44(10):576–583
122. Schlager D, Lazzareschi G, Whitten D, Sanders AB (1994) A prospective study of ultrasonography in the ED by emergency physicians. Am J Emerg Med 12(2):185–189
123. Blaivas M, Harwood RA, Lambert MJ (1999) Decreasing length of stay with emergency ultrasound examination of the gallbladder. Acad Emerg Med 6(10):1020–1023
124. Ross M, Brown M, McLaughlin K, Atkinson P, Thompson J, Powelson S, Clark S, Lang E (2011) Emergency physician-performed ultrasound to diagnose cholelithiasis: a systematic review. Acad Emerg Med 18(3):227–235
125. Scruggs W, Fox JC, Potts B, Zlidenny A, McDonough J, Anderson CL, Larson J, Barajas G, Langdorf MI (2008) Accuracy of ED bedside ultrasound for identification of gallstones: retrospective analysis of 575 studies. West J Emerg Med 9(1):1–5
126. Hilsden R, Leeper R, Koichopolos J, Vandelinde JD, Parry N, Thompson D, Myslik F (2018) Point-of-care biliary ultrasound in the emergency department (BUSED): implications for surgical referral and emergency department wait times. Trauma Surg Acute Care Open 3(1):e000164
127. Rosen CL, Brown DF, Chang Y, Moore C, Averill NJ, Arkoff LJ, McCabe CJ, Wolfe RE (2001) Ultrasonography by emergency physicians in patients with suspected cholecystitis. Am J Emerg Med 19(1):32–36
128. Summers SM, Scruggs W, Menchine MD, Lahham S, Anderson C, Amr O, Lotfipour S, Cusick SS, Fox JC (2010) A prospective evaluation of emergency department bedside ultrasonography for the detection of acute cholecystitis. Ann Emerg Med 56(2):114–122
129. Shekarchi B, Hejripour Rafsanjani SZ, Shekar Riz Fomani N, Chahardoli M (2018) Emergency department bedside ultrasonography for diagnosis of acute cholecystitis; a diagnostic accuracy study. Emergency 6(1):e11
130. Tootian Tourghabe J, Arabikhan HR, Alamdaran A, Zamani Moghadam H (2018) Emergency medicine resident versus radiologist in detecting the ultrasonographic signs of acute cholecystitis; a diagnostic accuracy study. Emergency 6(1):e19
131. Bektas F, Eken C, Soyuncu S, Kusoglu L, Cete Y (2009) Contribution of goal-directed ultrasonography to clinical decision-making for emergency physicians. Emerg Med J 26(3):169–172
132. Adhikari S, Morrison D, Lyon M, Zeger W, Krueger A (2014) Utility of point-of-care biliary ultrasound in the evaluation of emergency patients with isolated acute non-traumatic epigastric pain. Intern Emerg Med 9(5):583–587
133. Lahham S, Becker BA, Gari A, Bunch S, Alvarado M, Anderson CL, Viquez E, Spann SC, Fox JC (2018) Utility of common bile duct measurement in ED point of care ultrasound: a prospective study. Am J Emerg Med 36(6):962–966
134. Benabbas R, Hanna M, Shah J, Sinert R (2017) Diagnostic accuracy of history, physical examination, laboratory tests, and point-of-care ultrasound for pediatric acute appendicitis in the emergency department: a systematic review and meta-analysis. Acad Emerg Med 24(5):523–551
135. Nicole M, Desjardins MP, Gravel J (2018) Bedside sonography performed by emergency physicians to detect appendicitis in children. Acad Emerg Med. https://doi.org/10.1111/acem.13445
136. Lee SH, Yun SJ (2019) Diagnostic performance of emergency physician-performed point-of-care ultrasonography for acute appendicitis: a meta-analysis. Am J Emerg Med 37(4):696–705
137. Fields JM, Davis J, Alsup C, Bates A, Au A, Adhikari S, Farrell I (2017) Accuracy of point-of-care ultrasonography for diagnosing acute appendicitis: a systematic review and meta-analysis. Acad Emerg Med 24(9):1124–1136
138. Shahbazipar M, Seyedhosseini J, Vahidi E, Sheikh Motahar Vahedi H, Jahanshir A (2018) Accuracy of ultrasound exam performed by emergency medicine versus radiology residents in the diagnosis of acute appendicitis. Eur J Emerg Med. https://doi.org/10.1097/MEJ.0000000000000547
139. Sharif S, Skitch S, Vlahak D, Healey A (2018) Point-of-care ultrasound to diagnose appendicitis in a Canadian emergency department. CJEM 20(5):732–735
140. Corson-Knowles D, Russell FM (2018) Clinical ultrasound is safe and highly specific for acute appendicitis in moderate to high pre-test probability patients. West J Emerg Med 19(3):460–464
141. Riera A, Hsiao AL, Langhan ML, Goodman TR, Chen L (2012) Diagnosis of intussusception by physician novice sonographers in the emergency department. Ann Emerg Med 60(3):264–268
142. Lam SHF, Wise A, Yenter C (2014) Emergency bedside ultrasound for the diagnosis of pediatric intussusception: a retrospective review. World J Emerg Med 5(4):255–258
143. Chang Y-J, Hsia S-H, Chao H-C (2013) Emergency medicine physicians performed ultrasound for pediatric intussusceptions. Biomed J 36(4):175–178
144. Kim JH, Lee J-Y, Kwon JH, Cho H-R, Lee JS, Ryu J-M (2017) Point-of-care ultrasound could streamline the emergency department workflow of clinically nonspecific intussusception. Pediatr Emerg Care. https://doi.org/10.1097/PEC.0000000000001283
145. Becker BA, Lahham S, Gonzales MA, Nomura JT, Bui MK, Truong TA, Stahlman BA, Fox JC, Kehrl T (2019) A prospective, multicenter evaluation of point-of-care ultrasound for small-bowel obstruction in the emergency department. Acad Emerg Med. https://doi.org/10.1111/acem.13713
146. Unlüer EE, Yavaşi O, Eroğlu O, Yilmaz C, Akarca FK (2010) Ultrasonography by emergency medicine and radiology residents for the diagnosis of small bowel obstruction. Eur J Emerg Med 17(5):260–264
147. Jang TB, Schindler D, Kaji AH (2011) Bedside ultrasonography for the detection of small bowel obstruction in the emergency department. Emerg Med J 28(8):676–678
148. Frasure SE, Hildreth AF, Seethala R, Kimberly HH (2018) Accuracy of abdominal ultrasound for the diagnosis of small bowel obstruction in the emergency department. World J Emerg Med 9(4):267–271
149. Doniger SJ, Dessie A, Latronica C (2018) Measuring the transrectal diameter on point-of-care ultrasound to diagnose constipation in children. Pediatr Emerg Care 34(3):154–159
150. Hasani SA, Fathi M, Daadpey M, Zare MA, Tavakoli N, Abbasi S (2015) Accuracy of bedside emergency physician performed ultrasound in diagnosing different causes of acute abdominal pain: a prospective study. Clin Imaging 39(3):476–479
151. Bourcier J-E, Gallard E, Redonnet J-P, Majourau M, Deshaie D, Bourgeois J-M, Garnier D, Geeraerts T (2018) Diagnostic performance of abdominal point of care ultrasound performed by an emergency physician in acute right iliac fossa pain. Crit Ultrasound J 10(1):31
152. Johansen I, Grimsmo A, Nakling J (2002) Ultrasonography in primary health care—experiences within obstetrics 1983–99. Tidsskr Nor Laegeforen 122(20):1995–1998
153. Bratland SZ, Eik-Nes SH (1985) Ultrasonic diagnosis of pregnant women in general practice. Tidsskr Nor Laegeforen 105(28):1940–1946
154. Eggebø TM, Dalaker K (1989) Ultrasonic diagnosis of pregnant women performed in general practice. Tidsskr Nor Laegeforen 109(29):2979–2981
155. Ornstein SM, Smith MA, Peggs J, Garr D, Gonzales J (1990) Obstetric ultrasound by family physicians. Adequacy as assessed by pregnancy outcome. J Fam Pract 30(4):403–408
156. Rodney WM, Prislin MD, Orientale E, McConnell M, Hahn RG (1990) Family practice obstetric ultrasound in an urban community health center. Birth outcomes and examination accuracy of the initial 227 cases. J Fam Pract 30(2):163–168
157. Brunader R (1996) Accuracy of prenatal sonography performed by family practice residents. Fam Med 28(6):407–410
158. Keith R, Frisch L (2001) Fetal biometry: a comparison of family physicians and radiologists. Fam Med 33(2):111–114
159. Bailey C, Carnell J, Vahidnia F, Shah S, Stone M, Adams M, Nagdev A (2012) Accuracy of emergency physicians using ultrasound measurement of crown-rump length to estimate gestational age in pregnant females. Am J Emerg Med 30(8):1627–1629

160. Saul T, Lewiss RE, Rivera MDR (2012) Accuracy of emergency physician performed bedside ultrasound in determining gestational age in first trimester pregnancy. Crit Ultrasound J 4(1):22
161. Shah S, Teismann N, Zaia B, Vahidnia F, River G, Price D, Nagdev A (2010) Accuracy of emergency physicians using ultrasound to determine gestational age in pregnant women. Am J Emerg Med 28(7):834–838
162. Stein JC, Wang R, Adler N, Boscardin J, Jacoby VL, Won G, Goldstein R, Kohn MA (2010) Emergency physician ultrasonography for evaluating patients at risk for ectopic pregnancy: a meta-analysis. Ann Emerg Med 56(6):674–683
163. Beals T, Naraghi L, Grossestreuer A, Schafer J, Balk D, Hoffmann B (2019) Point of care ultrasound is associated with decreased ED length of stay for symptomatic early pregnancy. Am J Emerg Med 37(6):1165–1168
164. Strommen J, Masullo L, Crowell T, Moffett P (2017) First-trimester vaginal bleeding: patient expectations when presenting to the emergency department. Mil Med 182(11):e1824–e1826
165. Everett CB, Preece E (1996) Women with bleeding in the first 20 weeks of pregnancy: value of general practice ultrasound in detecting fetal heart movement. Br J Gen Pract 46(402):7–9
166. Varner C, Balaban D, McLeod S, Carver S, Borgundvaag B (2016) Fetal outcomes following emergency department point-of-care ultrasound for vaginal bleeding in early pregnancy. Can Fam Physician 62(7):572–578
167. Shah S, Adedipe A, Ruffatto B, Backlund BH, Sajed D, Rood K, Fernandez R (2014) BE-SAFE: bedside sonography for assessment of the fetus in emergencies: educational intervention for late-pregnancy obstetric ultrasound. West J Emerg Med 15(6):636–640
168. Gottlieb M, Holladay D, Peksa GD (2019) Point-of-care ocular ultrasound for the diagnosis of retinal detachment: a systematic review and meta-analysis. Acad Emerg Med. https://doi.org/10.1111/acem.13682
169. Jacobsen B, Lahham S, Lahham S, Patel A, Spann S, Fox JC (2016) Retrospective review of ocular point-of-care ultrasound for detection of retinal detachment. West J Emerg Med 17(2):196–200
170. Lahham S, Shniter I, Thompson M, Le D, Chadha T, Mailhot T, Kang TL, Chiem A, Tseeng S, Fox JC (2019) Point-of-care ultrasonography in the diagnosis of retinal detachment, vitreous hemorrhage, and vitreous detachment in the emergency department. JAMA Netw Open 2(4):e192162
171. Ojaghihaghighi S, Lombardi KM, Davis S, Vahdati SS, Sorkhabi R, Pourmand A (2019) Diagnosis of traumatic eye injuries with point-of-care ocular ultrasonography in the emergency department. Ann Emerg Med. https://doi.org/10.1016/j.annemergmed.2019.02.001
172. Ojaghi Haghighi SH, Morteza Begi HR, Sorkhabi R, Tarzamani MK, Kamali Zonouz G, Mikaeilpour A, Rahmani F (2014) Diagnostic accuracy of ultrasound in detection of traumatic lens dislocation. Emergency 2(3):121–124
173. Barbic D, Chenkin J, Cho DD, Jelic T, Scheuermeyer FX (2017) In patients presenting to the emergency department with skin and soft tissue infections what is the diagnostic accuracy of point-of-care ultrasonography for the diagnosis of abscess compared to the current standard of care? A systematic review and meta-analysis. BMJ Open 7(1):e013688
174. Subramaniam S, Bober J, Chao J, Zehtabchi S (2016) Point-of-care ultrasound for diagnosis of abscess in skin and soft tissue infections. Acad Emerg Med 23(11):1298–1306
175. Gaspari R, Dayno M, Briones J, Blehar D (2012) Comparison of computerized tomography and ultrasound for diagnosing soft tissue abscesses. Crit Ultrasound J 4(1):5
176. Greenlund LJS, Merry SP, Thacher TD, Ward WJ (2017) Primary care management of skin abscesses guided by ultrasound. Am J Med 130(5):e191–e193
177. Mower WR, Crisp JG, Krishnadasan A, Moran GJ, Abrahamian FM, Lovecchio F, Karras DJ, Steele MT, Rothman RE, Talan DA (2019) Effect of initial bedside ultrasonography on emergency department skin and soft tissue infection management. Ann Emerg Med. https://doi.org/10.1016/j.annemergmed.2019.02.002
178. Lam SHF, Sivitz A, Alade K et al (2018) Comparison of ultrasound guidance vs. clinical assessment alone for management of pediatric skin and soft tissue infections. J Emerg Med 55(5):693–701
179. Gaspari RJ, Sanseverino A (2018) Ultrasound-guided drainage for pediatric soft tissue abscesses decreases clinical failure rates compared to drainage without ultrasound: a retrospective study. J Ultrasound Med 37(1):131–136
180. Gaspari RJ, Sanseverino A, Gleeson T (2019) Abscess incision and drainage with or without ultrasonography: a randomized controlled trial. Ann Emerg Med 73(1):1–7
181. Lin MJ, Neuman M, Rempell R, Monuteaux M, Levy J (2018) Point-of-care ultrasound is associated with decreased length of stay in children presenting to the emergency department with soft tissue infection. J Emerg Med 54(1):96–101
182. Costantino TG, Satz WA, Dehnkamp W, Goett H (2012) Randomized trial comparing intraoral ultrasound to landmark-based needle aspiration in patients with suspected peritonsillar abscess. Acad Emerg Med 19(6):626–631
183. Adhikari S, Blaivas M, Lander L (2011) Comparison of bedside ultrasound and panorex radiography in the diagnosis of a dental abscess in the ED. Am J Emerg Med 29(7):790–795
184. Levine MC, Arroyo A, Likourezos A, Homel P, Dickman E (2018) The use of point of care ultrasound in the evaluation of pediatric soft tissue neck masses. Am J Emerg Med. https://doi.org/10.1016/j.ajem.2018.10.048
185. Friedman N, Tseng F, Savic R, Diallo M, Fathi K, Mclean L, Tessaro MO (2019) Reliability of neck mass point-of-care ultrasound by pediatric emergency physicians. J Ultrasound Med. https://doi.org/10.1002/jum.14993
186. Friedman DI, Forti RJ, Wall SP, Crain EF (2005) The utility of bedside ultrasound and patient perception in detecting soft tissue foreign bodies in children. Pediatr Emerg Care 21(8):487–492
187. Oguz AB, Polat O, Eneyli MG, Gulunay B, Eksioglu M, Gurler S (2017) The efficiency of bedside ultrasonography in patients with wrist injury and comparison with other radiological imaging methods: a prospective study. Am J Emerg Med 35(6):855–859
188. Lee SH, Yun SJ (2018) Point-of-care wrist ultrasonography in trauma patients with ulnar-sided pain and instability. Am J Emerg Med 36(5):859–864
189. Gün C, Unlüer EE, Vandenberk N, Karagöz A, Sentürk GO, Oyar O (2013) Bedside ultrasonography by emergency physicians for anterior talofibular ligament injury. J Emerg Trauma Shock 6(3):195–198
190. Lee SH, Yun SJ (2017) The feasibility of point-of-care ankle ultrasound examination in patients with recurrent ankle sprain and chronic ankle instability: comparison with magnetic resonance imaging. Injury 48(10):2323–2328
191. Wu TS, Roque PJ, Green J, Drachman D, Khor K-N, Rosenberg M, Simpson C (2012) Bedside ultrasound evaluation of tendon injuries. Am J Emerg Med 30(8):1617–1621
192. Mohammadrezaei N, Seyedhosseini J, Vahidi E (2017) Validity of ultrasound in diagnosis of tendon injuries in penetrating extremity trauma. Am J Emerg Med 35(7):945–948
193. Vieira RL, Levy JA (2010) Bedside ultrasonography to identify hip effusions in pediatric patients. Ann Emerg Med 55(3):284–289
194. Cruz CI, Vieira RL, Mannix RC, Monuteaux MC, Levy JA (2018) Point-of-care hip ultrasound in a pediatric emergency department. Am J Emerg Med 36(7):1174–1177
195. Adhikari S, Blaivas M (2010) Utility of bedside sonography to distinguish soft tissue abnormalities from joint effusions in the emergency department. J Ultrasound Med 29(4):519–526
196. Gottlieb M, Holladay D, Peksa GD (2019) Point-of-care ultrasound for the diagnosis of shoulder dislocation: a systematic review and meta-analysis. Am J Emerg Med 37(4):757–761
197. Lee SH, Yun SJ (2019) Efficiency of knee ultrasound for diagnosing anterior cruciate ligament and posterior cruciate ligament injuries: a systematic review and meta-analysis. Skel Radiol. https://doi.org/10.1007/s00256-019-03225-w
198. Weinberg ER, Tunik MG, Tsung JW (2010) Accuracy of clinician-performed point-of-care ultrasound for the diagnosis of fractures in children and young adults. Injury 41(8):862–868
199. Riera A, Chen L (2012) Ultrasound evaluation of skull fractures in children: a feasibility study. Pediatr Emerg Care 28(5):420–425
200. Parri N, Crosby BJ, Glass C, Mannelli F, Sforzi I, Schiavone R, Ban KM (2013) Ability of emergency ultrasonography to detect pediatric skull fractures: a prospective, observational study. J Emerg Med 44(1):135–141

201. Rabiner JE, Friedman LM, Khine H, Avner JR, Tsung JW (2013) Accuracy of point-of-care ultrasound for diagnosis of skull fractures in children. Pediatrics 131(6):e1757–e1764
202. Choi JY, Lim YS, Jang JH, Park WB, Hyun SY, Cho JS (2018) Accuracy of bedside ultrasound for the diagnosis of skull fractures in children aged 0 to 4 years. Pediatr Emerg Care. https://doi.org/10.1097/PEC.00000 00000001485
203. Parri N, Crosby BJ, Mills L, Soucy Z, Musolino AM, Da Dalt L, Cirilli A, Grisotto L, Kuppermann N (2018) Point-of-care ultrasound for the diagnosis of skull fractures in children younger than two years of age. J Pediatr 196:230–236.e2
204. Cross KP, Warkentine FH, Kim IK, Gracely E, Paul RI (2010) Bedside ultrasound diagnosis of clavicle fractures in the pediatric emergency department. Acad Emerg Med 17(7):687–693
205. Chien M, Bulloch B, Garcia-Filion P, Youssfi M, Shrader MW, Segal LS (2011) Bedside ultrasound in the diagnosis of pediatric clavicle fractures. Pediatr Emerg Care 27(11):1038–1041
206. Lee SH, Yun SJ (2019) Diagnostic performance of ultrasonography for detection of pediatric elbow fracture: a meta-analysis. Ann Emerg Med. https://doi.org/10.1016/j.annemergmed.2019.03.009
207. Rabiner JE, Khine H, Avner JR, Tsung JW (2015) Ultrasound findings of the elbow posterior fat pad in children with radial head subluxation. Pediatr Emerg Care 31(5):327–330
208. Chartier LB, Bosco L, Lapointe-Shaw L, Chenkin J (2017) Use of point-of-care ultrasound in long bone fractures: a systematic review and meta-analysis. CJEM 19(2):131–142
209. Hedelin H, Tingström C, Hebelka H, Karlsson J (2017) Minimal training sufficient to diagnose pediatric wrist fractures with ultrasound. Crit Ultrasound J 9(1):11
210. Rowlands R, Rippey J, Tie S, Flynn J (2017) Bedside ultrasound vs X-ray for the diagnosis of forearm fractures in children. J Emerg Med 52(2):208–215
211. Douma-den Hamer D, Blanker MH, Edens MA, Buijteweg LN, Boomsma MF, van Helden SH, Mauritz G-J (2016) Ultrasound for distal forearm fracture: a systematic review and diagnostic meta-analysis. PLoS ONE 11(5):e0155659
212. Sivrikaya S, Aksay E, Bayram B, Oray NC, Karakasli A, Altintas E (2016) Emergency physicians performed point-of-care-ultrasonography for detecting distal forearm fracture. Turk J Emerg Med 16(3):98–101
213. Tayal VS, Antoniazzi J, Pariyadath M, Norton HJ (2007) Prospective use of ultrasound imaging to detect bony hand injuries in adults. J Ultrasound Med 26(9):1143–1148
214. Neri E, Barbi E, Rabach I, Zanchi C, Norbedo S, Ronfani L, Guastalla V, Ventura A, Guastalla P (2014) Diagnostic accuracy of ultrasonography for hand bony fractures in paediatric patients. Arch Dis Child 99(12):1087–1090
215. Kozaci N, Ay MO, Akcimen M, Sasmaz I, Turhan G, Boz A (2015) The effectiveness of bedside point-of-care ultrasonography in the diagnosis and management of metacarpal fractures. Am J Emerg Med 33(10):1468–1472
216. Aksay E, Yesilaras M, Kılıc TY, Tur FC, Sever M, Kaya A (2015) Sensitivity and specificity of bedside ultrasonography in the diagnosis of fractures of the fifth metacarpal. Emerg Med J 32(3):221–225
217. Aksay E, Kilic TY, Yesılaras M, Tur FC, Sever M, Kalenderer O (2016) Accuracy of bedside ultrasonography for the diagnosis of finger fractures. Am J Emerg Med 34(5):809–812
218. Gungor F, Akyol KC, Eken C, Kesapli M, Beydilli I, Akcimen M (2016) The value of point-of-care ultrasound for detecting nail bed injury in ED. Am J Emerg Med 34(9):1850–1854
219. Kocaoğlu S, Özhasenekler A, İçme F, Pamukçu Günaydın G, Şener A, Gökhan Ş (2016) The role of ultrasonography in the diagnosis of metacarpal fractures. Am J Emerg Med 34(9):1868–1871
220. Kozaci N, Ay MO, Avci M, Turhan S, Donertas E, Celik A, Ararat E, Akgun E (2017) The comparison of point-of-care ultrasonography and radiography in the diagnosis of tibia and fibula fractures. Injury 48(7):1628–1635
221. Atilla OD, Yesilaras M, Kilic TY, Tur FC, Reisoglu A, Sever M, Aksay E (2014) The accuracy of bedside ultrasonography as a diagnostic tool for fractures in the ankle and foot. Acad Emerg Med 21(9):1058–1061
222. Tollefson B, Nichols J, Fromang S, Summers RL (2016) Validation of the Sonographic Ottawa Foot and Ankle Rules (SOFAR) study in a large urban trauma center. J Miss State Med Assoc 57(2):35–38
223. Ozturk P, Aksay E, Oray NC, Bayram B, Basci O, Tokgoz D (2018) The accuracy of emergency physician performed ultrasonography as a diagnostic tool for lateral malleolar fracture. Am J Emerg Med 36(3):362–365
224. Yesilaras M, Aksay E, Atilla OD, Sever M, Kalenderer O (2014) The accuracy of bedside ultrasonography as a diagnostic tool for the fifth metatarsal fractures. Am J Emerg Med 32(2):171–174
225. Kozaci N, Ay MO, Avci M, Beydilli I, Turhan S, Donertas E, Ararat E (2017) The comparison of radiography and point-of-care ultrasonography in the diagnosis and management of metatarsal fractures. Injury 48(2):542–547
226. Fagan TJ (1975) Letter: Nomogram for Bayes theorem. N Engl J Med 293(5):257

9

Cardiac point-of-care ultrasound reveals unexpected, life-threatening findings in two children

Stephanie J. Doniger[1*] and Nicholas Ng[2]

Abstract

Background: The diagnosis of pericardial effusion with cardiac tamponade can at times be elusive in pediatric patients since it is relatively uncommon. Point-of-care ultrasound (POCUS) can readily be performed at the bedside to assess for the presence of a pericardial effusion, tamponade, and can occasionally yield unexpected results.

Case presentation: Two cases where POCUS unexpectedly identified pericardial effusions, with one patient who also had an anterior mediastinal mass.

Conclusions: Though underutilized, cardiac POCUS in children can be immediately life-saving and drastically change the clinical management at the patient's bedside.

Keywords: Focused cardiac ultrasound, Point-of-care ultrasound, Pediatric emergency medicine, Pericardial effusion, Tamponade, Anterior mediastinal mass

Background

Point-of-care ultrasound (POCUS) is designed to answer very specific questions in real time. Additionally, it can help expeditiously make life-saving diagnoses, while avoiding unnecessary or potentially costly testing or imaging [1]. An important POCUS application in the emergency and critical care settings is the focused cardiac examination. The primary goal of focused cardiac POCUS is to identify pericardial effusions, tamponade, and asystole. Overall, the use of cardiac POCUS is underutilized in the pediatric patient population. This is presumably because the overall incidence of acquired (non-congenital) cardiac pathology in pediatric populations is quite low when compared with adult patient populations. Nonetheless, the identification of cardiac pathology in children can be immediately life-saving.

There exists a tremendous body of literature that supports the use of cardiac POCUS in diagnosing pericardial effusions in adult patient populations. Mandavia et al. [2] studied bedside cardiac POCUS performed by emergency medicine physicians in patients at high risk for pericardial effusions, with an overall accuracy of 98%, sensitivity of 96% and specificity of 98%. In patients with penetrating chest trauma and traumatic pericardial effusions, Plummer et al. [3] showed that cardiac POCUS improved outcomes when compared to those who did not receive cardiac POCUS, with shorter time to diagnosis (15.5 versus 42.4 min) and better overall survival (100% versus 57%).

There is limited literature on focused cardiac POCUS in pediatric patient populations. The majority of studies involving cardiac POCUS to identify pericardial effusions and tamponade in the pediatric ED setting are limited to case reports [4, 5]. However, in a prospective observational study of 70 pediatric emergency department patients, the overall sensitivity and specificity of cardiac POCUS in detecting diminished LV function, pericardial effusions, and abnormal IVC collapsibility, when

*Correspondence: sjdoniger@gmail.com
[1] Department of Pediatric Emergency Medicine, CHOC Children's Hospital of Orange County, Orange, CA, USA
Full list of author information is available at the end of the article

compared with comprehensive echocardiogram was 95% (95% CI 82–99%) and 83% (95% CI 64–93%), respectively [6].

Cardiac tamponade clinically presents as Beck's triad: jugular venous distension, muffled heart tones and hypotension [7]. However, only one-third of patients with tamponade will have all three features and 10% will not have any of them. POCUS can readily identify both pericardial effusions and sonographic tamponade [8]. The diagnosis of sonographic cardiac tamponade can be made before a patient becomes hypotensive or has clinical signs of tamponade. Signs of sonographic tamponade include a circumferential pericardial effusion, accompanied by poor filling and/or diastolic collapse of the right ventricle ("scalloping") due to increased intrapericardial pressure, which results in reduction of stroke volume and cardiac output [9, 10].

Pericardiocentesis is the definitive treatment for cardiac tamponade. Ultrasound-guidance for pericardiocentesis has been shown to improve success rates and decrease complications when compared with blind attempts [11]. Though it is a rare condition in the pediatric population, pericardiocentesis may be indicated after blunt or penetrating trauma, or after cardiac catheterization or cardiac surgery [12]. Tsang et al. showed that those pediatric patients who had ultrasound-guided pericardiocentesis, had a 99% success rate, with 93% on the first attempt, and 1% major and 3% minor complication rates [13].

The identification of cardiac masses is not the primary goal of POCUS. However, this may be an unexpected or incidental finding. Alternatively, in a child presenting with a widened mediastinum on chest radiograph, a focused cardiac POCUS may be expeditiously performed to evaluate for the presence of a mass at the bedside.

Case presentations

The following are two cases where POCUS unexpectedly identified pericardial effusions, with one patient who also had an anterior mediastinal mass.

Case 1

A 12-year-old male was admitted to the pediatric inpatient unit for treatment of pneumonia. After being in the hospital for 7 days without improvement of the pneumonia, the patient acutely developed progressively worsening chest pain, shortness of breath, and diaphoresis. The pediatric intensive care team was consulted overnight for evaluation of the patient, and the patient was noted to be ill appearing and sitting in an upright "tripod" position. He was afebrile with a respiratory rate (RR) 38, heart rate (HR) 122, blood pressure (BP) 118/70, pulse oximetry 95% on simple facemask. No electrocardiogram (EKG) had been performed during his hospital admission. A Pediatric Emergency Medicine (PEM) fellow with extensive POCUS training performed a POCUS examination, to evaluate the progression of the previously diagnosed pneumonia as the likely etiology of the patient's acute decompensation.

A lung ultrasound was initially performed to evaluate the progression of the previously diagnosed pneumonia. However, the normal lung artifacts were obliterated by a large anechoic structure. Therefore, a focused cardiac POCUS was performed, which revealed a large circumferential pericardial effusion. This heart exhibited a "swinging" movement within the large effusion (Fig. 1), and diastolic right ventricular collapse. The inferior vena cava (IVC) was visualized as being dilated without respiratory variation. As a result of these findings, the diagnosis of cardiac tamponade was made, and a pediatric cardiologist was immediately consulted. The pediatric cardiologist performed an emergent ultrasound-guided pericardiocentesis, yielding one liter of serosanguinous fluid.

Case 2

A 17-year-old male, presented to the Pediatric ED with a 4-month history of intermittent chest pain and progressively worsening shortness of breath for the past month. He was referred from a local urgent care facility with an "abnormal chest X-ray" (Fig. 2). Of note, the patient also had an "abnormal chest X-ray" 6 months prior, but was lost to follow-up. This prior X-ray was not available for review. On examination, he was diaphoretic, sitting upright in mild respiratory distress. His vital signs were:

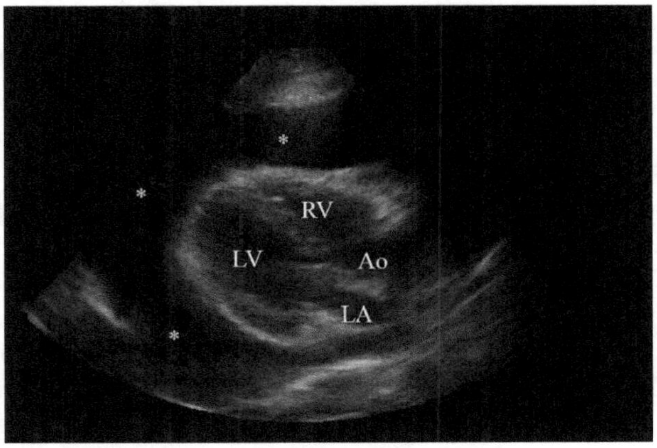

Fig. 1 POCUS, Case 1. Parasternal long-axis view of pericardial tamponade with a large circumferential pericardial effusion (*). The classic "swinging heart" was visualized in real-time ultrasonography. For orientation, the "emergency medicine" orientation was used for scanning. Structures visualized are: the left ventricle (LV), right ventricle (RV), left atrium (LA) and aortic outflow tract (Ao)

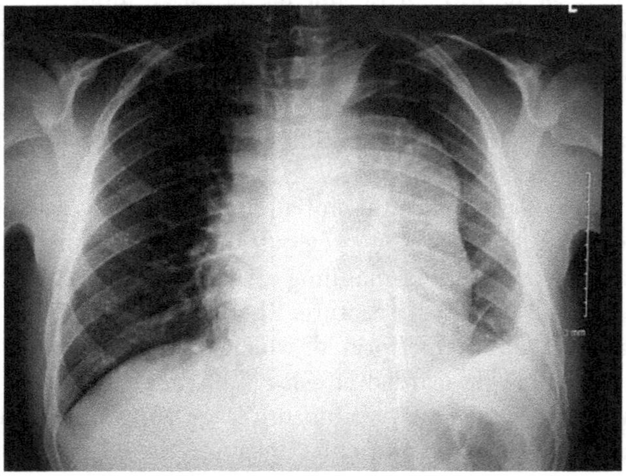

Fig. 2 Chest radiograph, Case 2. This AP chest radiograph exhibits a widened mediastinum, suggestive of a mediastinal mass

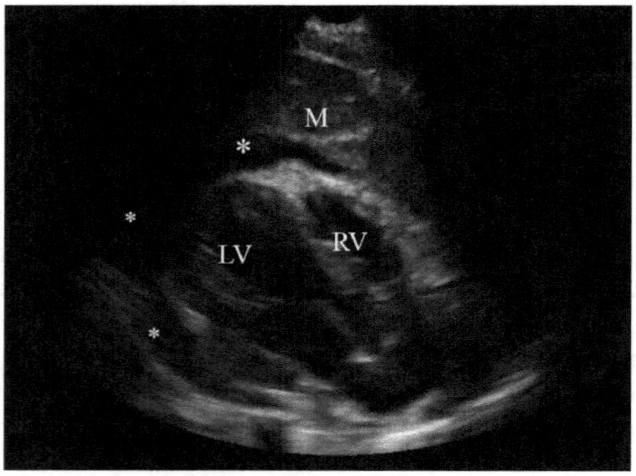

Fig. 3 POCUS, Case 2. Parasternal long-axis view, revealing a circumferential pericardial effusion (*) and an anterior mediastinal mass (M). For orientation, the left ventricle (LV) and right ventricle (RV) can be visualized in this view

98 F, RR 32, HR 102, BP 110/60, pulse oximetry 95% on room air. A PEM physician with extensive experience in POCUS performed the focused cardiac POCUS.

The focused cardiac POCUS showed a large mediastinal mass with a circumferential pericardial effusion, diastolic right ventricle collapse and a small left pleural effusion (Fig. 3). These findings were consistent with sonographic tamponade, which was unexpected, given that the patient did not yet exhibit clinical tamponade (BP and HR were noted to be within normal limits for age). Cardiothoracic surgery was consulted, and the patient was admitted to the cardiac intensive care unit. Due to the POCUS findings, computerized tomography (CT) of the chest was postponed due to the risk of cardiovascular collapse with supine positioning. Had there not been the information from the POCUS, a chest CT would have been performed. Ultimately a pericardiocentesis was performed by the cardiothoracic surgeons in the operating room. Surgical pathology revealed a B-cell lymphoma.

Conclusions

There remains a tremendous potential to study the utilization of cardiac POCUS in pediatric patients in the acute care setting. Overall, cardiac POCUS may be a useful adjunct to the clinical examination when radiologic and laboratory studies can be unreliable, non-specific, and not always timely. However, it is important to note that since it is a focused examination, it is not meant to replace comprehensive echocardiography [9]. The use of focused cardiac POCUS for suspected pericardial effusions, tamponade, and mediastinal masses presents an opportunity for pediatric emergency medicine, cardiology, and critical care services to collaborate and establish best practices for these, at times, elusive diagnoses.

Though relatively uncommon, it is important to consider cardiac etiologies in the differential diagnosis of a pediatric patient presenting with shortness of breath. The above cases illustrate how POCUS can help identify pericardial effusions, tamponade, and mediastinal masses when diagnostic clarity may be lacking.

Abbreviations

Ao: aortic outflow tract; BP: blood pressure; CXR: chest X-ray, radiograph; CT: computerized tomography; EKG: electrocardiogram; HR: heart rate; IVC: inferior vena cava; LA: left atrium; LV: left ventricle; PEM: pediatric emergency medicine; PICU: pediatric intensive care unit; POCUS: point-of-care ultrasound; RR: respiratory rate; RV: right ventricle; US: ultrasound.

Acknowledgements

The authors would like to acknowledge Aaron Kornblith, MD, who performed the point-of-care ultrasound and provided ultrasound images for the first case patient.

Authors' contributions

SJD performed the POCUS on the second case patient and was the major contributor in writing the manuscript. NN was a contributor in writing the manuscript. Both authors read and approved the final manuscript.

Author details

[1] Department of Pediatric Emergency Medicine, CHOC Children's Hospital of Orange County, Orange, CA, USA. [2] Department of Pediatric Critical Care, Morgan Stanley Children's Hospital of New York-Presbyterian, New York, NY, USA.

References

1. Marin J, Lewiss R (2015) Point-of-care ultrasonography by pediatric emergency physicians. Policy statement. Ann Emerg Med 65:472–478
2. Mandavia D, Hoffner R, Mahaney K et al (2001) Bedside echocardiography by emergency physicians. Ann Emerg Med 38:377–382
3. Plummer D, Brunette D, Asinger R et al (1992) Emergency department echocardiography improves outcome to penetrating cardiac injury. Ann Emerg Med 21:709–712

4. Miller A, Levy J, Rempell R, Nagler J (2017) Point-of-care ultrasound to diagnose postpericardiotomy syndrome in a child. Pediatr Emerg Care 33:700–702
5. Smith A, Watnick C, Ferre R (2017) Cardiac tamponade diagnosed by point-of-care ultrasound. Pediatr Emerg Care 33:132–143
6. Longjohn M, Wan J, Joshi V et al (2011) Point-of-care echocardiography by pediatric emergency physicians. Pediatr Emerg Care 27:693–696
7. Beck C (1935) Two cardiac compression triads. JAMA. https://doi.org/10.1001/jama.1935.02760090018005
8. ACEP (2016) Ultrasound guidelines: Emergency, point-of-care and clinical ultrasound guidelines in medicine. Ann Emerg Med 69:e27–e54
9. Doniger S (2010) Bedside emergency cardiac ultrasound in children. J Emerg Trauma Shock 3:282–291
10. Marin J, Abo A, Arroyo A et al (2016) Pediatric emergency medicine point-of-care ultrasound: summary of the evidence. Crit Ultrasound J 8:16
11. Tsang T, Freeman W, Sinak L et al (1998) Echocardiography guided pericardiocentesis: evolution and state-of-the-art technique. Mayo Clin Proc 73:647–652
12. Taylor R, Moore C (2013) Echocardiography. In: Cosby K, Kendall J (eds) Practial guide to emergency ultrasound, 2nd edn. Lippincott Williams & Wilkins, Philadelphia, pp 55–74
13. Tsang T, El-Naidawi E, Seward J et al (1998) Percutaneous echocardiographically guided pericardiocentesis in pediatric patients: evaluation of safety and efficacy. J Am Soc Echo 11:1072–1077

10

Tablet vs. station-based laptop ultrasound devices increases internal medicine resident point-of-care ultrasound performance: a prospective cohort study

Matt Glogoza[1], Jonathan Urbach[1], Terry K. Rosborough[1], Susan Olet[2], Catherine A. St. Hill[3], Claire S. Smith[3] and David M. Tierney[1*]

Abstract

Background: Point-of-care ultrasound (POCUS) is becoming an important part of internal medicine (IM) residency training. Achieving competency requires performing a large volume of clinical exams which can be difficult within the constraints of residency. Often-cited barriers include insufficient resident time and the interruption of daily workflow. Despite availability of hospital station-based laptop ultrasound machines, we hypothesized that the addition of ward team-based tablet ultrasound devices would lower barriers and increase clinical POCUS volume within an IM residency POCUS curriculum at a 670-bed, quaternary care, teaching hospital. IM resident POCUS volumes and characteristics during an 18-mo. baseline (station-based laptop devices only) period were compared to matched months during the intervention (station-based + tablet).

Results: Total patients examined with POCUS by 6 inpatient resident teams during the 18-mo. baseline and intervention periods were 1386 and 1853, respectively. Patients examined per month increased during the intervention by 34% (77 vs. 103, $p = 0.002$). The number of areas (e.g., abdominal, cardiac) and items (e.g., bladder, pericardial effusion) examined per month increased by 27% ($p = 0.021$) and 23% ($p = 0.073$), respectively.

Conclusions: A combined program infrastructure of station-based laptop and "in-the-pocket" tablet ultrasound devices lowered common POCUS barriers of inadequate time and workflow disruption for IM residents and resulted in a meaningful increase of exams within a longitudinal residency-based training program where station-based laptop devices already existed.

Keywords: Point-of-care ultrasound, Internal medicine, Medical education

Background

Point-of-care ultrasound (POCUS) significantly improves an internist's diagnostic ability at the bedside and is quickly becoming part of internal medicine (IM) residency training [1–3]. Recent position statements from the Society of Hospital Medicine, American College of Physicians, and Alliance for Academic Internal Medicine all endorse POCUS as an important tool for internists [3–6].

A goal of the American College of Physicians is to "define the educational curriculum needed to train residents and internists in the appropriate use of POCUS in internal medicine" [5]. An IM residency-based curriculum should be longitudinal and target POCUS competency which encompasses basic ultrasound knowledge, image acquisition and identification skills, and the ability to clinically integrate findings. A large volume of clinical

*Correspondence: david.tierney@allina.com
[1] Department of Graduate Medical Education #11135, Abbott Northwestern Hospital, 800 E. 28th Street, Minneapolis, MN 55407, USA
Full list of author information is available at the end of the article

exams is essential for residents to understand how to clinically integrate POCUS findings [3]. Barriers to performing clinical exams include lack of time and workflow disruption [7–9]. Successful IM residency POCUS curricula must adopt programmatic efficiencies to overcome these barriers—specifically those targeting clinical exam performance amongst residents' "own" patients.

The Internal Medicine Bedside Ultrasound (IMBUS) Program, a longitudinal, 3-year, IM residency-based POCUS curriculum began at our hospital in 2010. Portable, laptop ultrasound devices were initially stored in a locked closet in the residency office. In September 2013, cart-based laptop ultrasound devices were introduced to each hospital station. This correlated with an increase in ultrasound use amongst the residents. The objective of this study was to evaluate whether, even in the setting of widely available station-based devices, the addition of tablet ultrasound devices to the pockets of resident inpatient ward teams would further increase the volume of clinical POCUS exams being performed by residents.

Methods

Setting

This prospective cohort study took place within a 670-bed, quaternary-care, teaching hospital from 2015 to 2019. The hospital's 30-resident IM residency program has a long-standing in- and outpatient POCUS curriculum (IMBUS) started in 2010. Ward teams comprise a hospitalist attending, one first-year and one second-year resident, and 2 medical students. The IRB approved the study as non-human subject research (Allina Health IRB; Reference 1070078-1).

IMBUS curriculum and infrastructure

First-year IM residents participate in a 5-day, 40-h (70% hands-on) POCUS course in August. All resident-performed POCUS exams following that introductory course are mentored by a certified faculty member at the bedside until the resident is certified in the given exam area. Once the minimum quantity requirement within an exam area is obtained (Additional file 1: Digital Content S1. IMBUS Certification Criteria), the resident is assessed at the bedside for the other elements of POCUS competency within that specific area (i.e. interpretation and clinical integration). Once quantity of exams and bedside assessment of competency are achieved, the resident is deemed "certified" in that exam area [10]. First-year residents have a required 1-month ultrasound and procedure team rotation, which is a 1:1 intensive POCUS experience with 3 of our core faculty. Second-year residents participate in an advanced outpatient POCUS rotation in our main faculty primary care clinic [11]. Many of our residents select a 1-month POCUS elective during their 2nd or 3rd year of training.

Beginning July 2012, resident and faculty ultrasound exams have been prospectively tracked on a multi-platform, web-based application with an interface on all resident smartphones. The application records type of ultrasound device used, location of exam (hospital or clinics), exam areas and items observed, faculty mentor, etc. (Fig. 1). The data are collected in a database allowing residents real-time access, via the smartphone application, to their current volume of exams in each certification area.

There have been several changes within the IMBUS curriculum since it began in 2010. Many of these have impacted the motivation of and volume of exams being performed by residents and faculty in the program (Fig. 2). Station-based laptop ultrasound devices with dedicated central parking locations on each station were added in September 2013 (SonoSite EDGE devices with P21 [1-5 mHz] phased-array and L25 [13–6 mHz] linear transducers; FUJIFILM SonoSite Inc., Bothell, WA). The devices were available in significant excess of demand, and when a given device was in use, the adjacent station's device was likely available. A hospital-wide tracking system provided residents real-time, room-specific location data for all devices. A separate fleet of ultrasound devices are used for procedures and educational scanning so as not to tie up the station-based devices. In November 2015, IMBUS certification within the core areas (Additional file 1: Digital Content S1. IMBUS Certification Criteria) became a mandatory graduation requirement (Fig. 2).

In mid-August 2017, an 8-in. tablet able to fit into a white coat pocket (Huawei Technologies Co Ltd., model SHT-W09; Shenzhen, China) and a detachable sector array transducer (Philips Lumify S4-1 [4–1 mHz]; Philips Ultrasound Inc., Bothell, WA) were deployed on each of 6 resident ward teams. The intensive care unit-based resident team also received a linear transducer (Philips Lumify L12-4 [12–4 mHz]; Philips Ultrasound Inc., Bothell, WA). Residents on non-ward inpatient rotations did not have tablet ultrasounds, so continued to use the station-based laptop devices. Between December 2015 and May 2019, there were no other significant changes to the IMBUS curriculum/infrastructure, graduation requirements, resident individual or team characteristics, or inpatient population/census.

Baseline and intervention period definitions

Baseline data were collected starting after the introduction of graduation requirements in December 2015 through May 2017 (18 mo.), during which only station-based laptop ultrasound devices were available. Due to

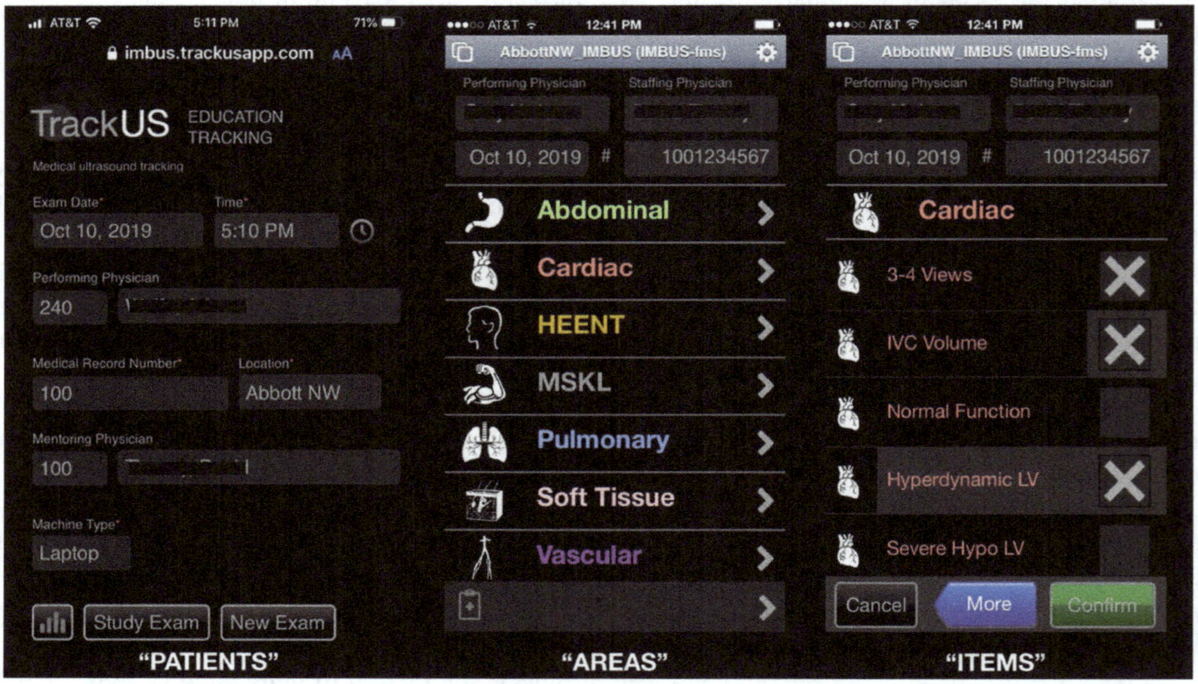

Fig. 1 Smartphone-based tracking application used to record "PATIENT" exams, "AREAS" examined on each patient, and "ITEMS" observed in each area

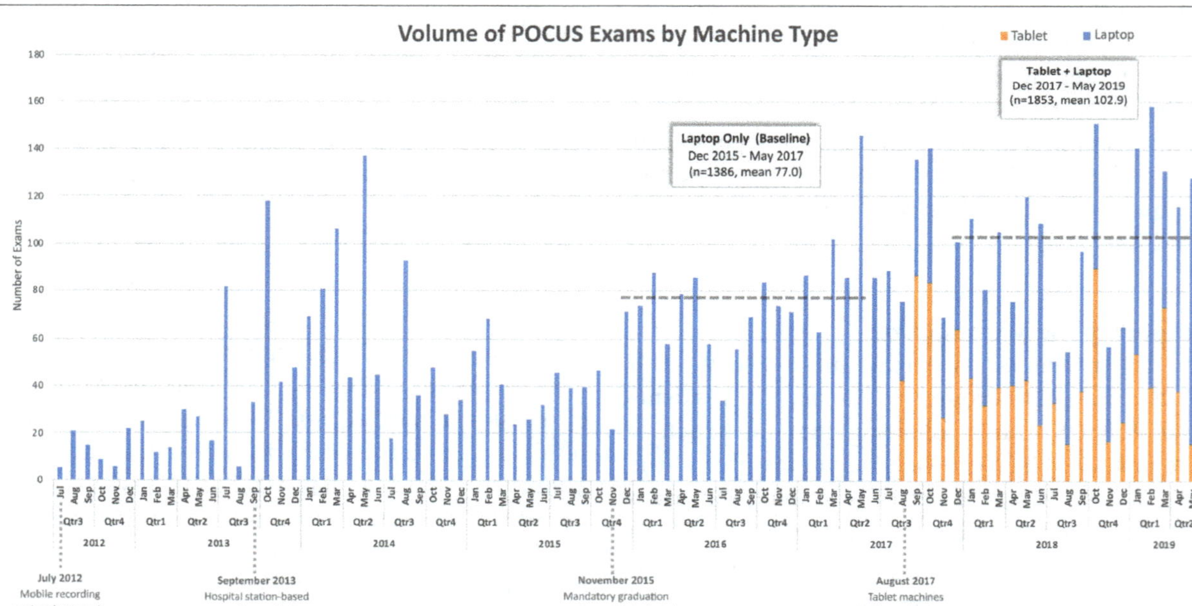

Fig. 2 Volume of POCUS exams by month within the IMBUS program, limited to those performed by residents on inpatient rotations. Baseline (station-based laptop ultrasound devices only) period (December 2015–May 2017) and intervention (station-based laptop devices + tablet devices) period (December 2017–May 2019) with horizontal dashed lines representing the mean number of exams for each period (77.0 vs. 102.9). Proportions of exams performed by device type from August 2017 through May 2019 are shown with orange (tablet) vs. blue (laptop) bars. The timeline shown annotates significant historical programmatic changes impacting volume of exams within the IMBUS program

the known seasonal variation in resident-performed POCUS within the IMBUS program, the intervention period did not include September through November of 2017 (the first 3 months after ward team tablet ultrasound devices were added), but rather included the 18 months with paired baseline data from December

2017 through May 2019 (Fig. 2). All data (including June–October 2017) from December 2015 through May 2019 was used for inflection point analysis.

Data analysis

The data are presented as counts and proportions for categorical variables and as mean ± standard deviation for continuous variables. A paired t test was used to assess whether there was a difference between total monthly exams performed during baseline and intervention periods. Using the iterative application of geometrical methods, a Unit Invariant Knee (UIK) point—an objective estimator for the "elbow point" was determined using inflection point analysis [12]. The "elbow point" is practically the point where a sharply diminishing or increasing curve starts to become 'flat enough'. All tests were performed at a 5% level of significance and the statistical analysis was done using SAS version 9.4 and R version 3.6.1 (2019-07-05).

Results

Total patients that underwent POCUS exams by 6 inpatient resident teams during the 18-mo. baseline and intervention periods were 1386 and 1853, respectively. There is a seasonal variation to the overall volume of POCUS exams performed by residents with predictable nadirs in July and August (prior to new first-year residents being trained, and new second-year residents in the team leader role), and peaks in September (the month after the week-long training course for first-year residents) and late spring (prior to resident advancement and graduation).

When analyzed by paired-month due to seasonal variation, the mean number of patients examined per month increased significantly during the intervention period by 34% (77 vs. 103, $p=0.002$). The number of areas (e.g., abdominal, cardiac) and items (e.g., bladder, pericardial effusion) examined per month increased by 27% ($p=0.021$) and 23% ($p=0.073$), respectively. There was no meaningful difference between baseline and intervention periods for the number of areas or items examined per patient exam, overall, or by ultrasound device type (i.e. laptop vs. tablet).

To further establish that the tablet ultrasound devices were responsible for the significant increase in monthly exam volume between baseline and intervention periods, instead of the observed difference being solely a result of an underlying positive trend present throughout the 39-month study period, two additional analyses were performed. Inflection point analysis [12] demonstrated two separate elbow points across the 39-month period from December 2015 to May 2019. The first occurred at the very large seasonal variation peak at the end of the baseline period in May of 2017 (Fig. 2). When accounting for the impact of May seasonal variation on the inflection analysis, a second observed elbow was identified in September of 2017, corresponding with the introduction of the tablet ultrasound devices. Additionally, monthly volume between the first and second halves of the baseline and subsequently between the first and second halves of the intervention periods were compared and showed no significant increase (or decrease) in volume within either study period (p value for differences $=0.275$ and 0.335, respectively).

During the timeframe when tablets were present on teams (September 2017–May 2019), 42% (926 vs. 1273) of patient exams were performed using the tablet ultrasound devices. Frequency of tablet vs. laptop utilization for exams areas where a low-frequency (sector) transducer was appropriate was 41.2% vs. 58.9% for pulmonary, 30.1% vs. 69.9% for cardiac, and 49.2% vs. 50.8% for the abdominal area (Fig. 3). The critical care team (the only team with a linear array transducer) had the ability to perform additional tablet-based exams that required a high-frequency transducer. This team accounted for all the tablet-performed exams within the exam areas of HEENT (6%), soft tissue (14%), musculoskeletal (19%), and vascular (8%). All exams in these areas performed by the other 5 ward teams (without linear transducers) were performed using the laptop ultrasound devices.

During the baseline period, an audit of 100 resident-performed exams showed an 87% recording rate. Because it was possible that resident recording of exams may have increased during the intervention period, an analysis theorizing a change to 100% recording during the intervention period was performed demonstrating a maintained 18% increase in exams ($p=0.048$).

Residents were asked to consider the previous barriers to regularly using laptop ultrasound devices. Frequent responses included: "it just wasn't on my mind while I was in the room", "the flow of taking a history and doing a physical exam is disrupted when I leave the room to get a device", and "I didn't have time". When asked why they performed more exams after the introduction of tablet ultrasound devices, resident comments were recorded and categorized into two major themes. The first theme encompassed the idea that a device you carry with you (like your stethoscope) feels more like an intrinsic part of being an internist, compared to getting a common device from the nursing station. A second theme centered around the often-forgotten impact of context shifting on quality and efficiency.

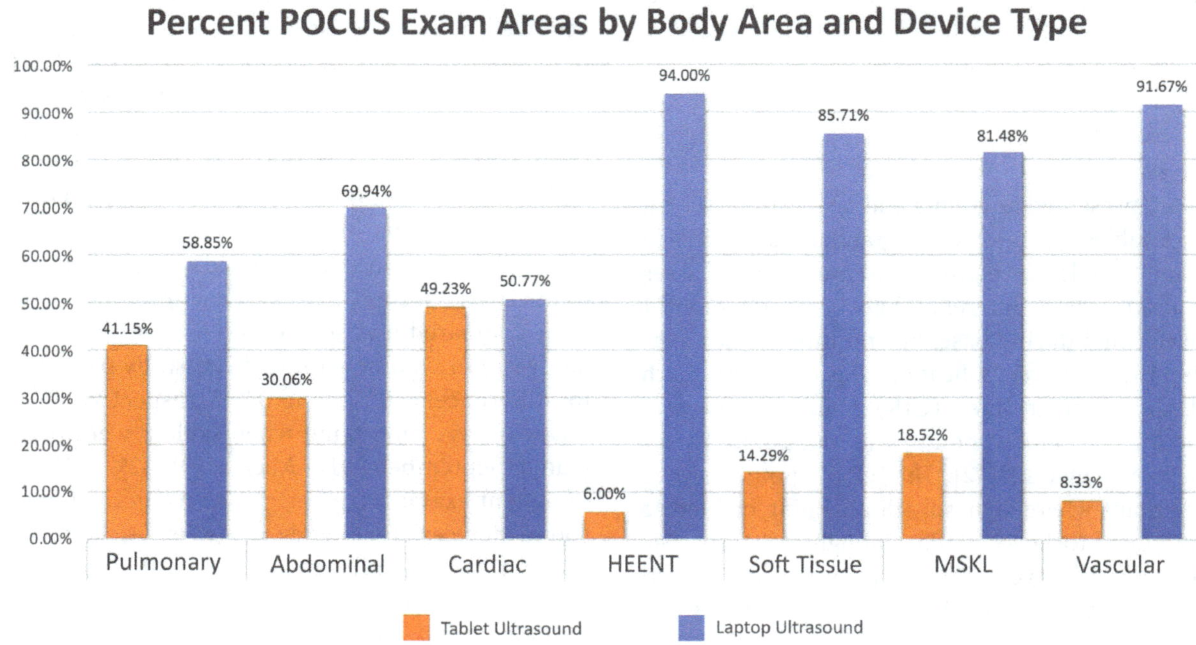

Fig. 3 Percent of POCUS exam areas ($n = 2901$) performed grouped by body area and ultrasound device type (tablet vs. laptop) from September 2017 through May 2019. HEENT = head, eyes, ears, nose, throat; MSKL = musculoskeletal

Discussion

The impact of POCUS on clinical quality and safety, system efficiency, patient and physician satisfaction, and medical education has resulted in a quickly growing rate of adoption within medical schools and IM residency programs [2–4, 13, 14]. However, fully realizing these benefits takes a significant investment in training. The most efficient training setting is within graduate medical education where mentorship, immersion, and condensed repetition can take place. Once programmatic aspects of a residency-based training curriculum are secured, the success of the program becomes dependent on volume of resident-performed clinical exams. That clinical volume is requisite for, but not sufficient for achieving and maintaining competency.

The results of this study show that the addition of "in their pocket" tablet ultrasound devices to 6 IM ward teams significantly increased volume of clinical POCUS exams even in a mature POCUS training environment with abundant station-based ultrasound devices. The IMBUS program trialed several incentive programs from 2012 to 2015 aimed at increasing resident daily POCUS volume. Other than the addition of a mandatory graduation requirement and moving devices from the residency offices to the inpatient stations, no other efforts significantly influenced volume.

The reason for the increased volume seen in this study is unlikely related solely to the few minutes saved by having the device in your pocket versus getting a machine from the nursing station. To fully understand why the addition of tablets impacted volume to the extent seen, it is helpful to consider the previous barriers to regularly using station-based US reported by the residents, but perhaps more insightful to reflect on their ideas behind why they performed more exams after the introduction of the tablet devices. One unanticipated theme, the idea that "a device you carry with you (like your stethoscope) feels more like an intrinsic part of being an internist", may have provided subtle but significant motivation to master the tool. A second theme, centered around the disruption of context shifting in a resident's daily workflow where partially completed tasks are frequently put on hold, was likely minimized by not having to leave a patient encounter to retrieve an ultrasound machine. We conjecture that these two impacts, beyond the actual time savings of having an ultrasound in your pocket, likely have a meaningful impact on a resident's likelihood of performing exams.

There are several reasons why residents did not use the tablet devices for all exams (Fig. 3). First, the tablet devices were only added to the hands of 12 residents (6 two-resident teams) performing POCUS in the hospital. While the vast majority of POCUS exams within the IMBUS program are performed on the inpatient resident ward teams, senior residents on non-ward rotations only had access to laptop devices providing a constant laptop background use across periods. If a resident carrying only a sector transducer (5 of the 6 teams) was going to perform a combined exam necessitating both sector and linear array transducers (e.g., cardiac and vascular exams), they would have likely used the station-based laptop cart. In an educational setting where an additional goal of POCUS is teaching patients, family members, and medical students, the larger screen size of a laptop device is more easily viewed and may be preferentially chosen. Finally, certain cardiac applications within the curriculum utilize spectral and tissue Doppler unavailable on these tablet devices.

Image quality was not directly compared between tablet and laptop devices in this study. However, the fact that only 12 patients (0.6%) initially examined with the tablet ultrasound device had a subsequent exam recorded using a laptop within the same exam area on the same day supports the anectdotal experience that the images obtained using the tablet ultrasound was rarely inadequate for answering the clinical POCUS question being asked. This conclusion is limited as residents may have chosen to initially use a laptop device for patients who they predicted would be inadequately imaged with the tablet or not recorded both exams.

In the current state of ultra-portable ultrasound devices, these study results support a rationale for a mixed fleet of devices in the inpatient setting. The cost and quality of ultra-portable tablet and phone-sized ultrasound devices vary considerably, however a program is often able to purchase 5–20 pocket-size devices for the cost of a cart-based laptop device. Thus, a combination of devices is often the most cost-effective approach, and this study would also support an educational rationale for this approach within an IM inpatient training environment. However, as ultra-portable devices evolve to deliver image quality equivalent to larger devices, features such as spectral Doppler, and the ability to display images on various screen sizes, their current benefits of significantly lower cost and impact on learner volume demonstrated in this study may result in a future rationale for a fleet including only tablet-sized devices in resident coat pockets.

This study has limitations. (1) It took place in a single center's, mature POCUS training program that has already moved beyond the programmatic barriers often encountered (e.g., faculty mentors, sufficient devices, training time, etc.). In a less mature program, or a program with a different baseline machine workflow, the relative impact of tablet device addition may differ. (2) The number of ultrasound devices available in the hospital increased from 14 to 20 with the addition of the tablet devices during the intervention period. Station-based devices were rarely unavailable during the baseline period, however, we cannot exclude that some of the increase in volume was due to machine availability. (3) Residents were not aware of this study, and even if there was a Hawthorne effect, the sustained > 18 month increase in volume makes an effect unlikely. Further, if the goal is to increase exam volume, these limitations do not necessarily detract from the study conclusions.

Conclusions

The addition of team-based tablet ultrasound devices in a setting with abundant station-based laptop ultrasound devices, significantly increased inpatient POCUS volume within a 3-year longitudinal, residency-based, IM POCUS curriculum. Especially in the initial training environment where volume of exams is often a limiting factor, the addition of "in your pocket" devices may provide motivation beyond just the time savings of "getting a device" and be an important element in efficiently achieving trainee competency.

Supplementary information

Additional file 1: Digital Content S1. "IMBUS Certification Areas & Items". Listing of exam items by area that are tracked within the IMBUS program for certification. Minimum number of exams required to be eligible for certification assessment within each exam item is listed. Achievement of minimum quantities is requisite for but not the only aspect required for certification in the item. Core elements noted are required for residency graduation.

Abbreviations

POCUS: Point-of-care ultrasound; IMBUS: Internal medicine bedside ultrasound; IM: Internal medicine.

Acknowledgements

Not applicable.

Authors' contributions

MG, JU, TR and DT all contributed to study design and manuscript preparation. SO, CSH, and CS provided study design and data analysis consultation and feedback. SO performed statistical analysis for the study. All authors read and approved the final manuscript.

Author details

[1] Department of Graduate Medical Education #11135, Abbott Northwestern Hospital, 800 E. 28th Street, Minneapolis, MN 55407, USA. [2] Clinical Research Informatics and Analytics, Allina Health, Minneapolis, MN, USA. [3] Department of Care Delivery Research, Allina Health, Minneapolis, MN, USA.

References

1. Moore CL, Copel JA (2011) Point-of-care ultrasonography. N Engl J Med 364:749–757
2. Bhagra A, Tierney DM, Sekiguchi H, Soni NJ (2016) Point-of-care ultrasonography for primary care physicians and general internists. Mayo Clin Proc 91:1811–1827
3. Soni NJ, Schnobrich D, Matthews BK, Tierny DM, Jensen TP, Dancel R, Cho J, Dversdal RK, Mints G, Bhagra A, Reierson K, Kurian LM, Liu GY, Candotti C, Boesch B, LoPresti CM, Lenchus J, Wong T, Johnson G, Maw AM, Franco-Sadud R, Lucas BF (2019) Point-of-care ultrasound for hospitalists: a position statement of the society of hospital medicine. J Hosp Med 14:E1–E6
4. LoPresti CM, Jensen TP, Dversdal RK, Astiz DJ (2019) Point-of-care ultrasound for internal medicine residency training: a position statement from the alliance of academic internal medicine. Am J Med 132:1356–1360

5. American College of Physicians. ACP Statement in Support of Point-of-Care Ultrasound in Internal Medicine. https://www.acponline.org/meetings-courses/focused-topics/point-of-care-ultrasound-pocus-for-internal-medicine/acp-statement-in-support-of-point-of-care-ultrasound-in-internal-medicine. Accessed 15 Nov 2019
6. Dubuque J. (2019) Barriers to implementation of point-of-care ultrasound in primary care. Family medicine clerkship student projects. 464. https://scholarworks.uvm.edu/fmclerk/464. Accessed 15 Nov 2019
7. Peh WM, Kang ML (2018) A pilot survey on an understanding of point of care bedside ultrasound (POCUS) among medical doctors in internal medicine: exposure, perceptions, interest and barriers to training. Proc Sing Healthc 27:85–95
8. Bellows B, Totten J, Shah S, Adedipe A (2015) Perceived barriers in the use of point-of-care ultrasound in the WWAMI Region. J Emerg Med Crit Care 1:4
9. Schnobrich DJ, Gladding S, Olson AP, Duran-Nelson A (2013) Point-of-care ultrasound in internal medicine: a national survey of educational leadership. J Grad Med Educ 5:498–502
10. Tierney D (2015) Competency cut-point identification derived from a mastery learning cohort approach: a hybrid model. Ultrasound Med Biol 41:S19
11. Rosborough TK, Tierney DM (2018) A late-career internist and point-of-care-ultrasound in a primary care clinic. South Med J 111:418–420
12. Christopoulos DT (2012) Developing methods for identifying the inflection point of a convex/concave curve. arXiv preprint arXiv:12065478 [mathNA]. https://arxiv.org/abs/1206.5478
13. Dinh VA, Fu JY, Lu S, Chiem A, Fox JC, Blaivas M (2016) Integration of ultrasound in medical education at united states medical schools: a national survey of directors' experiences. J Ultrasound Med 35:413–419
14. LoPresti CM, Schnobrich DJ, Dversdal RK, Schembri F (2019) A road map for point-of-care ultrasound training in internal medicine residency. Ultrasound J 11:10

11

Point-of-care ultrasound in resource-limited settings: the PURLS fellowship

Samuel L. Burleson[1*], David C. Pigott[1], John P. Gullett[1], Christopher Greene[1], Courtney B. Gibson[1], Scott Irvine[1] and Daniel Kaminstein[2]

Abstract

Background: The role of point-of-care ultrasonography (POCUS) is rapidly expanding in both resource-rich and resource-limited settings (RLS). One limitation to this rapid expansion has been the lack of educators adequately trained to teach this user-dependent skill. This is particularly true in RLS, where disease presentations, infrastructure limitations, and approach to medical education present unique challenges to the direct application of resource-rich emergency department POCUS curricula.

Objectives: We describe the point-of-care ultrasound in resource-limited settings (PURLS) fellowship, a novel curriculum designed to provide advanced training and expertise in clinical care and POCUS application and education in RLS.

Conclusion: Our curriculum design is one approach to create context-specific POCUS education for use in RLS, thereby improving patient care.

Keywords: Point-of-care ultrasound, Tropical infectious disease, Resource-limited settings, Fellowship

Introduction

Improvements in portability, image quality, and ease-of-use are driving the expansion of point-of-care ultrasound (POCUS) for screening, diagnosis, and procedural guidance [1]. Emergency clinicians employ a wide variety of POCUS applications to make rapid diagnoses, guide resuscitation, and improve procedural success and decrease complications [2, 3].

As POCUS use expands, accreditation bodies in the United States (USA) [4] and internationally [5] are requiring or recommending POCUS incorporation into emergency medicine training programs. In the USA, this training is primarily provided by emergency ultrasound (EUS) fellowship-trained faculty. The goal of fellowship training is to create leaders in POCUS education [6]. As a result of the increased use of POCUS there has been a proliferation of USA EUS fellowships, with 115 active programs at the time of this writing [7]. In addition, POCUS fellowships are developing in other specialties such as Internal Medicine, Pediatrics, and Critical Care. Few, if any, such training opportunities exist for clinicians living and working in resource-limited settings (RLS), or for those planning to.

The goal of the fellowship outlined below is to equip graduates to appropriately use and teach contextualized ultrasound skills in RLS. The benefits of POCUS in RLS are increasingly recognized. Maru et al. deem X-ray and ultrasound the "key" imaging modalities primary and emergency care in rural and RLS [8]. Unfortunately, traditional radiology modalities, even when available in RLS, require expensive equipment, maintenance, trained staff, and specialists to interpret images [9], and the costs of such studies or the distance of travel required may be prohibitive. Trained clinicians with POCUS may alleviate some of these limitations [10]. Portable hand-held ultrasound systems can be purchased for $2000 USD, adding a solar charger and external battery brings the total cost

*Correspondence: slburleson@uabmc.edu
[1] Department of Emergency Medicine, University of Alabama at Birmingham Hospital, Old Hillman Building Suite 251, 619 19th St S, Birmingham, AL 35249, USA
Full list of author information is available at the end of the article

for an ultrasound system that does not require a stable power supply to $2200 USD. While this is still expensive for any individual provider, it represents a dramatic drop in cost from the laptop-based systems costing tens of thousands of dollars that were the primary tool for providers in RLS up until a few years ago. Many clinicians with POCUS expertise have brought their skills to RLS, and while there has been a huge benefit of this expertise, there are reasons ultrasound use and training in these settings needs to become more context specific.

Many POCUS applications thought to have the highest utility in the RLS are familiar to developed-world clinicians. POCUS use in peripartum care, trauma, heart failure [11], undifferentiated hypotension or dyspnea [12, 13], and deep venous thrombosis [14] in RLS are all well-described. In settings lacking confirmatory diagnostics, POCUS may be even more valuable to a patient's clinical evaluation than in a developed setting. POCUS use in RLS may impact the clinical management of 50–70% patients [15, 16].

A growing body of literature documents POCUS use in the management of tropical infectious diseases including extrapulmonary tuberculosis in Human Immunodeficiency Virus (HIV), cystic echinococcosis, liver abscess, schistosomiasis, lymphatic filariasis, visceral leishmaniasis, and viral hemorrhagic fever [17, 18]. These applications are not included in most POCUS curricula and may yield unique ultrasound findings or apply traditional ultrasound exams to new contexts (such as the application of the FAST exam to extrapulmonary tuberculosis or dengue). Belard et al. conclude the potential of POCUS in tropical infectious disease management appears "huge and increasing", but high-quality training and standardized protocols are the keys to continued growth [17]. Becker and colleagues concur that the lack of POCUS-trained clinicians, specifically qualified instructors and educational opportunities, inhibits the broader implementation of ultrasound in RLS [15].

Many POCUS training strategies in RLS rely initially on external expertise, usually provided by clinicians with extensive POCUS experience requiring years to develop or by EUS fellowship-trained faculty. Unfortunately, resource limitations and tropical diseases create challenges when attempting direct translation of emergency POCUS to these settings. Van Hoving and Lamprecht describe discrepancies between the standardized South African POCUS curriculum (modeled after resource-rich settings) and the actual diseases seen by providers [19]. Salmon and colleagues note that the direct transfer of curricula to RLS "fails to acknowledge the unique challenges, needs, and disease burdens" of those settings [20]. Henwood et al. emphasize the importance of a needs assessment involving stakeholders at multiple levels to determine which applications should be included in any potential curriculum [21]. Burdick et al. note that training in International Emergency Medicine (IEM) or Global Health "needs to emphasize knowledge of both biologic and cultural aspects of care in specific environments" and recommend against applying resource-rich systems directly to RLS without careful analysis of actual effects and limitations [22]. The same could be said of the application of POCUS curricula.

Clinicians and especially educators in RLS therefore require expertise in tropical diseases and POCUS applications not included in USA EUS fellowship curricula. They also must understand regional differences in epidemiology, pathology, and resources. A structured fellowship curriculum can provide this expertise, while also developing the educational capacity to then provide training to other clinicians in RLS in a "train the trainer" model tailored to the needs of that particular setting [9, 11, 20]. We describe the point-of-care ultrasound in RLS (PURLS) fellowship, a novel Emergency Medicine fellowship. Conceptualized to meet the curricular guidelines of USA EUS fellowships [6] while providing clinical and ultrasound experience in RLS and tropical medicine, the curriculum develops fellows into effective clinicians in RLS and leaders in POCUS training in any clinical setting.

Discussion

Curriculum description

The PURLS fellowship is an 18-month curriculum integrating clinical faculty practice at an academic ED with clinical experience in a variety of RLS and international training sites. This includes advanced hands-on POCUS experience and teaching in both resource-rich and RLS. An overview of the curriculum is provided in Table 1. Table 2 details the PURLS timeline.

Clinical experience in the RLS is fluid by design to adapt to the aspirations of the individual fellow, and includes a combination of hospital work, primary care, and refugee/disaster medicine. Most clinical work will take place at sites or with organizations with established relationships with fellowship faculty, in order to facilitate a more coherent longitudinal experience for the fellow, faculty, local partners, and ongoing projects.

To improve clinical expertise and provide context for the expansion of ultrasound in tropical medicine and RLS, the fellow must complete a clinical tropical medicine course [23–26] and sit for the Diploma of Tropical Medicine and Hygiene (DTM&H) exam. This provides the framework on which fellows build their clinical and POCUS experience and allows fellows to better understand the diseases and health infrastructure in other settings. Fellows also have the opportunity to complete

Table 1 Overview of PURLS fellowship curriculum components

Content area	Frequency	Length
Emergency ultrasound		
Bedside scanning and teaching shifts with students and residents	Weekly	Longitudinal
Advanced scanning skills (cardiac, musculoskeletal, hepatic, OB/pelvic, procedural)	Monthly	Longitudinal
Image review, quality assurance, program administration	Weekly	Longitudinal
Tropical medicine and global health		
Diploma in tropical medicine and hygiene		9–12 weeks
Clinical experience in RLS	Variable	8–10 weeks
Global health conference	Every 2 weeks	Longitudinal
Humanitarian response or trip leadership course		2 weeks
Point-of-care ultrasound in resource-limited settings		
Clinical ultrasound in tropical infectious diseases course		2 weeks
Clinical and teaching experience in RLS	Variable	Longitudinal while abroad
Research		

Table 2 Summary of a fellow's international and domestic work

Timeline	Location	Description of work	Length
July–August	United States	Routine clinical and fellow duties	
September	Tanzania	POCUS scanning and education at an academic tert ary referral hospital	3 weeks
October–November	United States	Routine clinical and fellow duties	
December	The Gambia	Rural primary care clinics with no imaging besides POCUS	2 weeks
January–March	Peru	Clinical ultrasound in tropical infectious diseases course	1 week
		Diploma of tropical medicine and hygiene—POCUS on daily inpatient rounds	9 weeks
April	United States	Humanitarian response course	2 weeks
May–August	United States	Routine clinical and fellow duties	
September	Tanzania	POCUS scanning and education at an academic tertiary referral hospital	2 weeks
October–December	United States	Routine clinical and fellow duties	

courses in medical trip leadership or humanitarian response [27, 28].

Fellows participate with faculty in global health teaching discussions every 2 weeks, focused on tropical medicine case studies, trip planning, logistics, and refugee health. Time is also spent outlining research goals, and integrating clinical practice and POCUS into local patterns according to needs assessments or published guidelines. This teaching complements the clinical tropical medicine course and provides longitudinal mentorship focused on practice in RLS while the fellow works domestically. Conferences are also an opportunity to address topics not encountered by the fellow in their personal experience.

Fellows integrate POCUS into clinical practice in all settings. They participate in and teach advanced training courses [29] focusing on ultrasound in tropical infectious disease which emphasize the unique role of POCUS in both tropical infections and RLS. Fellows and faculty also train local providers in discrete basic POCUS protocols, such as the FASH or obstetric exams, or POCUS-guided vascular access. These education modules are driven by local needs assessments or by the requests of local partners. Fellows also complete a research project integrating POCUS, education, and practice in the RLS.

When working in the USA, fellows fulfill a traditional EUS fellowship role, including resident and medical student education, image review, QA, EUS program management, research, and advanced training in specific areas as directed by the needs of the fellow. Each aspect is intended to equip the fellow with the skills to implement a fully functioning POCUS training program. These roles allow faculty to evaluate the fellow's practical competencies and develop the teaching skills of the fellow prior to independent work in the RLS.

Advanced echocardiography training includes scanning sessions in the echocardiography laboratory and echocardiographic interpretation with a board-certified cardiologist. Pathology relevant to RLS is emphasized, such as rheumatic heart disease, pulmonary hypertension (often secondary to chronic parasitic infections such as schistosomiasis), and hypertensive heart disease, all of which are common in these settings [30–32], and often diagnosed in advanced stages [30, 32, 33].

Fellows have the opportunity to scan with expert ultrasound technicians in the resource-rich setting to gain experience with applications not often included in POCUS curricula, but frequently utilized in RLS, such as hepatic and splenic ultrasound [21]. Fellows may also work with an emergency and sports medicine physician in clinic to improve skills in diagnostic musculoskeletal POCUS, regional anesthesia, and ultrasound-guided procedures.

Faculty augment this training with supervised scanning in RLS, case studies, and image review over the course of the fellowship. With new technology, image review can be performed remotely and almost instantaneously, allowing fellows to consult faculty when encountering new pathology in the field. Fellows also participate in an ultrasound training course in RLS run by a faculty member with both expertise in tropical medicine and ultrasound. This provides the fellow an opportunity to participate in training other providers with limited ultrasound skills in a low-resource environment where tropical diseases are common.

Goals and objectives

The authors believe the combination of clinical experience and teaching in RLS, formal training in tropical infectious diseases, and training in advanced POCUS applications enables fellows to expertly obtain and interpret images, then apply those findings appropriately to the patient and the clinical context. The authors envision the PURLS curriculum producing graduates who are competent to provide excellent contextualized patient care in RLS, employ POCUS to improve the care of individual patients in RLS, and to train other providers to use the modality, both those from the resource-rich setting gaining new skills for global health work and those native to RLS. Focused teaching, research, and experience during the fellowship further equip graduates to develop appropriate curricula that address the assessed needs of patients and clinicians in a particular setting and implement curricula such that POCUS usage can become self-sufficient in regards to local expertise, quality assurance, and supplies.

The PURLS curriculum combines aspects of both EUS and IEM fellowships, inculcating fellows with both advanced ultrasonography skills and the flexibility, cultural competence, and knowledge of disease burdens in RLS. Our curriculum emphasizes the complementary aspects of both fellowships, providing a broader perspective and skill set than either fellowship alone.

Future changes

These conclusions and the limitations to follow represent the views of one fellow (SLB) and fellowship faculty upon completion of the fellowship. Future changes to the curriculum could include the development of hands-on short-term courses in a variety of settings and specialties to increase dissemination of the content and provide supervised settings for competency development in a greater number of learners. The development of a comprehensive, distributable, interactive, asynchronous educational resource would benefit the fellow and other learners, especially with rarer pathology, or that with limited geographic distribution. Finally, POCUS use in tropical infectious disease is growing rapidly, so new applications will likely need to be added to the curriculum continually.

Limitations

Limitations for our particular fellowship include the necessity of prior Emergency Medicine residency training, basic POCUS competency, and a broad knowledge base encompassing multiple subspecialties. The 18-month duration of the fellowship is a significant time commitment. The fellowship curriculum could potentially be applied to other specialties, such as internal, family, or critical care medicine, though the fellowship itself might require more time, since emergency medicine graduates have more extensive ultrasound training built into residency in the USA. One dual-boarded Internal Medicine and Pediatric physician has completed an earlier iteration of this fellowship model, so this concept has been trialed outside of Emergency Medicine.

Another limitation is that this fellowship and curriculum is based on model of advanced training that is primarily found in Canada and the United States. Other countries where specialty training and graduate medical education has a different structure will have trouble following the exact format of the fellowship and creating a financially viable model that is similar to what has been done here. We believe the primary concept of focused training that combines ultrasound with tropical medicine and an advanced knowledge of care delivery in RLS is achievable in most training settings, but may require modification of the timeline and cost specifics.

To allow adequate time for international and educational responsibilities, fellows work approximately half the clinical shifts of full-time academic faculty and are paid commensurate with the clinical work completed, which is consistent practice among all Emergency Medicine fellowships at our institution. Financial resources available to fellows for training and travel are also a potential limitation, but at our institution, a portion of the fellow salary from clinical work is withheld to pay for travel and other expenses, an arrangement acceptable to prior fellows.

The need for significant departmental resources, likely including a pre-existing EUS fellowship and either an IEM fellowship or faculty with extensive experience and professional contacts in the RLS may limit creation of similar fellowships in other contexts. At our institution, the PURLS fellowship is integrated alongside pre-existing IEM and EUS fellowships, and faculty from the IEM and EUS fellowships participate in PURLS fellow education according to their expertise. The authors with dedicated PURLS training (SLB and DK) focus on the specific applications of POCUS in RLS. Acquisition and maintenance of functioning ultrasound machines is a possible limitation for any institution utilizing POCUS. This is doubly true in the RLS, but many possible solutions exist, including newer "ultra-portable" machines, a variety of NGOs providing refurbished machines for short- or long-term use in RLS, and the increasing availability of ultrasound machines at institutions in the RLS.

Conclusion

POCUS plays an important role in clinical practice in many settings, but it is increasingly relevant in the RLS. There exists a significant lack of qualified educators to adequately train new providers in the unique applications of POCUS in RLS. The PURLS curriculum provides a model for producing clinician educators with context-specific expertise in tropical infectious disease, clinical practice in RLS, and ultrasound education who can practice effectively and can train other RLS clinicians in POCUS. We believe this novel fellowship can produce clinicians and educators with the knowledge and ability to help improve POCUS education and, ultimately, patient care, where it is needed most.

Abbreviations

PURLS: Point-of-care ultrasound in resource-limited settings; DTM&H: Diploma of Tropical Medicine and Hygiene; ED: Emergency Department; EUS: Emergency ultrasound; FASH: Focused assessment with sonography in HIV-associated TB; HIV: Human Immunodeficiency Virus; IEM: International Emergency Medicine; POCUS: Point-of-care ultrasonography; QA: Quality assurance; RLS: Resource-limited setting; USA: United States of America.

Acknowledgements

Not applicable.

Prior presentations

Not applicable.

Authors' contributions

SLB: primary manuscript author, fellowship planning and design, fellowship graduate. DCP: fellowship planning and design, manuscript editing. JPG: fellowship planning and design, manuscript editing. CG: fellowship planning and design, manuscript editing. CBG: fellowship planning and design, manuscript editing, director of US portion of fellowship. SI: fellowship planning and design, manuscript editing, director of IEM portion of fellowship, hands-on fellow education in RLS. DK: fellowship planning and design, manuscript editing, hands-on fellow education in RLS. All authors read and approved the final manuscript.

Author details

[1] Department of Emergency Medicine, University of Alabama at Birmingham Hospital, Old Hillman Building Suite 251, 619 19th St S, Birmingham, AL 35249, USA. [2] Department of Emergency Medicine, Augusta University, Augusta, GA, USA.

References

1. Moore CL, Copel JA (2011) Point-of-care ultrasonography. N Engl J Med 364:749–757
2. Whitson MR, Mayo PH (2016) Ultrasonography in the emergency department. Crit Care 20:227
3. Tirado A, Wu T, Noble E et al (2013) Ultrasound-guided procedures in the emergency department—diagnostic and therapeutic asset. Emerg Med Clin N Am 31:117–149
4. Accreditation Council for Graduate Medical Education (2016) Program requirements for graduate medical education in emergency medicine. Revised Common Program Requirements. https://www.acgme.org/Portals/0/PFAssets/ProgramRequirements/CPRs_2017-07-01.pdf Accessed 18 Jan 2018
5. Atkinson P, Bowra J, Lambert M et al (2015) International federation for emergency medicine point of care ultrasound curriculum. CJEM 17(2):161–170
6. American College of Emergency Physicians (2011) Emergency ultrasound fellowship guidelines. Emergency ultrasound section information paper https://www.acep.org/workarea/downloadasset.aspx?id=80954 Accessed 17 Jan 2018
7. Society of clinical ultrasound fellowships. https://eusfellowships.com/programs.php Accessed 17 Jan 2018
8. Maru DS, Schwarz R, Jason A et al (2010) Turning a blind eye: the mobilization of radiology services in resource poor regions. Glob Health 6:18
9. Stolz LA, Muruganandan KM, Bisanzo MC et al (2015) Point-of-care ultrasound education for non-physician clinicians in a resource-limited emergency department. Trop Med Int Health 20(8):1067–1072
10. Sippel S, Muruganandan K, Levine A et al (2011) Review article: use of ultrasound in the developing world. Int J Emerg Med 4:72
11. Henwood PC, Mackenzie DC, Rempell JS et al (2014) A practical guide to self-sustaining point-of-care ultrasound education programs in resource-limited settings. Annals Emerg Med 64:277–285
12. Becker TK, Tafoya CA, Osei-Ampofo M et al (2017) Cardiopulmonary ultrasound for critically ill adults improves diagnostic accuracy in a resource-limited setting: the AFRICA trial. Trop Med Int Health 22(12):1599–1608
13. Tafoya CA, Tafoya MJ, Osei-Ampofo M et al (2017) Sustainable resuscitation ultrasound education in a low-resource environment: the Kumasi experience. J Emerg Med 52(5):723–730
14. Heller T, Mtemang'ombe EA, Huson MAM et al (2017) Ultrasound for patients in a high HIV/tuberculosis prevalence setting: needs assessment and review of focused applications for sub-Saharan Africa. Int J Infect Dis 56:229–236
15. Becker DM, Tafoya CA, Becker SL et al (2016) The use of portable ultrasound devices in low- and middle-income countries: a systematic review of the literature. Trop Med Int Health 21(3):294–311

16. Stanley A, Wajanga BMK, Jaka H et al (2017) The impact of systematic point-of-care ultrasound on management in a resource-limited setting. Am J Trop Med 96(2):489–492
17. Belard S, Tamarozzi F, Bustinduy AL et al (2016) Point-of-care ultrasound assessment of tropical infectious diseases—a review of applications and perspectives. Am J Trop Med 94(1):8–21
18. Brunetti E, Heller T, Richter J et al (2016) Application of ultrasonography in the diagnosis of infectious disease in resource-limited settings. Curr Infect Dis Rep. 18:6
19. Van Hoving DJ, Lamprecht H (2016) Toward an appropriate point-of-care ultrasound curriculum: a reflection of the clinical practice in South Africa. J Med Ultrasound 24:18–24
20. Salmon M, Landes M, Hunchak C et al (2017) Getting it right the first time: defining regionally relevant training curricula and provider core competencies for point-of-care ultrasound education on the African continent. Ann Emerg Med 69(2):218–226
21. Henwood PC, Mackenzie D, Liteplo et al (2017) Point-of-care ultrasound use, accuracy, and impact on clinical decision making in Rwanda hospitals. J Ultrasound Med 36:1189–1194
22. Burdick WP, Hauswald M, Iserson KV (2010) International emergency medicine commentary. Acad Emerg Med 17(7):758–761
23. Gorgas diploma course in clinical tropical medicine. Lima https://www.uab.edu/medicine/gorgas/diploma-course Accessed 22 Jan 2018
24. London school of Hygiene and Tropical Medicine Professional Diploma in Tropical Medicine and Hygiene. London https://www.lshtm.ac.uk/study/courses/short-courses/DTMH. Accessed 21 June 2018
25. London School of Hygiene and Tropical Medicine Professional Diploma in Tropical Medicine and Hygiene (East Africa Partnership). Moshi, Tanzania. https://www.lshtm.ac.uk/study/courses/short-courses/DTMH Accessed June 21, 2018
26. Liverpool School of Tropical Medicine and Hygiene Diploma in Tropical Medicine and Hygiene. Liverpool https://www.lstmed.ac.uk/study/courses/diploma-in-tropical-medicine-hygiene. Accessed 21 June 2018
27. Humanitarian Response Intensive Course. Harvard Humanitarian Initiative. Cambridge https://www.humanitarianacademy.harvard.edu/education/workshops/hric. Accessed 22 Jan 2018
28. Health Emergencies in Large Populations. International Committee of the Red Cross. https://www.icrc.org/en/document/helpcourse. Accessed 21 June 2018
29. Clinical Ultrasound in Tropical Infectious Diseases. Augusta University and Universidad Peruana Cayetano Heredia. Lima https://www.augusta.edu/mcg/em/ed/fellowships/ultrasound/id.php. Accessed 31 Aug 2019
30. Mirabel M, Tafflet M, Noel B et al (2015) Newly diagnosed rheumatic heart disease among indigenous populations in the Pacific. Heart 101:1901–1906
31. Papamatheakis DG, Mocumbi AOH, Kim NH, Mandel J (2014) Schistosomiasis-associated pulmonary hypertension. Pulm Circ 4(4):596–611
32. Ogah OS, Stewart S, Falase AO et al (2014) Contemporary profile of acute heart failure in southern Nigeria. J Am Coll Cardiol HF 2:250–259
33. Zuhlke L, Engel ME, Karthikeyan G et al (2015) Characteristics, complications, and gaps in evidence based interventions in rheumatic heart disease: the Global Rheumatic Heart Disease Registry (the REMEDY study). Eur Heart J 36:1115–1122

12

Point-of-care ultrasound for the detection of hydronephrosis in emergency department patients with suspected renal colic

Stephanie Sibley[1*], Nathan Roth[2^], Charles Scott[3], Louise Rang[1], Heather White[1], Marco L. A. Sivilotti[1] and Eric Bruder[1]

Abstract

Background: Point-of-care ultrasound (PoCUS) by emergency physicians for renal colic has been proposed as an alternative to computed tomography (CT) to avoid ionizing radiation exposure and shorten emergency department length of stay. Previous studies have employed experienced or credentialed ultrasonographers or required advanced ultrasound skills. We sought to measure the diagnostic accuracy of PoCUS by physicians with varied experience using a simplified binary outcome of presence or absence of hydronephrosis. Secondary outcomes include assessment as to whether the presence of hydronephrosis on PoCUS is predictive of complications, and to evaluate possible causes for the reduced diagnostic accuracy such as body mass index (BMI) and time between PoCUS and formal imaging, and scanner experience.

Results: 413 patients were enrolled in the study. PoCUS showed a specificity of 71.8% [95% CI 65.0, 77.9] and sensitivity of 77.1% [95% CI 70.9, 82.6]. Hydronephrosis on PoCUS was predictive of complications (relative risk 3.13; [95% CI 1.30, 7.53]). The time interval between PoCUS and formal imaging, BMI, and scanner experience did not influence the accuracy of PoCUS.

Conclusions: PoCUS for hydronephrosis in suspected renal colic has moderate accuracy when performed by providers with varied experience for the binary outcome of presence or absence of hydronephrosis. Hydronephrosis on PoCUS is associated with increased rates of complications. PoCUS for hydronephrosis is limited in its utility as a stand-alone test, however this inexpensive, readily available test may be useful in conjunction with clinical course to determine which patients would benefit from formal imaging or urologic consultation.

ClinicalTrials.gov Identifier NCT01323842

Keywords: Hydronephrosis, PoCUS, Point-of-care ultrasound, Renal colic, Emergency department, BMI

Background

Renal colic is a common presentation in the ED with over 3.6 million visits in the United States between 2006 and 2009 [1]. While most attacks are self-limited, some patients benefit from urologic intervention, and others harbor a more dangerous cause for their pain. Since identifying such cases is largely based on formal imaging, especially computed tomography (CT), suspected renal colic is an important driver of advanced imaging, of prolonged or repeated emergency department utilization, and of direct and indirect costs related to patient care and lost work time [2–4].

Computed tomography remains the imaging modality of choice to confirm the diagnosis, prognosticate spontaneous stone passage, and rule out other causes of abdominal pain [5, 6]. A study of US emergency department

*Correspondence: stephanie.sibley@kingstonhsc.ca
^Nathan Roth: Deceased (19th September 2017)
[1] Department of Emergency Medicine, Queen's University, Kingston, ON, Canada
Full list of author information is available at the end of the article

visits for suspected renal colic reported very high rates of abdominal CT (> 80%) despite low rates of admission (< 20%) and urologic intervention (< 10%) [7]. Radiology ultrasound (radUS) has been proposed as the preferred test for patients at low risk for complications of urolithiasis [6]. When using this modality, the calculus is often not visualized and the identification of hydronephrosis due to ureteric obstruction becomes the salient finding. Point-of-care ultrasound (PoCUS) by emergency physicians has been widely adopted in emergency medicine [8] and has been proposed as a cost-effective, quick and radiation-free alternative to CT to aid in decision-making in cases of suspected renal colic [9–17]. Several studies have reported only moderate sensitivity and specificity of PoCUS for urolithiasis. These studies have been performed by either credentialed ultrasonographers [12] or attending emergency physicians [15] or have required physicians to perform complicated scans including grading the degree of hydronephrosis and identifying ureteric jets [10, 11, 14, 17]. Smith-Bindman et al. found no significant difference in high-risk diagnoses, return emergency visits, pain scores or hospitalizations when initial ultrasonography was compared to CT. However, there was no head-to-head comparison between PoCUS and CT in this comparative effectiveness study, the diagnosis of renal colic was dependent on passage of a stone or surgical intervention rather than formal imaging, and obese patients were excluded from this study, limiting its generalizability [18].

We performed a prospective, observational study to determine the diagnostic accuracy of PoCUS for hydronephrosis in patients with suspected renal colic. Our secondary outcome evaluated if hydronephrosis on PoCUS was predictive of patients who developed subsequent complications. This study adds to the current body of literature by addressing issues such as physician experience, generalized by having resident and attending emergency physicians with varied levels of ultrasound experience perform scans, and a simplified binary outcome of presence or absence of hydronephrosis as opposed to grading hydronephrosis or detecting ureteric jets. Additionally, the effect of body mass index (BMI), scanner experience and the time interval from formal imaging to PoCUS on the accuracy of this test was assessed.

Methods

This was a prospective observational study conducted in two academic emergency departments in Ontario (combined visits of ~ 110,000/year). The Queen's University Health Sciences Research Ethics Board approved this study, which accrued subjects over 30 months (April 2011–July 2013). All subjects provided written consent prior to enrollment.

Patients aged 16–65 years who had either CT or radUS ordered for suspected renal colic were screened for eligibility. The treating emergency physicians enrolled eligible patients 24 h a day, 7 days a week, assisted by dedicated research personnel during daytime to evening hours up to 7 days a week, which matched the availability of advanced imaging for this indication.

Patients were excluded for hemodynamic instability, fever, suspected urinary tract infection based on symptoms or urinalysis positive for leukocytes and nitrites, pregnancy, renal transplant, single functioning kidney, known abdominal aortic aneurysm or incarceration. Patients were ineligible if no formal imaging was ordered at the time of their emergency visit.

Attending or resident emergency physicians performed the PoCUS scans. To be eligible to perform study scans, physicians had to complete an accredited emergency department ultrasound course (such as those endorsed by the Canadian Point of Care Ultrasound Society) or the local, required, introductory point-of-care ultrasound course for emergency medicine residents focusing on focused assessment with sonography in trauma (FAST), aortic and obstetrical ultrasound skills. Scanning physicians had to attend a didactic lecture where the study was described and renal anatomy, ultrasound technique and several examples were reviewed. They attended a training session where physicians scanned live models with hydronephrosis. The newly trained physicians had to complete 25 observed renal ultrasounds with an expert physician (fellowship trained or additional training in renal ultrasound) prior to enrolling patients.

Other than undergoing PoCUS, subjects were treated according to usual practice. The decision and type of formal imaging was left entirely to the discretion of the treating physician, and potential subjects were approached by research staff only after formal imaging had been ordered. Scans were performed using a My Lab 5 (Esaote, Genoa Italy) ultrasound machine with a curvilinear 3.5-MHz probe. Scanning physicians performed a B-mode scan of the abdominal aorta and bilateral kidneys (short and long axis). The scanning physician recorded subject weight, height, if hydronephrosis was present/absent/indeterminate for each kidney, as well as the diameter of the abdominal aorta on a standardized form while blinded to any formal imaging. In cases where the formal imaging was performed prior to PoCUS, the scanning physician was directed not to look at images or the formal radiology report.

A radiologist (CS) blinded to the PoCUS reviewed all formal CT or radUS images to establish the degree of hydronephrosis, graded as absent, mild, moderate or severe [19]. The radiologist also documented the presence, position and size of any urinary calculus, signs suggestive of recent stone passage, as well as any alternative diagnosis that could account for the patient's symptoms and the presence of abdominal aortic aneurysm (AAA) on a standardized form.

Research assistants performed 30-day telephone follow-up and asked scripted standardized questions regarding urgent consultations with urologists, any interventions or hospitalizations. A chart review was performed at 30 days (NR and SS). Details of urologic consultations, interventions, hospitalizations, sepsis and death within the regional healthcare system were extracted from the record, recorded on standardized forms, and entered into a RedCap database. Patients were considered lost to follow-up if they could not be contacted by telephone and had no record of emergency room visit, urology intervention or hospital admission in the medical record.

The primary outcome measure was the sensitivity and specificity of PoCUS for the presence or absence of hydronephrosis compared to formal imaging in patients with suspected renal colic.

The secondary outcome was the association between PoCUS findings and complications within 30 days, defined as the composite of any urologic intervention (e.g., lithotripsy, stent, or percutaneous nephrostomy), sepsis, hospital admission or death. Urgent complications were defined as any of the composite outcomes that occurred within 7 days of initial emergency department visit. Urgent complications were assessed separately to differentiate patients who presented with an acute worsening of their symptoms versus patients who had urology follow-up and were scheduled for a surgical procedure within 30 days. The effects of BMI, time interval to formal imaging and physician scanning experience on the accuracy of PoCUS were analyzed.

For the primary analysis, indeterminate PoCUS scans were deemed negative for hydronephrosis, but reclassified as positive in a separate sensitivity analysis. The degree of severity of hydronephrosis on formal imaging was dichotomized at different cut points to determine the diagnostic accuracy of PoCUS when hydronephrosis was considered positive only when graded "mild, moderate and severe", "moderate and severe", or "severe". Patients who were lost to 30-day follow-up were excluded from the analysis for the secondary outcome of complications and no imputation was performed.

Statistical analysis was performed SAS software, version 9.4 (Cary, North Carolina). Baseline characteristics were summarized as means and standard deviations and medians and quartiles for continuous variables and proportions for binary and categorical variables. Sensitivity, specificity and likelihood ratios were calculated for detection of hydronephrosis with PoCUS using the formal radiology result as the reference standard. A Chi square test was used to compare risk of complications, and to assess for changes in accuracy for detection of hydronephrosis compared to formal imaging time between PoCUS and formal imaging, and BMI.

Results are reported in accordance with the STARD 2015 guidelines for studies of diagnostic accuracy [20].

We performed an a priori sample size calculation using estimates taken from Edmonds et al. [21], a retrospective chart review of patients undergoing formal ultrasound for the diagnosis of renal colic in emergency patients. These investigators reported that 0.6% of subjects with no abnormality on ultrasound received urologic intervention versus 6.2% of patients with a visualized stone and 6.8% of patients with ultrasounds suggestive of ureterolithiasis. Assuming a 7% versus 1% in complications/interventions between patients with and without hydronephrosis on PoCUS, two-tailed α of 5%, and a power of 80%, it was determined that 167 subjects would be required in each group. We estimated that this would provide 95% confidence bands of $\pm$ 10% around the point estimate of sensitivity and specificity for the primary outcome.

Results

A total of 955 unique patient encounters were screened for potential enrollment in the study. The total enrollment was 415 patients, and 413 patients completed formal imaging and represent the study cohort for the primary analysis of hydronephrosis. Total patients lost at 1-month follow-up totaled 69, leaving 344 patients in the analysis for the secondary outcome of urologic complications (Fig. 1).

Seventeen emergency physicians and residents were eligible to perform renal PoCUS for the study, including five physicians considered to be experts.

Baseline characteristics of the cohort are summarized in Table 1. Half (50.4%) were male, with mean age was 42.2 years and mean BMI was 29 kg/m^2. Most patients (85.0%) underwent formal imaging with a CT scan. Hydronephrosis on formal imaging was found in 51.0% of patients. Hydronephrosis on PoCUS was seen in 53.0% of patients, and 4.6% had indeterminate PoCUS scans. A small number of subjects had alternate diagnoses established on formal imaging, including ovarian cysts, diverticulitis and appendicitis (Table 2). Of those with an alternate diagnosis the detection of hydronephrosis with POCUS was rare and seen only in one case of pyelonephritis, one case of perforated diverticulitis, one ureteric stricture and one gynecological cancer. There were no cases of ectopic pregnancy or abdominal aortic aneurysm in the study cohort.

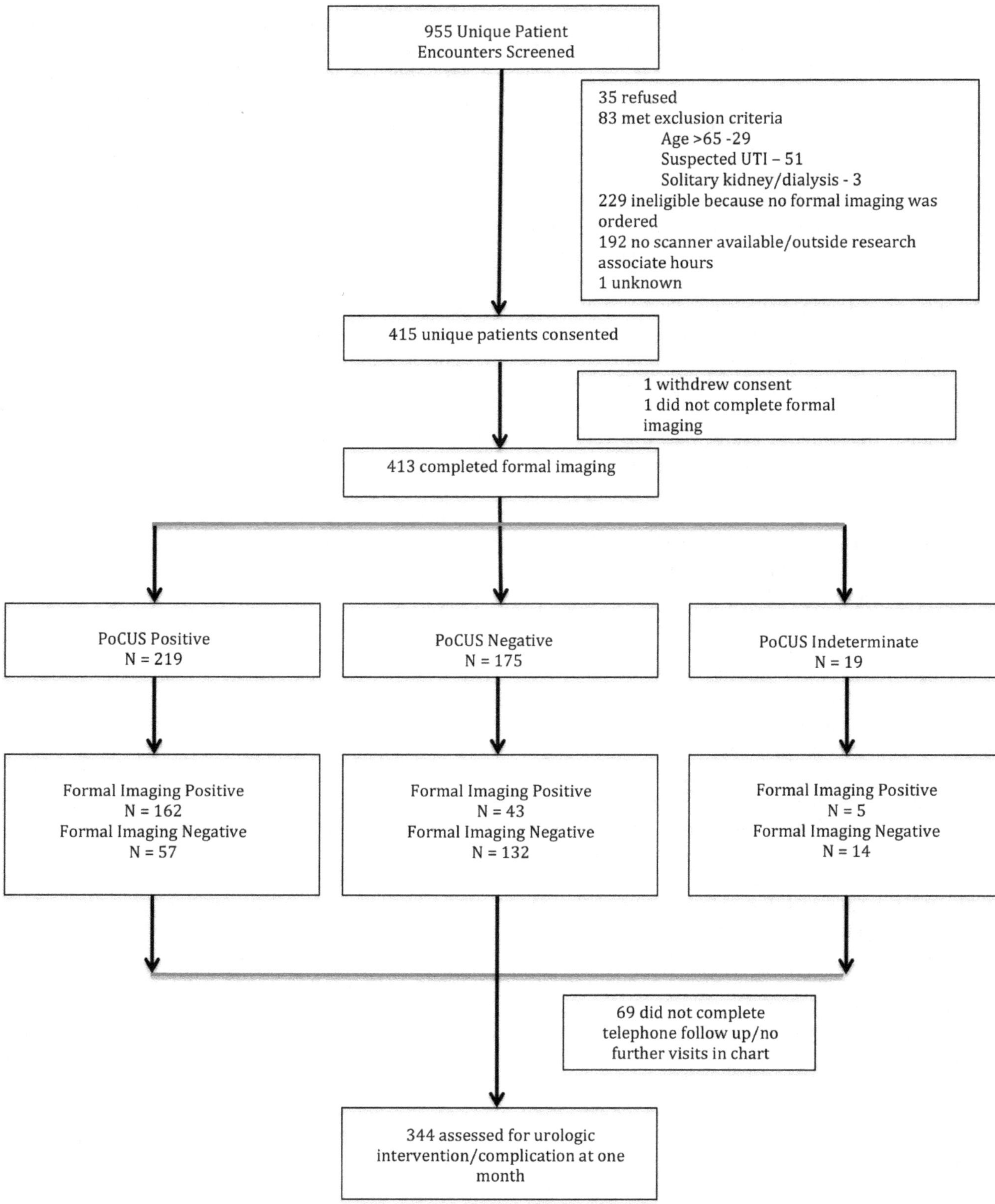

Fig. 1 STARD flow diagram of patient enrollment and follow-up

Table 1 Cohort characteristics

N	413
Male (%)	208 (50.4)
Age, years mean (SD)	42.2 (13.5)
BMI, mean (SD)	28.96 (11.2)
BMI category (%)	
< 20	27 (6.7)
20–24.9	111 (27.6)
25–29.9	126 (31.3)
30–34.9	76 (18.9)
> 35	62 (15.4)
Missing	10
Time from POCUS to formal imaging, min	
Mean (SD)	−31.81 (63.1)
Median	−40.50
25th percentile	−58.0
75th percentile	−24.0
Hydronephrosis present on POCUS	
No	175 (42.4)
Yes	219 (53.0)
Indeterminate	19 (4.6)
Formal imaging modality	
CT	350 (85.0)
US	63 (15.0)
Hydronephrosis on formal imaging	
Severe	19 (4.6)
Moderate	78 (19.0)
Mild	113 (27.4)
Absent	202 (49.0)
2nd ER visit for Imaging results (%)	49 (12)
Urologic Consult	60 (17.4)
Urologic intervention/complication	
Lithotripsy	15 (4.4)
Stent	20 (5.8)
Percutaneous nephrostomy	0
Sepsis	8 (2.3)
Hospital admission	17 (5.2)
Death	0
Stone or evidence of recent passage seen on formal imaging (%)	205 (50)

SD standard deviation, *BMI* body mass index, *CT* computed tomography, *US* ultrasound)

Table 2 Alternative diagnoses found on formal imaging

Ovarian cyst	6
Diverticulitis	4
Appendicitis	3
Pyelonephritis	3
Biliary colic/cholecystitis	3
Ovarian torsion/mass	2
Bony lesions/compression fracture	2
Epiploic appendagitis	2
Shingles	2
Uterine mass/cancer	2
Testicular torsion	1
Interabdominal carcinomatosis with metastatic disease to the liver	1
Pneumonia	1
Bowel obstruction	1
Ileitis	1
AAA	0
Ectopic pregnancy	0

AAA abdominal aortic aneurysm

Twenty-eight (6.8%) subjects developed the composite outcome at 30 days, with 19 (4.6%) deemed to be urgent within 7 days. There were no deaths.

The sensitivity of POCUS for the detection of hydronephrosis was 77.1% [95% CI 70.9, 82.6] and the specificity was 71.8% [95% CI 65.0, 77.9]. The sensitivity of PoCUS improved with worsening degrees of hydronephrosis. Two unplanned sensitivity analyses were performed. These measures did not improve appreciably for patients with confirmed stone or signs of recent stone passage on formal imaging (sensitivity 78.2 [95% CI 71.3, 84.1], specificity 74.2 [95% CI 55.4, 88.1]), or when considering only patients who had a CT scan (sensitivity 75.9 [95% CI 69.2, 81.8], specificity 72.3 [95% CI 64.7, 79.1]) (Table 3).

The presence of hydronephrosis on PoCUS was associated with increased complications (11.8% [95% CI 7.6, 17.4] versus 3.8% [95% CI 1.4, 8.0], relative risk of 3.1 [95% CI 1.3, 7.5]) (Table 4). The association between hydronephrosis on formal imaging and 30-day complications was somewhat stronger (14.5% [95% CI 9.7, 20.6] versus 1.21% [95% CI 0.2, 4.3], relative risk 11.98 [95% CI 2.9, 49.7]).

In a post hoc analysis, we considered only the subgroup of patients with urgent interventions. The presence of hydronephrosis on PoCUS was also associated with urgent interventions within 7 days (8.1% [95% CI 4.6, 13.0] versus 2.5% [95% CI 0.7, 6.3], relative risk of 3.2 [95% CI 1.1, 9.5]).

A sensitivity analysis was performed where indeterminate scans were considered positive, with little difference in complications (11.4% [95% CI 7.0, 15.7] vs 3.5% [95% CI 0.4, 6.6], relative risk 3.23% [95% CI 1.3, 8.3]).

The diagnostic accuracy of PoCUS for hydronephrosis did not appear to be strongly influenced by any of the pre-specified factors we examined. Almost all PoCUS scans were obtained within 1 h of formal imaging (Fig. 2). Most (86.2%) patients had PoCUS performed after being transferred back to the emergency department from formal imaging. The agreement did

Table 3 Sensitivity, specificity, positive-likelihood ratio and negative-likelihood ratio for detection of hydronephrosis with POCUS

	TP	TN	FP	FN	Sensitivity (95% CI)	Specificity (95% CI)	+LR (95% CI)	−LR (95% CI)
Hydronephrosis (mild/moderate/severe positive)[a]	162	146	57	48	77.1% (70.9, 82.6)	71.8% (65.0, 77.9)	2.73 (2.17, 3.48)	0.31 (0.24, 0.41)
Hydronephrosis (moderate/severe positive)[a]	85	182	134	12	87.6 (79.4, 93.4)	57.5 (51.8, 63.0)	2.05 (1.78, 2.39)	0.22 (0.13, 0.37)
Hydronephrosis (severe positive)[a]	18	193	201	1	94.7 (74.0, 99.9)	48.9 (43.8, 53.9)	1.85 (1.60, 2.14)	0.11 (0.02, 0.73)
Hydronephrosis (with confirmed stone on formal imaging)[b]	136	23	8	38	78.2 (71.3, 84.1)	74.2 (55.4, 88.1)	3.03 (1.66, 5.53)	0.29 (0.21, 0.42)
Hydronephrosis (patients undergoing CT scan)[c]	145	115	44	46	75.9 (69.2, 81.8)	72.3 (64.7, 79.1)	2.74 (2.11, 3.57)	0.33 (0.25, 0.44)

LR likelihood ratio, *TP* true positive, *TN* true negative, *FP* false positive, *FN* false negative)

[a] A positive test on formal imaging was dichotomized at various cut points (mild/moderate/severe, moderate/severe, severe)

[b] Sensitivity analysis with confirmed stone on formal imaging

[c] Senstivity analysis with the gold standard of CT scan

Table 4 Intervention/complication for POCUS and formal imaging

	Intervention/complication	No intervention/complication	Risk (95% CI)	Relative risk (95% CI)
POCUS				
Positive	22	163	11.83% (7.56, 17.36)	3.13 (1.30, 7.53)
Negative/indeterminate	6	153	3.77% (1.40, 8.03)	
POCUS				
Positive/indeterminate	23	179	11.39% (7.36, 16.59)	3.23 (1.26, 8.30)
Negative	5	137	3.52% (1.15, 8.03)	
Formal imaging				
Positive	26	153	14.53% (9.71, 20.55)	11.98 (2.89, 49.70)
Negative	2	163	1.21% (0.15, 4.31)	

Patients were positive for intervention/complication if they had any one of the following at 30 days follow-up—lithotripsy, stent, percutaneous nephrostomy, sepsis, hospital admission or death

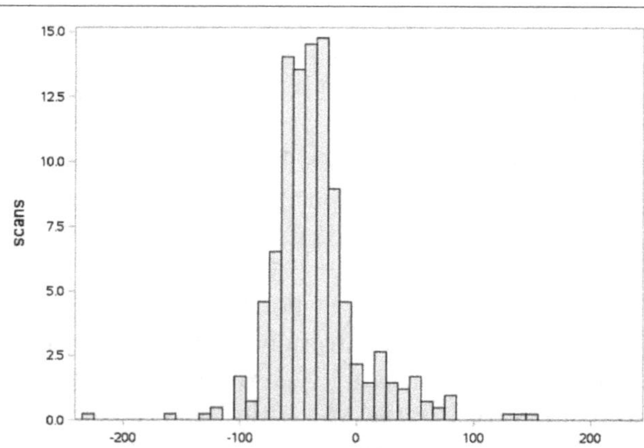

Fig. 2 Time distribution of POCUS to formal imaging (time = 0 − time of PoCUS exam)

not improve when the absolute value of the time interval between formal imaging and PoCUS was shorter. Agreement with formal imaging for each quartile was 76.2%, 78.1%, 76.5% and 67.3% ($p = 0.27$).

When performing PoCUS for the detection of hydronephrosis, expert scanners were comparable to non-experts (sensitivity 81.5% [95% CI 70.0, 90.1] vs 75.2% [95% CI 67.3, 82.0]), (specificity 65.4 [95% CI 50.9, 78.0] vs 74.2 [95% CI 66.4, 80.9]). There was no difference in agreement with formal imaging, with experts in agreement 66.7% [95% CI 57.4, 75.1] and non-experts in agreement 63.9% [95% CI 58.1, 69.3] ($p = 0.65$). Agreement between PoCUS and formal imaging did not improve with a physician's increased scanning experience within the study Agreement was 70.1% for 1–3

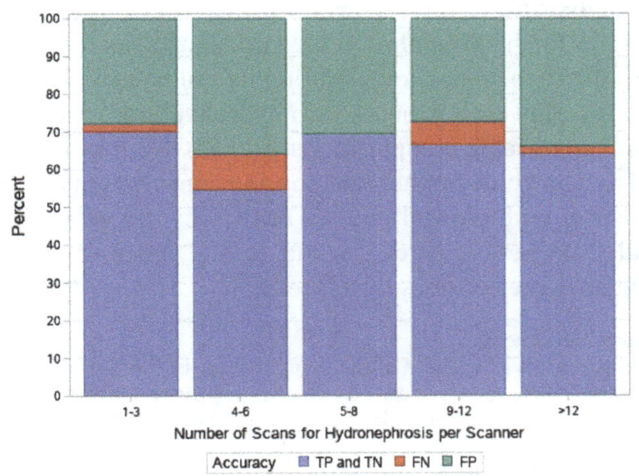

Fig. 3 Accuracy of POCUS with formal imaging with increasing scanning experience (*TP* true positive, *TN* true negative, *FP* false positive, *FN* false negative)

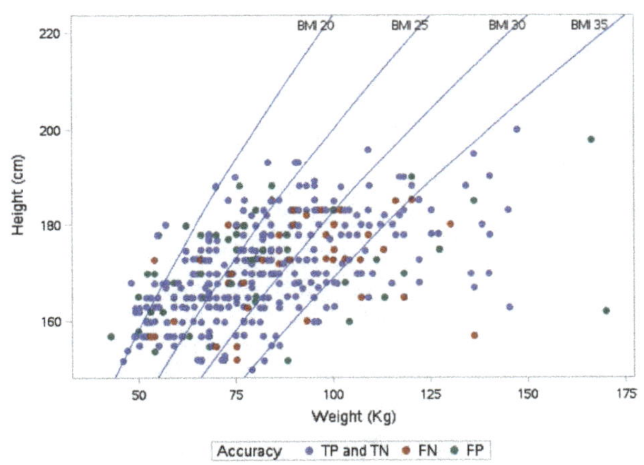

Fig. 4 Accuracy of POCUS for the detection of hydronephrosis relative to patient BMI (*TP* true positive, *TN* true negative, *FP* false positive, *FN* false negative)

scans, 54.8% for 4–6 scans, 69.4% for 10–12 scans, and 64.3% for > 12 scans (Fig. 3).

BMI did not influence the accuracy with agreement between PoCUS and formal imaging of 70.4%, 73.9%, 72.2% and 81.6% and 71.0% for BMI of < 20, 20–24.9, 25–29.9, 30–34.9 and > 30, respectively ($p = 0.56$) (Fig. 4).

Discussion

Our study reaffirms the modest sensitivity and specificity reported by previous studies which limits the utility of PoCUS as a stand-alone diagnostic tool for renal colic. PoCUS is predictive of complications and may help identify patients who require further imaging and urologic consultation.

Our study has similar results to a meta-analysis [9] by Wong et al. that demonstrated modest diagnostic accuracy for nephrolithiasis with moderate sensitivity (77.1%) and specificity (71.8%). They included high-quality studies ($N = 1773$) including two studies with scans performed by credentialed ultrasonographers [12] or attending emergency physicians [15] and four studies requiring physicians to perform more complicated scans [10, 11, 14, 17]. While these studies showed improved specificity, physician ability to grade hydronephrosis is moderate and limits sensitivity [22]. Our study demonstrated that physicians at all levels of training and experience can obtain similar sensitivity and specificity while performing a simplified scan for the presence or absence of hydronephrosis.

The presence of hydronephrosis on PoCUS was associated with an increased risk of subsequent urologic intervention or complication in our study. Fields et al. [11] performed a study of 77 emergency department patients to predict 30-day outcomes. Thirteen patients required admission to hospital, and all admitted patients had hydronephrosis on their PoCUS exam. Daniels et al. [10] performed a study to determine the ability of PoCUS to predict need for urologic intervention at 90 days and demonstrated that 22.8% of patients with hydronephrosis as opposed to 10% of those without required urologic intervention.

While PoCUS was associated with need for urologic intervention, it identified fewer patients than CT or radUS. This is in keeping with a study by Ganesan et al. suggesting 22% of patients would be inappropriately counseled for either observation or intervention if ultrasound was used alone to guide clinical decision-making [23].

Smith-Bindman et al. showed PoCUS has the advantage of being a readily available modality that has the potential to reduce the time from presentation to imaging in the emergency department and expedite clinical decision-making [18]. In this study, we hypothesized the modest sensitivity and specificity of PoCUS in previous studies may have been due to the length of time between PoCUS and formal imaging due to factors such as dehydration and fluid administration [24], and spontaneous stone passage [25]. PoCUS was performed as close to the formal imaging as possible to reduce the effect of these factors. Most of the PoCUS scans were performed within 1 h of formal imaging and there was no difference in agreement with shorter time intervals, indicating these factors had little influence on the sensitivity and specificity in this study.

There was no difference in accuracy between expert and non-expert scanners and no improvement with increased scanning experience which suggests the training session and 25 practice scans prior to enrolling patients in the study may be adequate to develop and retain the skill for detection of hydronephrosis. This is in contrast to Herbst et al. who found fellowship trained emergency physicians had greater accuracy than those without fellowship training [14]. This difference is likely a result of the differing definition of expert scanners and the outcome of graded hydronephrosis versus a simplified binary outcome. It is important to note the overall sensitivity (72.6%), specificity (73.3%) were similar.

Few PoCUS studies have assessed the relationship between diagnostic accuracy and BMI for detection of renal colic. BMI was not a predictor of accuracy of PoCUS for hydronephrosis in this study, and good-quality images were obtained in patients with BMI up to 35 kg/m^2. This is in keeping with findings using ultrasound by diagnostic imaging sonographers [23, 26], who found that detection of a renal stone was independent of BMI.

While PoCUS for hydronephrosis lacks the sensitivity and specificity for a stand-alone diagnostic test, it may be useful when combined with a clinical prediction tool to improve accuracy in diagnosis [10] or clinical score based on history and physical exam [27]. The ability to use this test in patients with increased risk factors such as older age, fever, leukocytosis, history of kidney disease or solitary kidney remains unclear.

Strengths and limitations

The strengths of this study are the inclusion of both resident and attending physicians with varied PoCUS experience and our comprehensive renal PoCUS training program which included practice scanning on patients with known hydronephrosis and observed scans by PoCUS experts. This study also included obese patients who were excluded from other large studies.

Limitations to our study include missed, potentially eligible patients due to lack of an available scanning physician which may have introduced a selection bias. As well, many patients had their PoCUS exam performed after their formal imaging was completed, however scanners were instructed not to look at any imaging prior to completing the PoCUS exam. Most of the PoCUS exams were completed within 1 h of the formal imaging, and it is unlikely the formal reports would be available prior to the completion of the PoCUS exam, mitigating this risk of unblinding. Finally, radUS is not considered a diagnostic gold standard for detection of renal stones or recent passage. 15% of patients had formal ultrasound as opposed to CT scanning, mainly young women. A sensitivity analysis was performed for patients who received a CT scan and little difference in sensitivity and specificity was noted.

Conclusion

PoCUS for hydronephrosis has moderate sensitivity and specificity for renal colic limiting its utility as a diagnostic test. However, patients with hydronephrosis are more likely to develop complications, and PoCUS may be useful to help guide further imaging and consultation in conjunction with clinical course. BMI, provider experience and time between PoCUS and formal imaging do not influence the accuracy of this test.

Acknowledgements

Special thanks to Dr. Andrew Day and Dr. Xiaoqun Sun for their assistance with statistical analysis, to Jane Reid and the research coordinators for screening for patients and to Dr. Heather Mackenzie and Dr. Arianne Buchan for support.

Authors' contributions

SS, LR, EB and MS conceived and designed the study, obtained funding and supervised the conduct of the study. SS, NR and HW performed chart reviews and data entry. CS performed the formal radiology assessments. SS performed the statistical analysis and drafted the manuscript with substantial input from MS. SS takes responsibility for the paper as a whole. All authors read and approved the final manuscript.

Author details

[1] Department of Emergency Medicine, Queen's University, Kingston, ON, Canada. [2] School of Medicine, Faculty of Health Sciences, Queen's University, Kingston, ON, Canada. [3] Department of Radiology, Queen's University, Kingston, ON, Canada.

References

1. Ghani KR, Roghmann F, Sammon JD et al (2014) Emergency department visits in the United States for upper urinary tract stones: trends in hospitalization and charges. J Urol 191:90–96
2. Saigal CS, Joyce G, Timilsina AR, Urologic Diseases in America P (2005) Direct and indirect costs of nephrolithiasis in an employed population: opportunity for disease management? Kidney Int 68:1808–1814
3. Eaton SH, Cashy J, Pearl JA, Stein DM, Perry K, Nadler RB (2013) Admission rates and costs associated with emergency presentation of urolithiasis: analysis of the Nationwide Emergency Department Sample 2006–2009. J Endourol 27:1535–1538
4. Pearle MS, Calhoun EA, Curhan GC, Urologic Diseases of America P (2005) Urologic diseases in America project: urolithiasis. J Urol 173:848–857
5. Brisbane W, Bailey MR, Sorensen MD (2016) An overview of kidney stone imaging techniques. Nat Rev Urol 13:654–662
6. Wang RC (2016) Managing urolithiasis. Ann Emerg Med 67:449–454
7. Schoenfeld EM, Pekow PS, Shieh MS, Scales CD Jr, Lagu T, Lindenauer PK (2017) The diagnosis and management of patients with renal colic across a sample of US Hospitals: high CT utilization despite low rates of admission and inpatient urologic intervention. PLoS ONE 12:e0169160
8. American College of Emergency P (2009) Emergency ultrasound guidelines. Ann Emerg Med 53:550–570
9. Wong C, Teitge B, Ross M, Young P, Robertson HL, Lang E (2018) The accuracy and prognostic value of point-of-care ultrasound for nephrolithiasis in the emergency department: a systematic review and meta-analysis. Acad Emerg Med 25(6):684–698
10. Daniels B, Gross CP, Molinaro A et al (2016) STONE PLUS: evaluation of emergency department patients with suspected renal colic, using a clinical prediction tool combined with point-of-care limited ultrasonography. Ann Emerg Med 67:439–448
11. Fields JM, Fischer JI, Anderson KL, Mangili A, Panebianco NL, Dean AJ (2015) The ability of renal ultrasound and ureteral jet evaluation to predict 30-day outcomes in patients with suspected nephrolithiasis. Am J Emerg Med 33:1402–1406
12. Gaspari RJ, Horst K (2005) Emergency ultrasound and urinalysis in the evaluation of flank pain. Acad Emerg Med 12:1180–1184
13. Goertz JK, Lotterman S (2010) Can the degree of hydronephrosis on ultrasound predict kidney stone size? Am J Emerg Med 28:813–816

14. Herbst MK, Rosenberg G, Daniels B et al (2014) Effect of provider experience on clinician-performed ultrasonography for hydronephrosis in patients with suspected renal colic. Ann Emerg Med 64:269–276
15. Moak JH, Lyons MS, Lindsell CJ (2012) Bedside renal ultrasound in the evaluation of suspected ureterolithiasis. Am J Emerg Med 30:218–221
16. Riddell J, Case A, Wopat R et al (2014) Sensitivity of emergency bedside ultrasound to detect hydronephrosis in patients with computed tomography-proven stones. West J Emerg Med 15:96–100
17. Watkins S, Bowra J, Sharma P, Holdgate A, Giles A, Campbell L (2007) Validation of emergency physician ultrasound in diagnosing hydronephrosis in ureteric colic. Emerg Med Australas 19:188–195
18. Smith-Bindman R, Aubin C, Bailitz J et al (2014) Ultrasonography versus computed tomography for suspected nephrolithiasis. N Engl J Med 371:1100–1110
19. Narita T, Hatakeyama S, Koie T et al (2017) Presence of transient hydronephrosis immediately after surgery has a limited influence on renal function 1 year after ileal neobladder construction. BMC Urol 17:72
20. Bossuyt PM, Reitsma JB, Bruns DE et al (2015) STARD 2015: an updated list of essential items for reporting diagnostic accuracy studies. BMJ 351:h5527
21. Edmonds ML, Yan JW, Sedran RJ, McLeod SL, Theakston KD (2010) The utility of renal ultrasonography in the diagnosis of renal colic in emergency department patients. Cjem 12:201–206
22. Pathan SA, Mitra B, Mirza S et al (2018) Emergency physician interpretation of point-of-care ultrasound for identifying and grading of hydronephrosis in renal colic compared with consensus interpretation by emergency radiologists. Acad Emerg Med 25:1129–1137
23. Ganesan V, De S, Greene D, Torricelli FC, Monga M (2017) Accuracy of ultrasonography for renal stone detection and size determination: is it good enough for management decisions? BJU Int 119:464–469
24. Morse JW, Hill R, Greissinger WP, Patterson JW, Melanson SW, Heller MB (1999) Rapid oral hydration results in hydronephrosis as demonstrated by bedside ultrasound. Ann Emerg Med 34:134–140
25. Perry KJ, Ko P, Mariani P, Ciaccio AJ (2010) Time course resolution of hydronephrosis with spontaneous ureteral stone passage. West J Emerg Med 11:105
26. Ulusan S, Koc Z, Tokmak N (2007) Accuracy of sonography for detecting renal stone: comparison with CT. J Clin Ultrasound 35:256–261
27. Aubrey-Bassler FK, Lee SD, Barter RB, Asghari S, Cullen R, Godwin M (2013) Utility of computed tomography and derivation and validation of a score to identify an emergent outcome in 2,315 patients with suspected urinary tract stone. CJEM 15:261–269

13

Value of point-of-care ultrasonography compared with computed tomography scan in detecting potential life-threatening conditions in blunt chest trauma patients

Amirhosein Jahanshir[1], Shida Mohajer Moghari[2], Ayat Ahmadi[3], Pejman Z. Moghadam[4] and Maryam Bahreini[5*]

Abstract

Background: Ultrasonography is a suitable modality that can potentially improve patient care, saving time and lives.

Purpose: This article has evaluated the caveats and pitfalls of point-of-care ultrasonography in the diagnosis of pneumothorax, hemothorax and contusion.

Materials and methods: This prospective study was performed in 157 patients with blunt chest trauma in 3 university hospitals. Ultrasonography was performed by 2 board-certified emergency medicine specialists and an emergency medicine resident PGY-3 after passing the training process successfully.

Results: The false-negative cases were not significantly correlated with accompanying traumatic injuries. Lung ultrasonography accompanied by chest physical examination show accuracy 91.8. Point-of-care ultrasonography (PoCUS) showed sensitivity 75.0%, specificity 100%, positive-predictive value (PPV) of 100% and a negative-predictive value (NPV) of 94.9% for the diagnosis of pneumothorax. For hemothorax, bedside PoCUS had a sensitivity of 45.4%, specificity of 100%, PPV of 100% and NPV of 91.8%. PoCUS was assessed 58.1% sensitive and 100% specific for detecting lung contusion with positive-predictive value (PPV) of 100% and a negative-predictive value (NPV) of 86.3%. Performing US resulted in no false-positive cases.

Conclusions: Point-of-care ultrasonography was highly sensitive to detect pneumothorax and can be beneficial for the disposition of stable patients and to detect PTX in unstable patients before transferring to the operating room. It is also moderately appropriate for the diagnosis of hemothorax and lung contusion compared to the gold standard, CT scan. It is essential to consider the false-negative and false-positive instances of lung ultrasound in various situations to enhance management and disposition of blunt thoracic injuries.

Keywords: Chest injury, Computed tomography, Emergency, Hemothorax, Lung injury, Pneumothorax, Predictive value of tests, Ultrasonography

Introduction

Background

Thoracic injuries account for 20 to 25% of the trauma mortality which can be preventable by timely diagnosis. Despite of undesirable low sensitivity, chest X-ray (CXR) has remained one of the adjuncts for evaluation of chest trauma. Bedside ultrasonography (US) has an important

*Correspondence: bahreinimaryam@gmail.com; m-bahreini@tums.ac.ir
[5] Department of Emergency Medicine, Sina Trauma and Surgery Research Center, Sina Hospital, Tehran University of Medical Sciences, Tehran, Iran
Full list of author information is available at the end of the article

role in primary and advanced trauma life support (ATLS) due to higher sensitivity and specificity to detect of pneumothorax (PTX) and hemothorax (HTX) [1–3]. However, lung contusion, a common injury in 30–75% of blunt chest trauma, may remain undiagnosed by radiography or ultrasonography depending on the extent and intensity [4]. Besides, computed tomography (CT) scan is the standard modality for the assessment of lung parenchymal injuries. Yet it is time-consuming, expensive and there are concerns about radiation exposure and patient hemodynamic instability during transfer [1]. In this context, multiple trauma patients often undergo CT scan in trauma centers; however, the presence of clinical injuries that require emergent operative management in unstable patients such as brain lateralizing signs, necessitates the use of extended focused assessment with sonography in trauma (eFAST) bedside exam and bypassing torso CT scan. This may also remain true for the stable and selective population of patients with high risk mechanism of injury to reduce the risk of radiation. Based on the possibility of diagnosing potential life-threatening conditions in traumatic injuries by US, revising the Advanced Trauma Life Support (ATLS) guidelines have been proposed to incorporate eFAST in the work-up of high-energy trauma patients [5].

Goals of investigation

Ultrasound may be overused without sufficient applicability in some situations. As the published papers were unable to find a unified answer for this issue, we discuss pitfalls and caveats to point-of-care lung ultrasound in various traumatic chest injuries, analyze false-negative and false-positive cases and highlight the growing topic of the point-of-care ultrasound (PoCUS) despite its common diagnostic limitations. Moreover, the diagnostic accuracy of ultrasonography was estimated in the detection of pneumothorax, hemothorax and contusion simultaneously in comparison with the gold standard, CT-scan.

Materials and methods

Selection of participants

Patients with blunt chest trauma were included if they were 18 years or older with acute chest trauma defined as the isolated blunt trauma to the chest or back and also multiple trauma patients involving chest trauma. All chest trauma patients were recruited in the study including unconscious or apneic patients, or individuals with open chest injuries. All participants consented to enter the study.

Patient with old chest trauma, past history of lung fibrosis or if they were not planned or assented to CT scan (except for clinically unstable patients who underwent chest tube insertion) were excluded.

Study design and setting

This longitudinal study was performed on 157 patients with blunt chest trauma in 3 university hospitals including a level I and 2 level II trauma centers with approximately 2200–3850 trauma patients per year. Bedside chest ultrasonography was performed by 2 board-certified emergency medicine specialists, certified from the Board Committee of Emergency Medicine of the country, and an emergency medicine resident PGY-3 (SM), in the third year of the residency program. The PGY-3 emergency medicine resident required to perform 50 successful ultrasound scans in this field prior to this study. These operators were blinded to the findings brought up by chest exam and radiography and were not involved in patient management. Patients were included by convenience sampling in the operators' clinical shifts 24/7 in the emergency department.

Interventions

As a common practice, the patients underwent the standard of care according to the ATLS guideline. Standard chest physical exam was performed routinely and documented consisting of tachypnea, abrasion or laceration, emphysema, rib tenderness or crepitation, hypotension, oxygen desaturation, stridor and other factors discussed in Table 1. Then, chest US was performed prior to imaging. Trauma patients commonly underwent supine CXR although in selected stable patients with definite intact spine, upright films might have been ordered up to the clinician's judgement and patient's condition. Chest X-ray was planned except for patients who were suspected for tension pneumothorax or massive hemothorax by physical exam and bedside ultrasonography. If rush of air or 100 ml of blood was detected during tube thoracostomy, the diagnosis became confirmed. These patients might undergo CT scan for further trauma evaluation if they became clinically and vitally stable; otherwise, because of the definite diagnosis, they were included in the study without CT scan. CTs were homogeneous by the technique applied and performed using 16-slice multidetector CT scanner (Philips Brilliance, Emotion, and Ingenuity) with slice width of 3 mm. Board-certified emergency physicians, who were blinded to the study, interpreted them.

Based on the discretion of the treating physician including clinical judgement in conjunction with the NEXUS chest trauma criteria, stable patients underwent chest computed tomography within 6 h of their trauma. As standard management in our setting, the time elapsed from the chest physical exam and CXR to chest

Table 1 The diagnostic findings applied to assess traumatic chest injuries in physical exam and ultrasonography

Assessment	Definition	Simple pneumothorax	Tension pneumothorax	Hemothorax	Massive hemothorax	Pulmonary contusion
Findings of physical examination						
Inspection	Chest expansion	Nl-↓	↓	↓	↓	Nl
	Trachea	Nl	Deviated	Nl	Deviated	Nl
	Jugular vein pressure	Nl	↑	Nl	↓	Nl
Percussion	The sound of striking 2 fingers on intercostal spaces	Nl-hyperresonance	Hyperresonance	Nl-dull	Dull	Nl
Auscultation	To hear both sides comparatively and note sounds' quality	↓	Nl-dull	Nl-↓	↓	Nl-crackles
Findings of ultrasonography						
Pleural sliding	The shimmering movement of parietal pleura during inspiration	Lost in injured zone	Lost	Nl	May be Nl	Maybe falsely ↓
Seashore sign	Normal lung M-mode of sandy appearance above and parallel lines below	Lost in injured zone	Lost	Nl	May be Nl	May be Nl
Barcode/stratosphere sign	Abnormal M-mode showing multiple parallel lines	+ in injured zone	+	-	-	May be falsely +
Lung point	The interface of normal lung and pneumothorax area in B-M mode	May be +	Often -	-	-	-
Sinusoid sign	The sinusoidal movement of the collapsed lung in the pleural fluid	-	-	+	+	-
V-line	Echogenic vertebral line with posterior shadow due to the transmission of ultrasound waves through the pleural fluid	-	-	May be +	+	-
B-lines/comet tails	Vertical echogenic artifact lines from the pleura to the screen edge, if multiple, resulting from alveolo-interstitial syndrome (rocket sign)	Lost	Lost	Nl	May be Nl	↑
Peripheral parenchymal lesions	Lung hepatization with subpleural hypoechoic foci and pleural line gap	-	-	-	-	+

CT was not more than 90 min. The chest trauma injuries were confirmed either by CT scan or by performing an emergent thoracostomy [6]. In our trauma centers, CT scan is frequently used and accessible 24/7. Generally, nearly asymptomatic patients with isolated occult PTX, small amount unilateral pneumothorax, hemothorax or contusion were observed to discharge without intervention according to our ED management protocols.

PoCUS protocol

PoCUS was performed by Medison 8 (SONOACE), SonoSite Edge II and Samsung UGEO HM70A and

Table 2 The diagnostic criteria of chest X-ray, US and CT scan to determine lung injuries in our settings

Diagnostic *criteria*	PTX	HTX	Contusion
Chest X-ray	A thin dense line as the visceral pleural edge separating from the parietal pleura, the distance between the 2 pleurae is radiolucent usually accumulating in the periphery and sometimes deep lucent lateral costo-phrenic angle	In the presence of sufficient amount of blood, the involved hemithorax is hazy. If upright film is performed, the costophrenic sulcus become blunted.	Alveolar infiltration, irregular patchy consolidation that usually evolve within the first 6 h
US	Absence of lung sliding and the presence of stratosphere sign and the absence of B lines with or without "lung point"	Dependent collection above diaphragm with or without the sinusoidal movement of collapsed lung in inspiration in the B and M mode scan, the presence of V line	Three B lines in at least 2 zone scans, alveolo-interstitial syndrome (AIS), peripheral parenchymal lesions (PPL) and punctiform hyperechoic lesions without respiratory alterations
CT scan	In the pulmonary window, the existence of air in pleural space that may collapse the adjacent lung	Blood in the pleural space with Hounsfield Unit of about 45–65 in the mediastinal window	An interstitial or alveolar lung injury, usually focal and non-segmental peripheral opacification in lung parenchyma in lower lobes

PTX pneumothorax, *HTX* hemothorax, *US* ultrasonography, *CT* computed tomography

3–8 MHZ and 7–15 MHZ transducers. Each lung was scanned at least in 4 spaces for the evidence of pneumothorax, hemothorax and lung contusion by B and M modes: the probe was placed in the 2nd to 4th intercostal spaces in midclavicular and parasternal lines and the 6th or 7th intercostal space in the mid-axillary line in the supine position.

Subsequently, the low-frequency probe was positioned in the 5th to 6th right anterior to mid-axillary region and 7th to 8th left mid to posterior axillary region to find hemothorax as part of the eFAST exam [7]. Each bedside scan was performed routinely in 3–5 min.

The detailed diagnostic findings of chest traumatic injuries including simple and tension PTX, simple and massive HTX and pulmonary contusion determined by ultrasonography and physical exam are presented in Table 1. Table 2 demonstrates how we conducted our study using CXR, ultrasonography (US) and CT scan for traumatic lung injuries.

Outcomes

This study aimed to widely assess the thoracic injuries by point-of-care ultrasonography in the emergency department compared to the computed tomography findings and interpreted false-positive and negative results.

A questionnaire was designed containing demographic data such as age, gender, trauma mechanism and detailed information on physical exam, ultrasonography and CT scan to detect thoracic injuries. As different scales are available to score injury severity with various accuracies and no definitive superiority, we report injuries according to the injury severity scale (ISS) [8, 9].

Analysis

Data were analyzed by SPSS, version 22.0. Chicago, IL, USA. Sensitivity, specificity, positive-predictive value (PPV) and negative-predictive value (NPV) of different diagnostic modalities were assessed. Besides, univariate regression analysis was performed to assess single factors that are correlated with false-negative results including some related injuries or multisystem injuries. The type-I error 0.05 was considered significant and the confidence intervals (CI 95%) were reported. Sample size calculation met 80% power for 95% sensitivity. False-negative episodes were analyzed with regard to the results of physical examination, CT scan and outcome details to assess whether they were clinically significant or not. In this context, false-negative cases are categorized by findings such as occult PTX, subcutaneous emphysema, which was analyzed in these cases as a confounder to ultrasound results, and also the clinical decision for placing tube thoracostomy.

Ethical considerations

The protocol of study has been reviewed and approved by the University of Medical Sciences Institutional Review Board and the ethical committee. All procedures were in accordance with the ethical standards of the institutional and national research committee and with the 1964 Helsinki declaration and its later ethical standards. Informed consent was obtained from the conscious participants and the relatives of critically ill patients.

Results

Characteristics of study subjects

In this study, of 160 patients, 157 agents with blunt chest trauma were enrolled after obtaining informed consent, of which 134 (85.4%) were men. Three patients were excluded, 1 was underaged and 2 were not willing to undergo the study. The mean age was 38.3 (SD: 18.57) years. Motor vehicle collision ($n=42$, 26.8%) and falling ($n=43$, 27.4%) were the most common injury mechanisms. Among all patients, 94 (59.87%) cases had injury severity score 10–50 while 19 (12.10%) cases had ISS more than 50. Furthermore, 56 (35.6%) of patients had pneumothorax ($n=21$, 13.3%), hemothorax ($n=10$, 6.3%) or contusion ($n=25$, 15.9%). The Venn diagram of samples of different diagnoses by PoCUS is presented in Fig. 1.

Main results

The sensitivity, specificity, PPV, NPV and accuracy of point-of-care ultrasonography for the diagnosis of blunt pneumothorax, hemothorax and pulmonary contusion are shown in Table 3. The US results for pneumothorax was 75.0% (CI 55.1–89.0), while it was 45.4% (CI 24.4–67.8) and 58.1% (CI 42.1–73.3) for hemothorax and pulmonary contusion, respectively. Performing US resulted in no false-positive cases (specificity = 100%), but when it was combined with physical examination, 9 cases were falsely diagnosed as positive (negative false-positive rate = 9.2%). Rib fracture was present in 25 patients (15.9%). Three patients (1.9%) were intubated as a result of other traumatic injuries. None needed resuscitative or urgent thoracotomy.

Description of false-negative cases

To elucidate why US missed PTX in 7 cases, false-negative results were reviewed. Of 157 enrolled participants, 28 (17.83%) patients had pneumothorax in CT scan. Seven patients were not diagnosed by US of whom, 3 patients had concomitant subcutaneous emphysema and another 2 had occult PTX ($P=0.000$). Regarding false-negative patient outcomes, 2 (of 7 false-negative results) were discharged with follow-up, 5 patients including

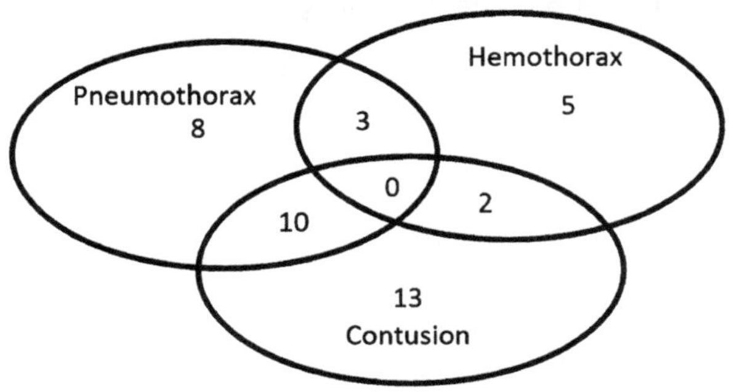

Fig. 1 The Venn diagram of the positive samples for pneumothorax, hemothorax and lung contusion detected by ultrasonography

those with subcutaneous emphysema required tube thoracotomy and 4 out of those 5 patients were suspected to have pneumothorax on physical exam. Ultrasound was not helpful to diagnose hemothorax in 12 out of 21 CT confirmed patients. Besides, CT scan confirmed lung contusion in 43 patients but 18 cases were not diagnosed by bedside ultrasonography of whom, 8 individuals had definite concomitant pneumothorax. There were too few false-negative cases to quantitatively appraise its correlated determinant factors in univariable and multivariable (logistic regression) analysis. However, occult pneumothorax and also the presence of concomitant hemothorax or lung contusion were more frequently seen among false-negative results than the state of clinical instability or the presence of multisystem injuries. Overall, 2 patients were not cooperative to undergo lung US and CT scan and were excluded. Only 3 patients acquired Glasgow Coma Scale under 9.

Furthermore, the diagnostic performance of ultrasound alone and positive physical exam in conjunction with ultrasound was assessed in comparison with CT scan and exhibited in Table 3.

There was no false-positive case in our study for traumatic lung injuries. The possible causes for false results of ultrasonography are shown in Table 4.

Discussion

The concrete indications for chest imaging have not yet been well established. There are some exclusion criteria for reducing CXR requests [10]. Here, we discussed the accuracy of chest PoCUS to delineate its uses in various settings to detect traumatic lung injuries simultaneously which is less discussed in previous studies. Furthermore, the false-negative results are discussed to ascertain the ambiguous situations when decision-making is critical to determine patient disposition in obviously stable or severely unstable patients.

Table 3 Sensitivity, specificity, PPV, NPV and the accuracy and point-of-care ultrasound in the diagnosis of blunt chest injuries

Type of injury	Diagnostic tool	Analysis	Point estimate	95% CI[a]
Pneumothorax	Sonography	Sensitivity, %	75.0	55.1–89.0
		Specificity, %	100	97.2–100
		PPV%	100	83.9–100
		NPV%	94.9	89.7–97.9
		Accuracy%	95.5	91.0–98.2
Hemothorax		Sensitivity, %	45.4	24.4–67.8
		Specificity, %	100	97.3–100
		PPV%	100	69.2–100
		NPV%	91.8	86.2–95.7
		Accuracy%	92.4	87.0–96.0
Contusion		Sensitivity, %	58.1	42.1–73.3
		Specificity, %	100	96.8–100
		PPV%	100	86.3–100
		NPV%	86.3	79.3–91.7
		Accuracy%	88.5	82.5–93.1
Pneumothorax, hemothorax and contusion	Physical exam and sonography	Sensitivity, %	91.5	81.3–97.2
		Specificity, %	90.8	83.3–95.7
		PPV	85.7	74.6–93.3
		NPV	94.7	88.0–98.3
		Accuracy	91.8	85.5–95.0

[a] Binomial exact calculation

Table 4 Possible suggested causes for false-positive and negative results of bedside ultrasonography for the diagnosis of traumatic chest injuries

Traumatic chest injury	Missed diagnoses	Causes
Pneumothorax	False positive	Achalasia
		Pleural adhesions
		Phrenic nerve palsy
		Pulmonary fibrosis
		Pulmonary atelectasis
		Cardiopulmonary arrest
		Congestive heart failure
		Right main bronchus intubation
		Subcutaneous chest emphysema
		Acute respiratory distress syndrome
		Significant concomitant lung contusion
		Bullous emphysema/pulmonary blebs
		Chronic obstructive pulmonary disease
		High positive end expiratory pressure-ventilated patients
	False negative	Lung remained in contact with the chest wall despite PTX
		Operator, machine or transducer conditions
		Cardiac movement with left lung sliding
		Subcutaneous chest emphysema
		Occult small pneumothorax
Hemothorax	False positive	Pleural effusion differential diagnoses
	False negative	Minimal amount hemothorax
		Subcutaneous emphysema
Lung contusion	False positive	Pulmonary fibrosis
		Cardiogenic pulmonary edema
		Acute respiratory distress syndrome
	False negative	Subcutaneous emphysema
		Inaccessible to ultrasound (retrosternal, paravertebral, etc.)

PTX pneumothorax

Analysis of false-negative results and other shortcomings of lung US

Pneumothorax

In this study, US sensitivity was lower though closely consistent with other studies suggesting that point-of-care ultrasonography is an acceptable modality to detect pneumothorax. Hyancinthe et al. retrospectively assessed the diagnostic accuracy of US and reported that it can detect PTX and contusion although it was not superior to CXR and chest exam [11]. Furthermore, a review article evaluated US sensitivity in blunt trauma patients and concluded that US is a sensitive screening test to assess PTX [12]. Ianniello et al. estimated the accuracy of US as the first diagnostic modality in major chest trauma patients and found a sensitivity, specificity, PPV and NPV of 77%, 99.8%, 98.5% and 97%, respectively [13]. Lichtenstein et al. showed that the absence of pleural sliding alone has the highest sensitivity (100%) and the presence of lung point provide 100% specificity to detect pneumothorax although Markota has recognized the false-positive absence of pleural sliding due to high positive end expiratory airway pressure [14, 15].

Although the presence of subcutaneous emphysema can be a clue to suspect PTX, it is known to be disruptive to lung ultrasound, scattering US signals [16]. Occult PTX, defined as a very small PTX that can only be found by CT scan, may not be clinically significant [17]. It is not thoroughly evident whether ultrasonography may miss clinically unimportant pneumothorax. However, there are some data to suggest that ultrasound does not miss clinically important PTX [18].

Several studies have discussed the pitfalls of chest sonography to discover pneumothorax. Some researchers described cases with clinically significant pneumothorax who were not diagnosed by chest ultrasonography due to the uneven distribution of pneumothorax in the pleural cavity with pulmonary adhesions to the chest wall with or without lung contusion. Moreover, "double lung point sign" as reported, may under or overestimate the PTX size by ultrasonography [4, 7, 19]. The extent of PTX was estimated by Blaivas et al. assessing the pleural sliding in several intercostal spaces and identified fair correlation with CT scan findings. They also evaluated pleural sliding by standard scan areas of "Power Doppler" to detect the fine pleural shimmering that may be difficult to detect due to resolution limitations [20, 21]. Some suggested differential diagnoses of dyspnea account for the most false-positive pneumothoraces in intensive care units including lung cancer, significant pulmonary infiltration or contusion, pleural or pulmonary adhesions and thoracic surgery, and in other settings such as achalasia [7, 22], many of which are grouped in Table 4.

Hemothorax

US has provided high specificity despite lower sensitivity in our study compared with other studies in the assessment of hemothorax that can be due to small insignificant amounts of HTX. In this context, Hyacinthe et al. reported that missed hemothoraces can be due to minimal amounts of blood or those located posteriorly. They mentioned two missed cases suffering from concomitant subcutaneous emphysema and thus reported a modest accuracy for US to assess hemothorax, nearly similar to CXR [11]. Chest X-ray has been known to have low sensitivity in clinically significant injuries [23]. Besides, hemothorax can be falsely recognized in cases of pleural effusion of other causes. However, ultrasonography has shown appropriate sensitivity (92%) and specificity (100%) in the evaluation of hemothorax in trauma patients by Brooks et al. [24]. Also, Atkinson showed that US has sensitivity 92–100% and specificity 100% to detect hemothorax in intensive care settings [25]. Table 4 shows the possible suggested causes of false US results.

Pulmonary contusion

The sensitivity of PoCUS was rather low in our study that may be caused by the inclusion of other lung injuries simultaneously. Leblanc D et al. showed that PoCUS can predict acute respiratory distress syndrome by detecting lung contusion in the first 72 h after trauma (receiving operator characteristic curve – area under the curve = 0.78 [95% CI 0.64–0.92]). The extent of contusion diagnosed by US had fair correlation with the corresponding clinical findings [26]. Trying to find various signs of lung contusion can improve the US diagnostic sensitivity. Some researchers reported high accuracy of the US in detecting alveolo-interstitial syndrome (AIS) (95.4%), although the diagnostic accuracy was estimated to be 65.9% in peripheral parenchymal lesions (PPL) [27]. Moreover, Helmy et al. assessed lung contusion by US to have 97.5% sensitivity, 90% specificity, PPV 97.5% and NPV 90% detecting AIS and PPL images [4]. Lung contusion may be falsely diagnosed in patients with acute respiratory distress syndrome (ARDS) and cardiogenic pulmonary edema by ultrasonography. In other words, ultrasonography may not be decisive to definitely distinguish pulmonary contusion and ARDS as contusion may be a predisposing factor and a severity determinant for acute respiratory distress syndrome and further complications [28–31]. The mechanism, severity and the time elapsed from the injury may be clinically helpful [32]. Further studies can address this issue as the current evidence require larger sample sizes [33]. Contusion can be falsely interpreted in the presence of a large PTX due to the presence of a collapsed lung. In addition, the falsely missed lung injuries did not correlate with concomitant systemic injuries in poly-trauma patients if it serves as a distracting factor for the US operator and this issue was consistent with our findings. Also, subcutaneous emphysema and injury in zones not accessible by US may lead to underdiagnose contusion [11]. Soldati et al. reported two patients with documented pulmonary fibrosis among the missed lung contusions in ultrasonography [27].

Overall, considering several criteria for the detection of pneumothorax increase the accuracy of ultrasonography rather than each, including pleural sliding, seashore sign, and normal A and B lines. It seems that the false-negative results of ultrasonography for the diagnosis of traumatic pneumothorax can be compensated by the findings of positive physical examination especially chest wall pain, decreased lung sounds and subcutaneous emphysema. Nonetheless, ultrasonography alone did not show convincing results regarding the false-negative cases of hemothorax and contusion. The possible cause may be the small amounts of blood or pulmonary contusion which can be well-defined in CT scan. Of note, the clinical significance of the detection of small PTX, HTX or contusion is questionable. The beneficial information added by PoCUS to clinical findings serves as a valuable diagnostic guide in emergency situations. In hemodynamically unstable patients not responding to resuscitation, PoCUS can be a useful guide to discover the source of instability. Non-massive hemothorax and contusion can be evaluated and treated after life-threatening conditions are obviated even if missed in the very first critical patient presentation. Additionally, in perfectly stable patients for whom CT scan may be safely deferred, it is beneficial to apply PoCUS as a screening tool to discharge patients safely without the need for CT scan.

Recommendations and limitations

The accuracy of bedside ultrasonography may vary between intercostal spaces in the diagnosis of pneumothorax. Clinically significant lung injuries were difficult to follow as the subgroup analysis did not acquire sufficient sample size to reach desirable power. Occasionally, the small size of positive samples cause wide confidence intervals that can be further studied with larger sample sizes. This stratification of results based on the ISS, intubated patients, and decreased level of consciousness were not adequately powered and reliable.

The extent of lung contusion can be further studied regarding the hospital observation and long-term outcomes. Furthermore, the lung injuries leading to admission usually coincide with other traumatic injuries that also deserve close monitoring, hospital admissions, surgery or intubation and the differentiation between the exact leading causes was often difficult. In addition, there is a concern about a simple pneumothorax to expand and evolve into tension pneumothorax due to positive pressure ventilation and this issue can be addressed comparing US and CT scan in the future.

Conclusion

The diagnostic performance of point-of-care ultrasonography was sensitive for blunt pneumothorax and can be beneficial for making disposition of stable patients and helpful in detecting PTX in unstable patients. POCUS was a moderately appropriate modality for diagnosing hemothorax and lung contusion compared to the gold standard, CT scan. Physical exam and ultrasonography augment the diagnostic accuracy of detecting traumatic lung injuries. Pitfalls and caveats should be considered to interpret lung ultrasound in specific situations regarding false-negative and false-positive instances.

Abbreviations

PGY-3: Post-graduate year-3; PoCUS: Point-of-care ultrasonography; PPV: Positive-predictive value; NPV: Negative-predictive value; CI: Confidence interval; ATLS: Advanced trauma life support; PTX: Pneumothorax; HTX: Hemothorax; CT: Computed tomography; CXR: Chest X-ray; eFAST: Extended focused assessment with sonography in trauma; AIS: Alveolo-interstitial syndrome; PPL: Peripheral parenchymal lesions; US: Ultrasonography; ARDS: Acute respiratory distress syndrome.

Acknowledgements

None.

Authors' contributions

Concept and design: MB, SM, AJ, Data collection: SM, MB, AJ, Writing the article: MB, SM, AJ, AH, PZ, Critical revision of the article: MB, SM, AJ, AH, PZ. All authors read and approved the final manuscript.

Author details

[1] Emergency Department, Shariati Hospital, Tehran University of Medical Sciences, Tehran, Iran. [2] Tehran University of Medical Sciences, Tehran, Iran. [3] Knowledge Utilization Research Center, Tehran University of Medical Sciences, Tehran, Iran. [4] Trust ST1/2 in Emergency Medicine, Mid Essex NHS Trust Broomfield Hospital, Chelmsford, Essex, UK. [5] Department of Emergency Medicine, Sina Trauma and Surgery Research Center, Sina Hospital, Tehran University of Medical Sciences, Tehran, Iran.

References

1. Kline JP, Dionisio D, Sullivan K, Early T, Wolf J, Kline D (2013) Detection of pneumothorax with ultrasound. AANA J. 81:265–271
2. Broderick SR (2013) Hemothorax: etiology, diagnosis, and management. Thorac Surg Clin. 23(89–96):6–7
3. Ludwig C, Koryllos A (2017) Management of chest trauma. J Thorac Dis. 9:S172
4. Helmy S, Beshay B, Abdel Hady M, Mansour A (2015) Role of chest ultrasonography in the diagnosis of lung contusion. Egypt J Chest Diseases and Tuberc. 64:469–475
5. Ianniello S, Piccolo CL, Trinci M, Ajmone Cat CA, Miele V (2019) Extended-FAST plus MDCT in pneumothorax diagnosis of major trauma: time to revisit ATLS imaging approach? J Ultrasound 22:461–469
6. Rodriguez RM, Anglin D, Langdorf MI et al (2013) NEXUS chest: validation of a decision instrument for selective chest imaging in blunt trauma. JAMA Surg. 148:940–946
7. Kaya S, Cevik AA, Acar N, Doner E, Sivrikoz C, Ozkan R (2015) A study on the evaluation of pneumothorax by imaging methods in patients presenting to the emergency department for blunt thoracic trauma. Ulusal travma ve acil cerrahi dergisi 21:366–372
8. Baker SP, Oneill B, Haddon WJ, Long WB (1974) The injury severity score: a method for describing patients with multiple injuries and evaluating emergency care. J Trauma Acute Care Surg. 14:187–196
9. Tohira H, Jacobs I, Mountain D, Gibson N, Yeo A (2012) Systematic review of predictive performance of injury severity scoring tools. Scand J Trauma Resusc Emerg Med. 20:63
10. Forouzanfar MM, Safari S, Niazazari M et al (2014) Clinical decision rule to prevent unnecessary chest X-ray in patients with blunt multiple traumas. Emerg Med Australas. 26:561–566
11. Hyacinthe AC, Broux C, Francony G et al (2012) Diagnostic accuracy of ultrasonography in the acute assessment of common thoracic lesions after trauma. Chest 141:1177–1183
12. Wilkerson RG, Stone MB (2010) Sensitivity of bedside ultrasound and supine anteroposterior chest radiographs for the identification of pneumothorax after blunt trauma. Acad Emerg Med 17:11–17
13. Ianniello S, Di Giacomo V, Sessa B, Miele V (2014) First-line sonographic diagnosis of pneumothorax in major trauma: accuracy of e-FAST and comparison with multidetector computed tomography. Radiol Med (Torino) 119:674–680
14. Markota A, Golub J, Stozer A et al (2016) Absence of lung sliding is not a reliable sign of pneumothorax in patients with high positive end-expiratory pressure. Am J Emerg Med 34:2034–2036
15. Lichtenstein DA, Meziere G, Lascols N et al (2005) Ultrasound diagnosis of occult pneumothorax. Crit Care Med 33:1231–1238
16. Kubodera T, Adachi YU, Hatano T, Ejima T, Numaguchi A, Matsuda N (2013) Subcutaneous emphysema and ultrasound sonography. J Intensive care. 1:8
17. Yadav K, Jalili M, Zehtabchi S (2010) Management of traumatic occult pneumothorax. Resuscitation. 81:1063–1068
18. Helland G, Gaspari R, Licciardo S et al (2016) Comparison of four views to single-view ultrasound protocols to identify clinically significant pneumothorax. Acad Emerg Med 23:1170–1175
19. Aspler A, Stone MB (2014) Pitfalls in the ultrasound diagnosis of pneumothorax: the authors respond. Am J Emerg Med 32:1127
20. Blaivas M, Lyon M, Duggal S (2005) A prospective comparison of supine chest radiography and bedside ultrasound for the diagnosis of traumatic pneumothorax. Acad Emerg Med 12:844–849
21. Cunningham J, Kirkpatrick AW, Nicolaou S et al (2002) Enhanced recognition of "lung sliding" with power color Doppler imaging in the diagnosis of pneumothorax. J Trauma 52:769–771
22. Jahanshir AH, Seyed Hosseini J, Bahreini M (2014) Misinterpretation of achalasia as a pneumothorax in transthoracic ultrasonography. J Emerg Med Case Rep. 5:2149–9934
23. Ojaghi Haghighi SH, Adimi I, Shams Vahdati S, Sarkhoshi Khiavi R (2014) Ultrasonographic diagnosis of suspected hemopneumothorax in trauma patients. Trauma Mon. 19:e17498
24. Brooks A, Davies B, Smethhurst M, Connolly J (2004) Emergency ultrasound in the acute assessment of haemothorax. Emerg Med J. 21:44–46
25. Atkinson P, Milne J, Loubani O, Verheul G (2012) The V-line: a sonographic aid for the confirmation of pleural fluid. Crit Ultrasound J. 4:19

26. Leblanc D, Bouvet C, Degiovanni F et al (2014) Early lung ultrasonography predicts the occurrence of acute respiratory distress syndrome in blunt trauma patients. Intensive Care Med 40:1468–1474
27. Soldati G, Testa A, Silva FR, Carbone L, Portale G, Silveri NG (2006) Chest ultrasonography in lung contusion. Chest 130:533–538
28. Watkins TR, Nathens AB, Cooke CR et al (2012) Acute respiratory distress syndrome after trauma: development and validation of a predictive model. Crit Care Med 40:2295–2303
29. Miller PR, Croce MA, Bee TK et al (2001) ARDS after pulmonary contusion: accurate measurement of contusion volume identifies high-risk patients. J Trauma 51:223–228
30. Bakowitz M, Bruns B, McCunn M (2012) Acute lung injury and the acute respiratory distress syndrome in the injured patient. Scand J Trauma Resus Emerg Med. 20:54
31. Haider T, Halat G, Heinz T, Hajdu S, Negrin LL (2017) Thoracic trauma and acute respiratory distress syndrome in polytraumatized patients: a retrospective analysis. Minerva Anestesiol 83:1026–1033
32. Copetti R, Soldati G, Copetti P (2008) Chest sonography: a useful tool to differentiate acute cardiogenic pulmonary edema from acute respiratory distress syndrome. Cardiovasc Ultrasound. 6:16
33. Daabis R, Banawan L, Rabea A, Elnakedy A, Sadek A (2014) Relevance of chest sonography in the diagnosis of acute respiratory failure: comparison with current diagnostic tools in intensive care units. Egypt J Chest Dis Tuberc. 63:979–985

14

Point-of-care lung ultrasound imaging in pediatric COVID-19

Eliana P. C. Giorno[1*], Milena De Paulis[2,3], Yoshino T. Sameshima[4], Kirstin Weerdenburg[5,6], Paulo Savoia[4,7], Danilo Y. Nanbu[1,3], Thomaz B. Couto[1], Fernanda V. M. Sa[1,3], Sylvia C. L. Farhat[1], Werther B. Carvalho[8], Marcela Preto-Zamperlini[1] and Claudio Schvartsman[1]

Abstract

Background: There has been limited data regarding the usefulness of lung ultrasound (US) in children with COVID-19.

Objective: To describe lung US imaging findings and aeration score of 34 children with COVID-19.

Methods: This study included 0–16-year-old patients with confirmed COVID-19, who were admitted between April 19 and June 18, 2020 in two hospitals in the city of Sao Paulo, Brazil. Lung US was performed as part of the routine evaluation by a skilled Pediatric Emergency physician. Clinical and laboratory data were collected and severity classifications were done according to an available clinical definition. The lung US findings were described for each lung field and a validated ultrasound lung aeration score was calculated. Data obtained was correlated with clinical information and other imaging modalities available for each case.

Results: Thirty-four confirmed COVID-19 patients had a lung US performed during this period. Eighteen (18/34) had abnormalities on the lung US, but eight of them (8/18) had a normal chest radiograph. Ultrasound lung aeration score medians for severe/critical, moderate, and mild disease were 17.5 (2–30), 4 (range 0–14), 0 (range 0–15), respectively ($p = 0.001$). Twelve patients (12/34) also had a chest computed tomography (CT) performed; both the findings and topography of lung compromise on the CT were consistent with the information obtained by lung US.

Conclusion: Point-of-care lung US may have a key role in assessing lung injury in children with COVID-19.

Keywords: COVID-19, Lung ultrasound, Point-of-care, Children

Introduction

Since its initial identification in December 2019, the coronavirus disease 2019 (COVID-19) has infected millions of people and has led to thousands of deaths worldwide as of July 2020 [1]. Although reports from adults suggest that this disease can have a more severe course in as many as 18.5% of infected people, in children it seems to be milder with an estimated incidence of severe cases of 4–6% and a lower case-fatality ratio reported [1–3]. Previous studies regarding the clinical aspects of COVID-19 in children described symptoms that followed a similar pattern as in adults [3], but recent reports have identified an emerging novel spectrum of the disease in children, which includes a multisystem inflammatory condition with overlapping features of toxic shock syndrome [4]. Up to now, the absolute number of those cases with prominent cardiovascular compromise is still low and respiratory symptoms remains the main reason for Pediatric Intensive Care Unit (PICU) admissions for COVID-19 [5].

Efforts have been made to create guidelines for the diagnosis, treatment, and prevention of COVID-19 in children [6, 7]. Of particular concern is which imaging

*Correspondence: eliana.giorno@gmail.com
[1] Emergency Department, Instituto da Criança da FMUSP, University of Sao Paulo, Av. Dr. Enéas Carvalho de Aguiar, 647, Cerqueira César, Sao Paulo, SP CEP-05403.000, Brazil
Full list of author information is available at the end of the article

modality is most suitable to assess the extension of lung involvement. Historically, chest radiograph has been the imaging modality of choice for most lower respiratory illnesses in children, but data from adult studies have shown that for COVID-19 it is of limited value and is not recommended as the first choice for imaging modalities [8]. Often, only the severe cases show abnormalities on chest radiographs [6]. In earlier stages of the infection, it frequently fails to show the typical features of COVID-19 that are found with chest computed tomography (CT) [9, 10].

Chest CT is undoubtedly the best imaging modality to accurately assess lung involvement in most respiratory illnesses including COVID-19, but the cost and possible harmful effects that radiation can have on a growing child's body must not be ignored, as even low-dose ionizing radiations may increase cancer risk in exposed children [11].

Lung ultrasound (US) is an ionizing radiation-free imaging modality that promptly provides bedside diagnosis of many pulmonary conditions in the emergency department. It has been reported to be highly accurate and reliable in diagnosing pneumonia, pleural effusion, and pneumothorax [12–14]. In patients who are mechanically ventilated, lung US enables clinicians to monitor lung aeration and its variations. It has been found that different US patterns correspond to different degrees of aeration loss, which led to the creation of a score that was subsequently validated to quantify lung aeration as a whole or in a given area of interest [15]. Compared to chest CT as the gold standard, the aforementioned lung US score has been useful in monitoring aeration in the settings of Acute Respiratory Distress Syndrome (ARDS) and Ventilator-Associated Pneumonia [16, 17].

Given the already widely acknowledged usefulness of lung US to detect several lung pathologies in acutely ill patients and its ability to estimate lung aeration, we decided to incorporate this imaging modality into our Pediatric Emergency Department (PED) observation unit as part of the routine evaluation of children admitted with confirmed COVID-19. In this study, we describe the lung US findings in these patients with COVID-19 and correlate it with clinical severity.

Methods

Design, setting and participants

This study included 0–16-year-old patients with laboratory-confirmed COVID-19 infection, who were admitted to two academic hospitals in the city of Sao Paulo, Brazil, between April 19 and June 18, 2020. The participating hospitals included one secondary care center and one tertiary care center, both from the University of Sao Paulo. The latter participating hospital has become a reference for the management of moderate and severe cases of COVID-19 in the state of Sao Paulo.

A confirmed case of COVID-19 was defined by a positive result on the RT-PCR assay of a specimen collected from a nasopharyngeal swab or a positive IgG and IgM antibodies specific for SARS-Cov-2, titled using the viral nucleoprotein as the antigen in an ELISA test in-house.

Point-of-care lung US is part of the routine evaluation carried out for children with respiratory illnesses in the PED of these institutions and is present on the evaluation flowchart of COVID-19 children as an option for an imaging assessment. When a patient had confirmed COVID-19, lung US was performed regardless of the symptoms reported. Patients with chronic lung disease or lung metastasis who had undergone a lung US were not included in this study. Patients with other chronic diseases or cancer without lung metastasis were not excluded.

We collected data on age, sex, clinical symptoms, and signs at presentation, coexisting or chronic conditions, laboratory and radiologic results, and the support needed during hospital admission. Patients were classified as mild, moderate, severe, or critical according to a clinical definition suggested by Qiu et al. [18] Laboratory and other imaging tests that were also performed, including chest radiograph and chest CT were requested based on each institution's guidelines and at the discretion of the treating physician.

Point-of-care lung ultrasound. It was performed by one of the five trained Pediatric Emergency (PEM) Physicians with more than 100 lung scans performed, using B-mode imaging, basic preset, adjusting depth, and 2D-gain according to each patient biotype. A high-frequency linear transducer (15 MHz) was used and the technique was similar to that described by Copetti and Catarossi [19] in which all intercostal spaces of the upper and lower parts of the anterior, lateral, and posterior regions of the left and right chest are examined, making a total of 12 regions. To describe the findings and to calculate the lung US aeration score, the worst US finding was considered in each examined region. To evaluate interobserver reproducibility, images of 25 patients enrolled were reviewed and scored by a different PEM of the team, who was blinded to the clinical information.

Four validated US patterns were defined and a score given for each: [16, 17] (1) normal aeration: presence of lung sliding and artifactual horizontal A-lines (0 points); (2) loss of lung aeration resulting from the scattered foci of bronchopneumonia or interstitial syndrome: presence of multiple well-defined vertical B-lines extending from the pleural line or a small subpleural consolidation (1 point); (3) loss of lung aeration resulting from alveolar-interstitial edema that corresponds to the CT imaging entity of the ground-glass: multiple confluent vertical B-lines extending from the pleural line or a small subpleural consolidation (2 points); (4) lung consolidation characterizing extensive bronchopneumonia: presence of a tissue structure containing hyperechoic punctiform images representative of air bronchograms (3 points). A global lung US aeration score ranging from 0 to 36 was obtained by summing the individual scores of all the regions.

All medical investigation procedures described were conducted as part of the standard clinical care. This research was part of a longitudinal study approved by the local ethics board.

Statistical analysis

The baseline patient characteristics were expressed as absolute and relative frequencies for qualitative variables and as median, minimum, maximum, mean and standard deviation for quantitative variables. The non-parametric Kruskal–Wallis *H*-test was applied to compare the lung US scores in relation to severity classification. In addition, we performed a post hoc analysis using the Bonferroni multiple comparison procedure. Interobserver agreements in lung aeration score determined for each region of interest were assessed using the kappa coefficient test. The significance level was fixed at 5% for all the tests. Statistical analyses were performed using IBM SPSS Statistics version 23.0 (IBM Corp., Armonk, NY, USA) and R software version 3.5 (R Foundation for Statistical Computing, Vienna, Austria).

Results

Clinical and laboratory characteristics of the patients

From April 19 to June 18, 2020, 34 admitted patients with confirmed COVID-19 had a lung US performed and were included in the study. During this period, a total of 51 pediatric patients with COVID-19 diagnosis were admitted. Lung US was performed depending on the availability of a skilled PEM physician in the PED observation unit or PICU. Of these 34 patients that were scanned, 33 had a positive RT-PCR assay and one had positive serology in a context of clinical suspicion. A summary of the clinical features is detailed in Table 1. The mean duration of symptoms in days before lung US was performed was 3.74 ± 1.76 and median 3 (range 1–8). The most common symptom was fever, followed by cough and shortness of breath. Five patients had critical disease (15%) and required respiratory and hemodynamic support. Three were classified as severe (9%), eight (23%) as moderate, and the remaining presented with mild disease (53%) but were admitted due to underlying chronic conditions or their young age.

The critical/severe group was composed of eight children, all of them with prominent respiratory disease. Seven out of these eight patients had echocardiography performed by a cardiologist or a focused cardiac exam performed by an intensive care physician. Systolic dysfunction was initially found in only two patients who also had consolidations on lung US and CT. The remaining five had a normal biventricular systolic function at the time of lung US, but three of them later developed shock probably due to worsening disease and elevated pressures on mechanical ventilation. Three critical patients have died. One due to cardiac failure and two due to ARDS.

Baseline medical conditions were common in our population and were present in 18 patients (53%); eight of them with cancer (8/18—44%), the remaining patients had chronic liver, kidney or neurologic/genetic disease. D-Dimer, a severity marker, was collected in 20/34 (59%) patients with a median of 2250.5 (190–54,153); 17 of them (17/20—85%) had elevated values, although symptoms were mild in seven out of these 17 (41%).

Imaging findings

Lung US abnormalities were found in 18 (53%) patients and these findings are described in Table 2. Of the 18 patients with lung US abnormalities, eight had severe/critical disease (44%), five had moderate disease (28%) and five (28%) had mild disease. All the patients with lung US abnormalities but who had a mild disease were previously healthy infants under 6 months of age (mean 1.24 ± 0.89), with fever and mild respiratory symptoms. Three of them were also tested for other 17 viruses, with negative results. Their median lung US aeration score was 12 (3–15).

Seventeen (17/18—94%) patients had confluent vertical B-lines on at least one posterior region; this pattern was found bilaterally in the posterior lung fields in 9/18 (50%) patients. Six out of 18 (33%) patients also had lung consolidations > 0.5 cm. Each patient's lung US aeration scores are depicted in Table 2. Mean lung US scores for severe/critical, moderate and mild cases were 16.75 ± 8.16, 5.25 ± 5.55 and 2.78 ± 5.36, respectively. When multiple comparisons were made, only mild versus severe/critical met statistical significance ($p < 0.0001$). Interobserver agreement was good, as attested by kappa coefficient of 0.71 ($p < 0.001$).

Chest radiograph was obtained in 25/34 patients (73%); only six with severe/critical disease and one with moderate disease showed pulmonary opacities; the remaining 18 were declared to be normal by the treating physician. Eight patients with lung abnormalities on lung US had a normal chest radiograph, but no patients with normal lung US had abnormalities on the chest radiograph.

Table 1 Summary of the clinical features of the patients

Variables studied	Clinical classification			
	Mild (*n*:18)	**Moderate (*n*:8)**	**Severe/critical (*n*:8)**	**Total (*n*:34)**
Epidemiological data				
Age, months Median (range)	23 (0.46–192)	4 (1–132)	29 (0.3–132.16)	13 (0,3–192)
Male sex *n* (%)	14 (78)	4 (50)	3 (37)	21 (62)
Chronic medical condition *n* (%)	9 (50)	6 (75)	3 (37)	18 (53)
Symptoms *n* (%)				
Fever	18 (100)	7 (87)	7 (87)	32 (94)
Rhinorrhea	5 (27)	4 (50)	0	9 (26)
Cough	5 (27)	5 (62)	7 (87)	17 (50)
Dyspnea	0	8 (100)	7 (87)	15 (44)
Nausea/vomiting	2 (11)	0	2 (25)	4 (12)
Respiratory failure	0	0	7 (87)	7 (20)
Shock	0	0	5 (62)	5 (15)
Hypoxemia	0	0	8 (100)	8 (23)
Early cardiac failure[a]	0	0	2 (25)	2 (6)
Pulmonary edema	0	0	1(12)	1 (3)
Laboratorial data				
D-Dimer (ng/mL) Median (range)	1251 (306–5809)	1990 (190–4127)	18,536 (1932–54,153)	2250 (190–54,153)
C-Reactive Protein (mg/L) Median (range)	5.4 (0.3–130)	3 (0.5–114)	185.5 (0.3–447)	20 (0.3–447)
Intensive care support *n* (%)				
Mechanical ventilation	0	0	5 (62)	5 (15)
Vasoactive drug	0	0	5 (62)	5 (15)
Imaging data *n* (%)				
Chest RX performed	12(66)	6 (75)	7 (87)	25 (73)
Chest RX abnormality	0	1/6 (16)	6/7(85)	7/25 (28)
Chest CT performed	3 (16)	3 (37)	6 (75)	12 (35)
Chest CT abnormality	1/3 (33)	3/3 (100)	6/6 (100)	10/12 (83)
Lung US score[b] Median (range)	0 (0–15)	4 (0–14)	17 (2–30)	2,5 (0–30)

[a] Present early after hospital admission, at the time lung US was performed

[b] *p* value < 0.001

Chest CT was performed in 12 patients (12/34—35%). Ten had abnormalities and two were normal. The most common feature was bilateral ground-glass opacities. After being carefully reviewed by two experienced radiologists, both findings and topography of the abnormalities on lung US were found to be similar to those of CT. More details on the CT findings and the corresponding lung US findings are described in Table 2. The time that elapsed from lung US and chest CT was less than 24 h for eight patients and more than 24 h for four patients; one of these four patients was unstable and could not be transported to the radiology suite earlier.

Figures 1, 2 and 3 and Additional file 1: Figure S1) show images from four cases in which lung US had provided information on lung injury due to COVID-19.

Discussion

Since the first reports on COVID-19 pneumonia, emphasis has been given to the role and impact of thoracic imaging for accurate assessment of lung compromise and timely detection of complications. Chest CT has gained an important role in this setting, because chest radiograph is of limited value for COVID-19 diagnosis, with a reported sensitivity of only 69% [95% CI 56–80%] [20].

Table 2 Summary of lung the US findings, lung US aeration score, and CT findings

Patient	Severity	Lung US Day[a]	Lung US main findings	Lung US score	CT Day[a]	CT finding
1	Mild	Day 3	Multiple well-defined B-lines in all the regions bilaterally; Confluent B-lines in the anterior and lateral bases and posterior upper right lobe; confluent B-lines on the lateral left base with pleural disruption	15		–
2	Mild	Day 3	Normal	0		–
3	Critical	Day 5	Consolidations > 0.5 cm in the anterior, lateral and posterior right lung, superior and inferior; Multiple confluent B-lines in the anterior base, lateral and posterior left lung with consolidation .0,5 cm in the posterior left base; Bilateral pleural effusion	30	Day 15	Foci of consolidation sometimes rounded, associated with multifocal ground-glass opacities seen bilaterally predominantly of peripheral distribution Small pleural effusion
4	Moderate	Day 5	Posterior right upper lobe subpleural consolidation < 0.5 cm with confluent B-lines	4	Day 4	Ground-glass opacity on the posterior right upper lobe
5	Mild	Day 3	Normal	0		–
6	Moderate	Day 2	Normal	0		–
7	Mild	Day 4	Normal	0		–
8	Mild	Day 4	Multiple well-defined B-lines bilaterally. Confluent B-lines in posterior left lung with pleural disruption and subpleural consolidations < 0.5 cm	12	Day 6	Multiple lung opacities and scarce foci of consolidation bilaterally, predominantly of peripheral distribution and in the left lower lobe
9	Critical	Day 7	Confluent B-lines on the lateral lung field bilaterally Consolidations > 0.5 cm of the posterior lung field bilaterally Bilateral pleural effusion	20	Day 7	Multiples ground-glass opacities, with interlobular septum thickening and multiple areas of consolidation, predominantly of peripheral distribution and in the posterior and inferior lung fields bilaterally Bilateral pleural effusion
10	Mild	Day 2	Normal	0		–
11	Mild	Day 2	Normal	0		–
12	Mild	Day 2	Normal	0	Day 3	Normal
13	Critical	Day 6	Scarce multiple well-defined B-lines in the anterior and lateral right lung; confluent B-lines and subpleural consolidation in the posterior right lung. Confluent B-lines in the posterior left lung	12	Day 7	Consolidation and centrilobular opacities with ground-glass attenuation in the upper and lower lobe of the right lung. Parenquimatous band in the left lower lobe
14	Moderate	Day 2	Confluent B-lines in the posterior bases bilaterally, with < 0.5 cm subpleural consolidation	4		–
15	Mild	Day 4	Multiple well-defined B-lines in the right posterior upper lobe; Confluent B-lines in the posterior right lower lobe	3		–
16	Mild	Day 4	Multiple well-defined B-lines on the right lung and anterior left lung; Confluent B-lines on the lateral left base and posterior left lung	15		–
17	Mild	Day 3	Normal	0		–
18	Mild	Day 3	Multiple well-defined B-lines on the anterior bases bilaterally; Consolidation > 0.5 cm in the left upper posterior lung	5		–
19	Moderate	Day 8	Multiple well-defined B-lines in the right lung Confluent B-lines and consolidation > 0.5 cm in the posterior left base	8	Day 14	Parenquimatous band in the upper lobes and inferior left lobe, with a small consolidation on the left base
20	Mild	Day 4	Normal	0	Day 5	Normal

Table 2 (continued)

Patient	Severity	Lung US Day[a]	Lung US main findings	Lung US score	CT Day[a]	CT finding
21	Mild	Day 1	Normal	0		–
22	Moderate	Day 2	Confluent B-lines and <0.5 cm subpleural consolidations in the right posterior upper and lower lung. Multiple well-defined B-lines and pleural disruption on the left lung, confluent B-lines on left lung base	14	Day 3	Ground-glass opacities with consolidation and atelectasis bilaterally, more prominent in the right posterior upper and lower lung
23	Mild	Day 2	Normal	0		–
24	Mild	Day 7	Normal	0		–
25	Critical	Day 3	Multiple well-defined B-lines in the lateral and posterior right lung; confluent B-lines on anterior upper right lung; Multiple well-defined B-lines on the left lung with consolidations >0.5 cm in the lateral and posterior upper left lobe	15		–
26	Moderate	Day 3	Multiple well-defined B-lines in all the lung fields bilaterally	12		–
27	Mild	Day 2	Normal	0		–
28	Moderate	Day 5	Normal	0		
29	Severe	Day 7	Multiple well-defined B-lines in the anterior lung fields bilaterally. Confluent B-lines on posterior lung fields bilaterally and lateral right base; <0.5 cm subpleural consolidations in the posterior right lung	14	Day 9	Ground-glass opacities bilaterally; few small consolidations on the right lung, upper and inferior lobes
30	Severe	Day 5	Confluent B-lines in the posterior upper right lobe	2		
31	Mild	Day 4	Normal	0		
32	Moderate	Day 3	Normal	0		
33	Critical	Day 2	Multifocal confluent B-lines and consolidations >0.5 cm on posterior and lateral lung fields bilaterally	20	Day 3	Multiple ground-glass opacities and scattered foci of consolidations, predominantly of peripheral distribution in the posterior lung fields bilaterally
34	Severe	Day 5	Confluent B-lines and <0.5 cm consolidations on anterior lateral and posterior lung fields bilaterally	21	Day 6	Multiples ground-glass opacities, with interlobular septum thickening and multiple areas of consolidation, predominantly of peripheral distribution

[a] Time elapsed, since the symptoms began

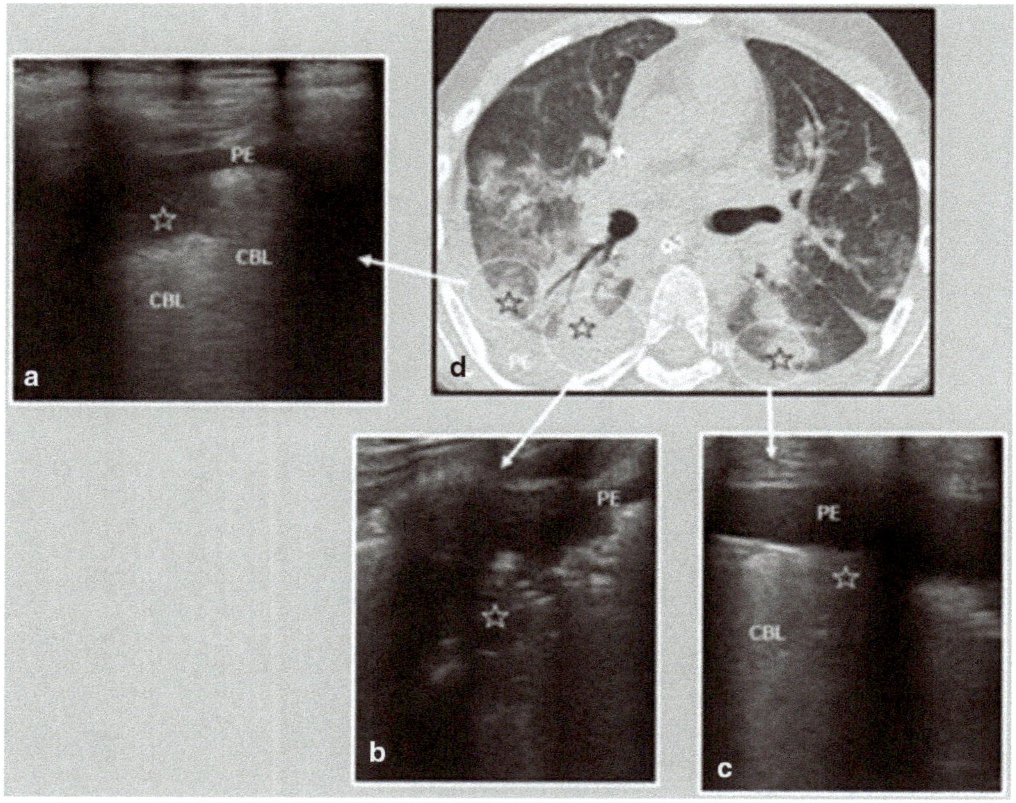

Fig. 1 Eleven-year-old male with respiratory failure and shock. Lung US (**a–c**) was performed on the 5th day after symptom onset and chest CT (**d**) on the 15th day. There was a pleural effusion (PE in **a–d**) and subpleural consolidations (stars in **a–d**). Confluent B-lines (CBL in **a** and **c**) were also present in the lung US, corresponding to the chest CT ground-glass pattern

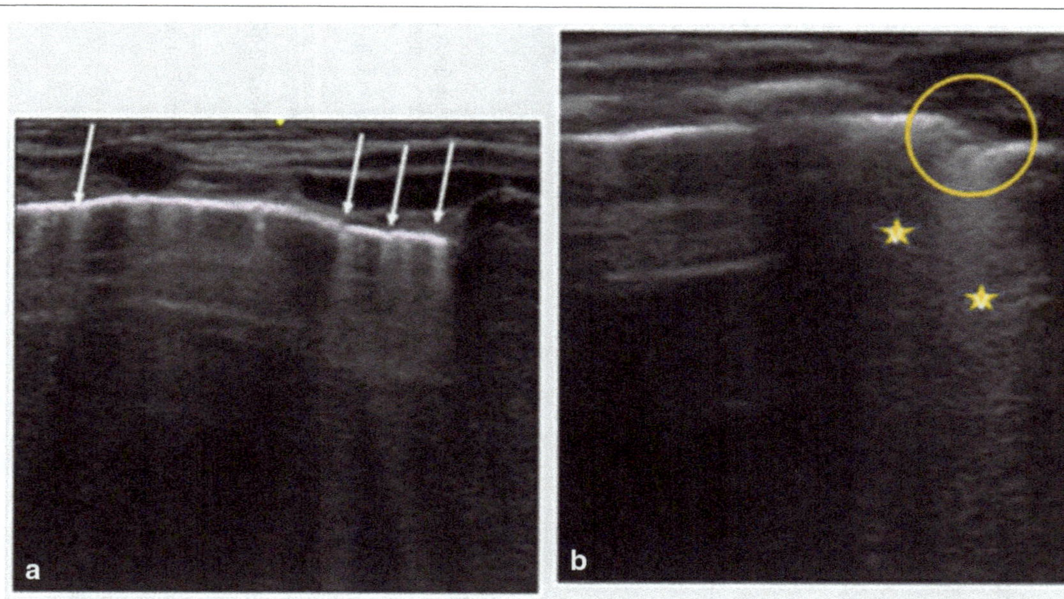

Fig. 2 Two-week-old male full-term newborn with fever and mild respiratory symptoms. Lung US showed multiple vertical B-lines on all the lung fields bilaterally (arrows in **a**). Coalescent B-lines could be seen on the posterior and inferior lung fields (stars in **b**), as well as an irregularity of the pleural line and a tiny subpleural consolidation (circle in **b**)

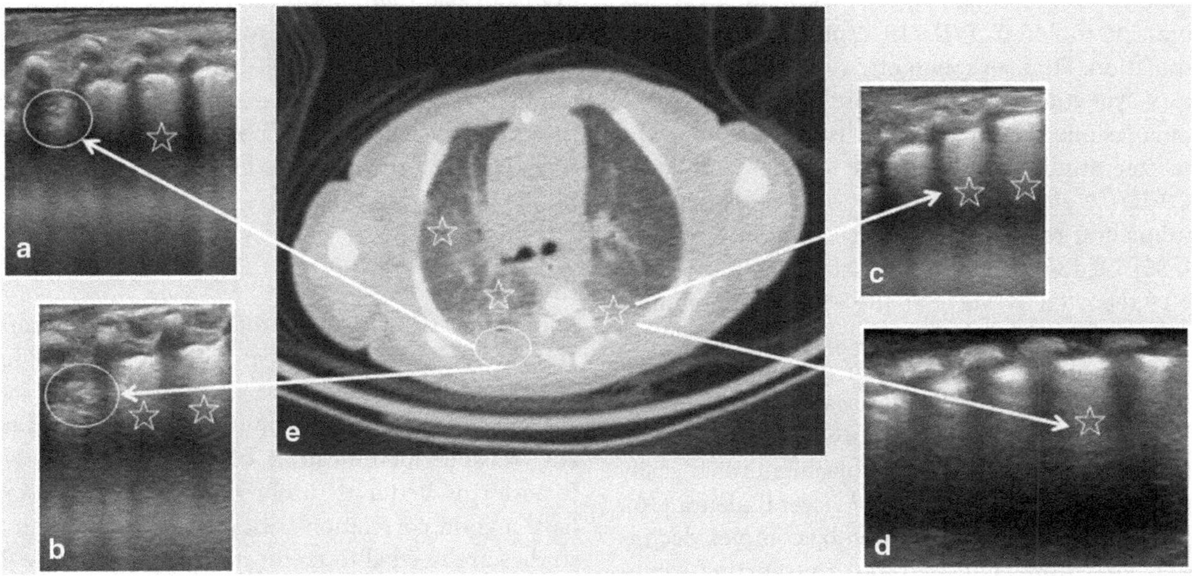

Fig. 3 Thirteen-day-old male preterm newborn, presented with hypoxemia, tachypnea and high D-dimer level. Lung US (**a–d**) showed irregularities of the pleural line and small subpleural consolidations in the posterior right lung field (circles in **a**, **b**). Confluent B-lines (stars in **a–d**) were also present in the bilateral posterior and inferior lung fields corresponding to the chest CT (**e**) ground-glass pattern (stars in **e**). Chest CT showed good correlation with lung ultrasound findings (arrows in **a–e**)

Lung US has an already established accuracy and reliability in diagnosing many lung pathologies, but up to now, only few studies have been published on its applicability in COVID-19. For pneumonia and ARDS, it is an excellent method of diagnosis and monitoring and has been found to detect lesions not seen on the chest radiograph, especially those localized in the retro-cardiac or juxta-diaphragmatic region [21–23].

Preliminary lung US studies on adult patients with COVID-19 identified numerous B-lines and subpleural pulmonary consolidations in an asymmetric multilobar distribution, involving mainly the lower lobes. What seems to be characteristic of COVID-19 in a positive epidemiological context is the bilateral patchy distribution of multiform clusters alternating with spared areas. Those findings were highly consistent with the findings on CT [24–29]. The first few case reports and case series published in children with COVID-19 showed lung US findings similar to what was described in adults [30–32].

Our findings are in accordance with previous small pediatric reports and adult studies and we also found an apparently good consistency between lung US and CT in terms of findings and topography. Confluent B-lines were later seen as consolidations on a chest CT performed the following day only in two specific zones. We cannot say whether it was a misdiagnosis or an early sonographic identification of organizing pneumonia. This could be clarified only by a study aiming to compare lung US and CT when both are performed simultaneously. Even though some comparisons were made between CT and lung US, this study was not designed to pair up these imaging modalities due to ethical concerns about unnecessarily exposing children to ionizing radiation.

As far as we know, our study was the first in pediatric COVID-19 population to analyze lung US aeration scores. Most of our patients that classified as moderate and severe/critical, had major abnormalities on lung US, and consequently higher lung US aeration scores. Due to the small sample size, we do not have statistical power to confirm the lung US aeration score as a disease severity predictor, but this preliminary result is an important finding that suggests that this score might be an additional tool to help clinicians in risk stratification and resource allocation. Two patients with moderate disease and normal US had an obstructive airway disease reversed with corticosteroids and bronchodilators.

Despite the apparent good association with disease severity, five of our children had significant lung US abnormalities, elevated scores, but few or no respiratory symptoms. All of them were under 6 months of age and four also had elevated D-dimers, which is believed to be a severity marker of disease in adult patients [33]. One of them, a 2 week-old newborn with fever, also had a chest CT that confirmed lung involvement. The reason why these young infants with confirmed lung involvement on imaging and elevated D-dimer have such a mild disease is yet to be clarified as many other clinical aspects of COVID-19 in children.

There are several reasons why we believe lung US may be a promising tool in COVID-19, especially in the pediatric population. First, although other viruses such as the respiratory syncytial virus and parainfluenza virus cause pneumonia lesions that are mostly distributed along the bronchial tree, studies addressing CT findings in children with COVID-19 showed that the periphery of the lung in the subpleural region is the most commonly affected area [34, 35]. Of 43 patients with CT abnormalities due to COVID-19 reported by Ma et al. [3], 95% had a predominance of lesions in the subpleural area and in the lower lung lobes (65%), especially in the posterior segment (78%). Given that the subpleural area seems to be the target for COVID-19, lung US may assume a key role in the early detection of these lung involvements as it easily identifies infections extending to the visceral pleura [16]. Second, chest CT should be followed by complex decontamination procedures and requires transporting sometimes critically ill patients to the radiology suite, while lung US can be performed at the bedside and given its smaller size, would be easier to decontaminate [35]. Of note, two of our critically ill patients were too unstable to leave the PICU and initial lung imaging assessments were made by lung US. Third, while US is radiation-free, CT scan exposes pediatric patients to harmful ionizing radiation during a time at which they are believed to be most at risk of harm [11].

Limitations of this imaging modality still exist, including an inability to visualize centrally located consolidation, inability to differentiate consolidation from atelectasis, and possibly some degree of overdiagnosis, as US can detect even small consolidations of unlikely significance [36–38]. Moreover, the aforementioned assumption from adult studies that lung US in COVID-19 may have characteristic features has not yet been extrapolated to children, as they more frequently have lower respiratory tract disease caused by a variety of viruses that may have a similar pattern. Further studies are needed to better understand this.

Our study also has some limitations. It is a descriptive study with a small number of patients included; however, given the scarcity of available data on lung US findings in COVID-19 pediatric patients, the information provided by our study is relevant and may provide a better understanding of this topic. Sonographers were not blinded to clinical information, because lung US assessment is performed on a regular basis as an extension of the physical examination in our institution. Also, even though the lung US score applied in our patients have been used in many lung pathologies, it is not specific to COVID-19 lung disease as the one proposed by Soldati et al. [39]. Lastly, we could not reliably compare lung US with the gold standard chest CT, since not all patients had both exams or had them performed at the same time. Despite these limitations, as far as we know our study on point-of-care lung US findings in children with COVID-19 is the first to include a more extensive number of pediatric patients. We believe our report adds important information regarding the utility of lung US in pediatric population with COVID-19.

Conclusion

Point-of-care lung US is a reliable tool that is capable of accurately diagnosing and monitoring many pulmonary conditions. Our study shows that it might also have a key role in children affected by COVID-19, providing early and reliable identification of pulmonary involvement. It performs better than chest radiograph and seems to have a good correlation with chest CT, although further studies are needed to confirm this. Integrated with clinical evaluation, lung US allows a better and rapid characterization of the disease, without ionizing radiation exposure.

Supplementary information

Additional file 1: Figure S1. Female, 11-year-old child with multisystem inflammatory syndrome in children (MIS-C) related to COVID-19 who developed cardiac failure and died. Post-mortem analysis detected SARS-CoV-2 RNA in cardiac and pulmonary tissues by RT-PCR and microthrombotic disease on lungs. Lung ultrasound (LUS—A and C) and Chest computed tomography (CT—B) were performed. There was pleural effusion (PE in A and B) and subpleural consolidation (star in A and B). Confluent B-lines (CBL in C) were also present in LUS in correspondence to the chest CT ground-glass pattern (GGP in B).

Abbreviations

COVID-19: Coronavirus disease 2019; US: Ultrasound; CT: Computed tomography; PICU: Pediatric Intensive Care Unit; RT-PCR: Reverse-transcriptase-polymerase-chain-reaction; ARDS: Acute Respiratory Distress Syndrome; PED: Pediatric Emergency Department; PEM: Pediatric Emergency.

Acknowledgements

We sincerely thank all the children, parents, nurses and physicians who helped make this study possible and we also thank Drs. Maria Augusta Bento Cicaroni and Marcela Malheiro Santos and Physiotherapist Carla Marques Nicolau for their assistance during data collection and performance of lung US.

Authors' contributions

EPCG conceptualized and designed the study, performed lung ultrasound, collected data, drafted the initial manuscript, and reviewed and revised the manuscript. MDP conceptualized the study, performed lung ultrasound, collected data, and reviewed and revised the manuscript. YTS and PS carried out the imaging analyses, designed the figures, and reviewed and revised the manuscript. DYN, TBC, and FVMS performed lung ultrasound, collected data, performed interobserver agreement, and reviewed and revised the manuscript. SCLF, KW, and WBC critically reviewed the manuscript for important intellectual content. MP-Z and CS coordinated and supervised data collection and critically reviewed the manuscript for important intellectual content. All authors approved the final manuscript as submitted and agree to be accountable for all aspects of the work. All authors read and approved the final manuscript.

Author details
[1] Emergency Department, Instituto da Criança da FMUSP, University of Sao Paulo, Av. Dr. Enéas Carvalho de Aguiar, 647, Cerqueira César, Sao Paulo, SP CEP-05403.000, Brazil. [2] Emergency Department, Hospital Universitario, University of Sao Paulo, Sao Paulo, Brazil. [3] Emergency Department, Hospital Israelita Albert Einstein, Sao Paulo, Brazil. [4] Radiology Department, Hospital Israelita Albert Einstein, Sao Paulo, Brazil. [5] Dalhousie University, Halifax, NS, Canada. [6] IWK Health Centre, Halifax, NS, Canada. [7] Radiology Department, Radiology Institute, University of Sao Paulo, Sao Paulo, Brazil. [8] Pediatric Intensive Care, Children's Institute, University of Sao Paulo, Sao Paulo, Brazil.

References

1. John Hopkins University of medicine. COVID-19 dashboard by the Center for Systems Science and Engineering (CSSE) at John Hopkins University (JHU). https://coronavirus.jhu.edu/map.html. Accessed 11 July.
2. Dong Y, Mo X, Hu Y et al (2020) Epidemiology of COVID-19 among children in China. Pediatrics. https://doi.org/10.1542/peds.2020-070202 (**Published online ahead of print, 2020 Mar 16**)
3. Ma H, Hu J, Tian J et al (2020) A single-center, retrospective study of COVID-19 features in children: a descriptive investigation. BMC Med 18(1):123. https://doi.org/10.1186/s12916-020-01596-9
4. Mahase E (2020) Covid-19: concerns grow over inflammatory syndrome emerging in children. BMJ 369:m1710
5. Shekerdemian LS, Mahmood NR, Wolfe KK et al (2019) Characteristics and outcomes of children with coronavirus disease 2019 (COVID-19) infection admitted to US and Canadian Pediatric Intensive Care Units. JAMA Pediatr. https://doi.org/10.1001/jamapediatrics.2020.1948
6. Shen KL, Yang YH, Jiang RM et al (2020) Updated diagnosis, treatment and prevention of COVID-19 in children: experts' consensus statement (condensed version of the second edition). World J Pediatr. https://doi.org/10.1007/s12519-020-00362-4 (**Published online ahead of print, 2020 Apr 24**)
7. Zimmermann P, Curtis N (2020) Coronavirus Infections in children including COVID-19: an overview of the epidemiology, clinical features, diagnosis, treatment and prevention options in children. Pediatr Infect Dis J 39(5):355–368. https://doi.org/10.1097/INF.0000000000002660
8. Dennie C, Hague C, Lim RS et al (2020) Canadian Association of Thoracic Radiology/Canadian Association of Radiologists Consensus statement regarding chest imaging in suspected and confirmed COVID-19. Can Assoc Radiol J. https://doi.org/10.1177/0846537120924606
9. Xia W, Shao J, Guo Y, Peng X, Li Z, Hu D (2020) Clinical and CT features in pediatric patients with COVID-19 infection: different points from adults. Pediatr Pulmonol 55(5):1169–1174. https://doi.org/10.1002/ppul.24718
10. Duan Y, Zhu Y, Tang L et al (2020) CT features of novel coronavirus pneumonia (COVID-19) in children. Eur Radiol. https://doi.org/10.1007/s00330-020-06860-
11. Hong JY, Han K, Jung JH, Kim JS (2019) Association of exposure to diagnostic low-dose ionizing radiation with risk of cancer among youths in South Korea. JAMA Netw Open 2(9):e1910584. https://doi.org/10.1001/jamanetworkopen.2019.10584
12. Pereda MA, Chavez MA, Hooper-Miele CC et al (2015) Lung ultrasound for the diagnosis of pneumonia in children: a meta-analysis. Pediatrics 135(4):714–722. https://doi.org/10.1542/peds.2014-2833
13. Lichtenstein DA, Mezière G, Lascols N et al (2005) Ultrasound diagnosis of occult pneumothorax. Crit Care Med 33(6):1231–1238. https://doi.org/10.1097/01.ccm.0000164542.86954.b4
14. Yousefifard M, Baikpour M, Ghelichkhani P et al (2016) Screening performance characteristic of ultrasonography and radiography in detection of pleural effusion; a meta-analysis. Emerg (Tehran) 4(1):1–10
15. Bouhemad B, Mongodi S, Via G, Rouquette I (2015) Ultrasound for "lung monitoring" of ventilated patients. Anesthesiology 122(2):437–447. https://doi.org/10.1097/ALN.0000000000000558
16. Bouhemad B, Liu ZH, Arbelot C et al (2010) Ultrasound assessment of antibiotic-induced pulmonary reaeration in ventilator-associated pneumonia. Crit Care Med 38(1):84–92. https://doi.org/10.1097/CCM.0b013e3181b08cdb
17. Bello G, Blanco P (2019) Lung ultrasonography for assessing lung aeration in acute respiratory distress syndrome: a narrative review. J Ultrasound Med 38(1):27–37. https://doi.org/10.1002/jum.14671
18. Qiu H, Wu J, Hong L, Luo Y, Song Q, Chen D (2019) Clinical and epidemiological features of 36 children with coronavirus disease 2019 (COVID-19) in Zhejiang, China: an observational cohort study. Lancet Infect Dis. https://doi.org/10.1016/S1473-3099(20)30198-5
19. Copetti R, Cattarossi L (2008) Ultrasound diagnosis of pneumonia in children. Radiol Med 113(2):190–198. https://doi.org/10.1007/s11547-008-0247-8
20. Wong HYF, Lam HYS, Fong AH et al (2019) Frequency and distribution of chest radiographic findings in COVID-19 positive patients. Radiology. https://doi.org/10.1148/radiol.2020201160 (**Published online ahead of print, 2019 Mar 27**)
21. Iorio G, Capasso M, Prisco S et al (2018) Lung ultrasound findings undetectable by chest radiography in children with community-acquired pneumonia. Ultrasound Med Biol 44(8):1687–1693. https://doi.org/10.1016/j.ultrasmedbio.2018.04.007
22. Soummer A, Perbet S, Brisson H et al (2012) Ultrasound assessment of lung aeration loss during a successful weaning trial predicts postextubation distress*. Crit Care Med 40(7):2064–2072. https://doi.org/10.1097/CCM.0b013e31824e68ae
23. Algieri I, Mongodi S, Chiumello D et al (2014) CT scan and ultrasound comparative assessment of PEEP-induced lung aeration changes in ARDS. Crit Care 18(suppl 1):285
24. Fiala MJ (2020) A brief review of lung ultrasonography in COVID-19: is it useful? Ann Emerg Med. https://doi.org/10.1016/j.annemergmed.2020.03.033 (**Published online ahead of print, 2020 Apr 8**)
25. Huang Y, Wang S, Liu Y, et al. A preliminary study on the ultrasonic manifestations of peripulmonary lesions of non-critical novel coronavirus pneumonia (COVID-19). https://doi.org/10.2139/ssrn.3544750. Accessed 26 Feb 2020.
26. Peng QY, Wang XT, Zhang LN, Chinese Critical Care Ultrasound Study Group (CCUSG) (2020) Findings of lung ultrasonography of novel corona virus pneumonia during the 2019–2020 epidemic. Intensive Care Med 46(5):849–850. https://doi.org/10.1007/s00134-020-05996-6
27. Poggiali E, Dacrema A, Bastoni D et al (2020) Can lung US help critical care clinicians in the early diagnosis of novel coronavirus (COVID-19) pneumonia? Radiology 295(3):E6. https://doi.org/10.1148/radiol.2020200847
28. Volpicelli G, Gargani L (2020) Sonographic signs and patterns of COVID-19 pneumonia. Ultrasound J 12(1):22. https://doi.org/10.1186/s13089-020-00171-w
29. Volpicelli G, Lamorte A, Villén T (2020) What's new in lung ultrasound during the COVID-19 pandemic. Intensive Care Med. https://doi.org/10.1007/s00134-020-06048-9 (**Published online ahead of print, 2020 May 4**)
30. Denina M, Scolfaro C, Silvestro E et al (2020) Lung ultrasound in children with COVID-19. Pediatrics. https://doi.org/10.1542/peds.2020-1157 (**Published online ahead of print, 2020 Apr 21**)
31. Musolino AM, Supino MC, Buonsenso D et al (2020) Lung ultrasound in children with COVID-19: preliminary findings. Ultrasound Med Biol 46(8):2094–2098. https://doi.org/10.1016/j.ultrasmedbio.2020.04.026
32. Gregorio-Hernández R, Escobar-Izquierdo AB, Cobas-Pazos J et al (2020) Point-of-care lung ultrasound in three neonates with COVID-19. Eur J Pediatr 179:1279–1285. https://doi.org/10.1007/s00431-020-03706-4
33. Garcia-Olivé I, Sintes H, Radua J, Capa JA, Rosell A (2020) D-dimer in patients infected with COVID-19 and suspected pulmonary embolism. Respir Med. https://doi.org/10.1016/j.rmed.2020.106023 (**Published online ahead of print, 2020 May 13**)
34. Virkki R, Juven T, Rikalainen H, Svedström E, Mertsola J, Ruuskanen O (2002) Differentiation of bacterial and viral pneumonia in children. Thorax 57(5):438–441. https://doi.org/10.1136/thorax.57.5.438
35. Smith MJ, Hayward SA, Innes SM, Miller ASC (2020) Point-of-care lung ultrasound in patients with COVID-19 - a narrative review. Anaesthesia. https://doi.org/10.1111/anae.15082 (**Published online ahead of print, 2020 Apr 10**)
36. Lissaman C, Kanjanauptom P, Ong C, Tessaro M, Long E, O'Brien A (2019) Prospective observational study of point-of-care ultrasound for diagnosing pneumonia. Arch Dis Child 104(1):12–18. https://doi.org/10.1136/archdischild-2017-314496
37. Stadler JAM, Andronikou S, Zar HJ (2017) Lung ultrasound for the diagnosis of community-acquired pneumonia in children. Pediatr Radiol 47(11):1412–1419. https://doi.org/10.1007/s00247-017-3910-1

38. Cheung JCH, Lam KN (2020) POCUS on COVID-19: pearls and pitfals. Lancet Resp Med. https://doi.org/10.1016/S2213-2600(20)30166-1
39. Soldati G, Smargiassi A, Inchingolo R et al (2020) Proposal for international standardization of the use of lung ultrasound for patients with COVID-19: a simple, quantitative, reproducible method. J Ultrasound Med 39(7):1413–1419. https://doi.org/10.1002/jum.15285

15

Life after a point-of-care ultrasound course: setting up the right conditions!

T. J. Olgers[1*], N. Azizi[1], H. R. Bouma[1,2] and J. C. ter Maaten[1]

Abstract

Background: Point-of-care Ultrasound (POCUS) is becoming an important diagnostic tool for internal medicine and ultrasound educational programs are being developed. An ultrasound course is often included in such a curriculum. We have performed a prospective observational questionnaire-based cohort study consisting of participants of a POCUS course for internal medicine in the Netherlands in a 2-year period. We investigated the usefulness of an ultrasound course and barriers participants encountered after the course.

Results: 55 participants (49%) completed the pre-course questionnaire, 29 (26%) completed the post-course questionnaire, 11 participants (10%) finalized the third questionnaire. The number of participants who performs POCUS was almost doubled after the course (from 34.5 to 65.5%). Almost all participants felt insufficiently skilled before the course which declined to 34.4% after the course. The majority (N = 26 [89.7%]) stated that this 2-day ultrasound course was sufficient enough to perform POCUS in daily practice but also changed daily practice. The most important barriers withholding them from performing ultrasound are lack of experts for supervision, insufficient practice time and absence of an ultrasound machine.

Conclusions: This study shows that a 2-day hands-on ultrasound course seems a sufficient first step in an ultrasound curriculum for internal medicine physicians to obtain enough knowledge and skills to perform POCUS in clinical practice but it also changes clinical practice. However, there are barriers in the transfer to clinical practice that should be addressed which may improve curriculum designing.

Keywords: POCUS, Point-of-care ultrasound, Ultrasound curriculum, Acute internal medicine, Ultrasound course, Barriers for ultrasound

Background

Point-of-care Ultrasound (POCUS) is an important diagnostic tool for medical decision making and resuscitation of patients used by many specialists around the world. The reliability of the POCUS exam is largely operator dependent and, therefore, requires a solid ultrasound training system [1]. For internal medicine, it is a relatively new skill and ultrasound curricula are being developed to ensure correct use of POCUS for safe patient care [2–4]. In ultrasound curriculum designing, the first step is choosing the core applications which are relevant for that specific specialty and providing the core knowledge of these applications [2, 5]. This first step is called the initial introduction and usually consists of taking an ultrasound course, ranging from several hours to several days. The second step is gaining experience, followed by the third step which is achieving competency. If the initial introduction is not followed by the next, the usefulness of a course is questionable. Gaining experience by practicing under supervision is necessary to become competent, as is taking driving lessons after learning how to control a car. In our previous research, we have already shown that one important barrier for internal medicine residents to perform POCUS is the lack of experts to provide supervision [6]. To investigate the impact of an ultrasound

*Correspondence: t.j.olgers@umcg.nl
[1] Dept Internal Med, Univ Groningen, Univ Med Ctr Groningen, 9700 RB Groningen, The Netherlands
Full list of author information is available at the end of the article

course and the barriers to clinical implementation of POCUS after the course, we have performed a questionnaire-based study among ultrasound course participants.

Methods

Since 2017, a 2-day ultrasound course specifically designed for internal medicine (DEUS course: Dutch Emergency UltraSound for internists) is being held 2–3 times a year. This is one of the two largest ultrasound courses for internal medicine in the Netherlands. These two courses are similar in content, educational tools, practice time and participants and both courses have a theoretical and practical exam. The number of participants in the DEUS course varies from 20 to a maximum of 24. We have invited all participants from 5 courses ($N=112$), held in 2018 and 2019, to complete a questionnaire 1 week before the ultrasound course, 1–2 weeks after the ultrasound course, and 3 months after the course. The questionnaire included demographic data, questions about POCUS training and practice, and questions about the perceived usefulness and limitations. The survey was distributed by the course secretary board using an online survey tool (http://www.thesistoolpro.com). Participants were only invited once. Missing data were excluded from analysis for that specific questionnaire and for the returned questionnaires descriptive statistics was used. Participants provided written informed consent to participate in this study. SPSS statistics 23 was used for descriptive statistics.

Results

55 participants (49%) completed the pre-course questionnaire, 29 (26%) completed the post-course questionnaire. Unfortunately, only 11 participants (10%) finalized the third questionnaire. Most participants were female (52.7%), and half of participants were aged between 30 and 39 (Table 1).

The majority were internal medicine residents (56.4%), and a significant amount were attending internists (41.8%). The participants perceived that ultrasound was used by internists in their hospital in the minority (38.2%) of hospitals, in contrast to ultrasound use by emergency physicians (83.6%). The experience and practice of POCUS before and after the ultrasound course is shown in Table 2.

Most participants indicated they have never performed any ultrasound in clinical practice prior to the course (65.5%), which decreased after the course (34.5%). If they have performed POCUS after the course, it was largely done under supervision. After the course, more participants use POCUS and the number of POCUS performed also increased. This effect seems to persist after 3 months, notwithstanding the low number of respondents. Strikingly, nearly all participants (98%) indicated they were insufficiently skilled to perform POCUS in their own situation, but after the course this number decreased to 34.4%.

Of all post-course respondents, the majority stated that this 2-day ultrasound course was sufficient enough to perform POCUS in daily practice (Table 2). The majority also experienced that this ultrasound course influenced their clinical practice for various reasons. The most mentioned were that they felt more secure about performing ultrasound and they practiced ultrasound more, they have a better understanding of the value of POCUS for clinical decision making and POCUS increased their confidence of fluid status assessment. After 3 months, despite the low number of respondents, these percentages are roughly the same. Finally we have asked them for perceived barriers for performing POCUS (Table 3).

This shows that lack of knowledge is substantially reduced by following this ultrasound course. A significant amount of participants do not have access to an ultrasound machine. The majority were not able to practice under supervision due to lack of experts (58.6%) and/or practice time (41.4%). These two were perceived as the most important barriers to use POCUS.

Discussion

We have shown that a 2-day hands-on ultrasound course is a solid first step in an ultrasound curriculum for internal medicine. Participants perceive they have sufficient knowledge and skills to perform POCUS in real practice, which is in line with the effect of other ultrasound courses and ultrasound curricula [7–10]. It should be noted that the number of post-course responders is lower as compared to pre-course responders, which possesses a high risk of bias. The second step in the curriculum, which is gaining experience, is difficult to fulfill if the conditions are not set properly. The largest remaining barriers in the Netherlands after following an ultrasound course, are lack of an ultrasound machine, lack of experts for supervision and lack of practice time. These barriers for learning POCUS are also seen in other specialties [11]. It is essential that we create a learning and training environment that is safe for patient care with enough experts available for supervision. Skills including ultrasound skills may subside quickly if ultrasound is not performed on a regular basis, especially by novel sonographers [12–14]. This implies that before an ultrasound course is offered as a start for the ultrasound curriculum, the conditions should be optimized for participants to complete all necessary steps in achieving and maintaining competency and not only the initial introduction [15, 16]. For example in the Netherlands, POCUS has been made

Table 1 Demographics of respondents

Demographics	Pre-course $N=55$ (%)	Post-course 2 weeks $N=29$ (%)	Post-course 3 months $N=11$ (%)
Age			
18–29	13 (23.6)	6 (20.7)	2 (18.2)
30–39	27 (49.1)	15 (51.7)	6 (54.5)
40–49	8 (14.5)	5 (17.2)	2 (18.2)
50–59	7 (12.7)	3 (10.3)	1 (9.1)
Gender			
Male	26 (47.3)	12 (41.4)	4 (36.4)
Residency (year)			
1	5 (9.1)	1 (3.4)	2 (18.2)
2	5 (9.1)	4 (13.8)	2 (18.2)
3	13 (23.6)	6 (20.7)	1 (9.1)
4	4 (7.3)	2 (6.9)	0 (0)
5	2 (3.6)	1 (3.4)	1 (9.1)
6	2 (3.6)	2 (6.9)	0 (0)
None (student)	1 (1.8)	0 (0)	0 (0)
None (attending)	23 (41.8)	13 (44.9)	5 (45.4)
(Sub)specialty			
General internal medicine	19 (34.5)	12 (41.4)	5 (45.5)
Nephrology	4 (7.3)	3 (10.3)	1 (9.1)
Hemato-oncology	8 (14.5)	4 (13.8)	3 (27.3)
Acute internal medicine	13 (23.6)	4 (13.8)	1 (9.1)
Other	11 (20.0)	6 (20.7)	1 (9.1)
Workplace			
University hospital	14 (25.5)	9 (31.0)	5 (45.5)
Large Teaching hospital	37 (67.3)	19 (65.5)	4 (36.4)
Rural hospital	4 (7.3)	1 (3.4)	2 (18.2)
Ultrasound performed in hospital by			
Internists	21 (38.2)	12 (41.4)	5 (45.5)
Emergency physicians	46 (83.6)	25 (86.2)	7 (63.6)
US-machine available	49 (89.1)	25 (86.2)	8 (72.7)

Data presented as absolute number and percentage ()

a mandatory skill for internal medicine residents by the Dutch Internal Medicine Federation (NIV). This obliged educators and hospitals to include ultrasound machines in their budget and to create focus groups for further development of POCUS educational programs. However, with increasing amounts of affordable handheld devices with good quality images, budget problems may become less of an issue. It required investing time and money to educate and train experts in the teaching hospitals for supervision of residents and to guarantee safe patient care. Addressing these issues are at least as important as sending staff or residents to an ultrasound course. In this way an ultrasound courses will not only be just a pleasant experience but a real start of an ultrasound curriculum.

Limitations

This survey has some potential limitations. The first questionnaire response rate was 49%, the post-course survey 26% and the 3-month response rate was only 10%. Most web-based data collection have a mean response rate of 27.6% [17]. The low response rate may have influenced the interpretation of the results. Especially the 3rd questionnaire must be seen as indicative due to the low number of respondents. Theoretically, if all post-course non-responders represent participants that did not benefit from the course in terms of knowledge, the number of participants with insufficient knowledge may have only decreased from 60 to 51%, although this is very unlikely. In addition, responders may be more enthusiastic about ultrasound and can

Table 2 Effect of ultrasound course on performing POCUS

	Pre-course $N = 55$ (%)	Post-course 2 weeks $N = 29$ (%)	Post-course 3 months $N = 11$ (%)
Performs POCUS			
No	36 (65.5)	9 (31.0)	2 (18.2)
Yes, mainly independent	8 (14.5	8 (27.6)	3 (27.3)
Yes, mainly supervised	11 (20.0)	12 (41.4)	6 (54.5)
Frequency of POCUS			
(Almost) daily	1 (1.8)	3 (10.3)	2 (18.2)
Multiple days a week	2 (3.6)	2 (6.9)	1 (9.1)
1 day a week	2 (3.6)	6 (20.7)	6 (54.5)
A few times per month	9 (16.4)	8 (27.6	2 (18.2)
(Almost) never	41 (74.5)	10 (34.5)	0 (0)
Number of POCUS performed[a]	**Before course**	**After course**	**After course**
0	36 (65.5)	9 (31.0)	2 (18.2)
1–20	12 (21.8)	20 (69.0)	7 (63.6)
21–60	4 (7.3)	0 (0)	2 (18.2)
61–100	2 (3.6)	0 (0)	0 (0)
101–200	0 (0)	0 (0)	0 (0)
> 200	1 (1.8)	0 (0)	0 (0)
Do you feel skilled			
No	46 (83.6)	1 (3.4)	3 (27.3)
Mostly not	8 (14.5)	9 (31.0)	3 (27.3)
Mostly yes	1 (1.8)	18 (62.1)	5 (45.5)
Yes	0 (0)	1 (3.4)	0 (0)
POCUS course sufficient to perform POCUS in daily practice?			
Yes	NA	26 (89.7)	10 (90.9)
No		3 (10.3)	1 (9.1)
Did following the course influenced your daily practice?			
Yes	NA	20 (69.0)	8 (72.7)
No		9 (31.0)	3 (27.3)

POCUS Point-of-care ultrasound, *NA* not applicable

[a] for post-course 2 weeks and post-course 3 months only number after the course; Data presented as absolute number and percentage ()

Table 3 Perceived barriers for performing POCUS

Perceived barriers	Pre-course $N = 55$ (%)	Post-course $N = 29$ (%)
Insufficient knowledge	33 (60.0)	2 (2.9)
Lack of adequate course	4 (7.3)	1 (3.4)
Insufficient experts/supervisors	22 (40.0)	17 (58.6)
Lack of US machine	12 (21.8)	13 (44.8)
Insufficient practice time	30 (54.5)	12 (41.4)
Insufficient opportunity for training under supervision	27 (49.1)	18 (62.1)
Resistance from other specialties	15 (27.3)	4 (13.8)
Lack of national guideline or from own profession	6 (10.9)	1 (3.4)
Other	3 (5.5)	3 (10.3)
None	3 (5.5)	0

Data presented as absolute number and percentage (); Post-course only including 2-week post-course

have different ideas than non-responders. Furthermore, responders may feel more confident about their knowledge after a course than non-responders which may have influenced the low percentage of the barrier lack-of-knowledge. Finally, participants may overestimate their own knowledge, a well-known psychological phenomena in unskilled participants called the Dunning–Kruger effect, although we do not know if this is applicable for our study population [18]. We think an ultrasound course might even have the opposite effect if participants have become more aware of their shortcomings (conscious incompetence) and underestimate their skills. We have shown an increase in their perceived knowledge. How this course actually increase ultrasound skills was beyond the scope of this research as we only asked participants for their perceived skills. Half of the respondents were residents and half were attending physicians, there also was a variability in their corresponding internal subspecialties but selection bias cannot be excluded. We did not contact a subgroup of non-responders nor did we sent structured reminders to complete the survey which could have increased the response rate. We omitted open questions on most topics so specific important issues not addressed in our questionnaire may be missed. This research represents the course participants perceived skills and knowledge but we did not test them afterwards for ultrasound skills. We only invited participants of one of the two ultrasound courses. These courses are very similar and faculty of both courses are also members of the Dutch taskforce developing the ultrasound curriculum in the Netherlands and some teach in both courses. We would expect the same results if we invited all participants.

Conclusion

This study shows that a 2-day hands-on ultrasound course is a sufficient first step in an ultrasound curriculum for internal medicine physicians. However, the conditions should be optimized to prevent loss of this knowledge and skills so course participants can proceed to the necessary consecutive steps which are gaining experience and achieving competency. The most important barriers to overcome are lack of experts for supervision and insufficient practice time, both problems should be addressed before attending an ultrasound course to increase the yield.

Acknowledgements
Not applicable.

Authors' contributions
All authors have substantially contributed to the conception of the study, interpretation of the results and critically appraised the previous and final version of the manuscript. All authors read and approved the final manuscript.

Author details
[1] Dept Internal Med, Univ Groningen, Univ Med Ctr Groningen, 9700 RB Groningen, The Netherlands. [2] Dept of Clinical Pharmacy and Pharmacology, Univ Groningen, Univ Med Ctr Gron ngen, 9700 RB Groningen, The Netherlands.

References

1. Bhagra A, Tierney DM, Sekiguchi H, Soni NJ (2016) Point-of-care ultrasonography for primary care physicians and general internists. Mayo Clin Proc 91:1811–1827
2. Olgers TJ, Azizi N, Blans MJ, Bosch FH, Gans ROB, Ter Maaten JC (2019) Point-of-care Ultrasound (PoCUS) for the internist in Acute Medicine: a uniform curriculum. Neth J Med 77(5):168–176
3. Mellor TE, Junga Z, Ordway S, Hunter T, Shimeall WT, Krajnik S, Tibbs L, Mikita J, Zeman J, Clark P (2019) Not just hocus POCUS: implementation of a point of care ultrasound curriculum for internal medicine trainees at a large residency program. Mil Med 184(11–12):901–906
4. LoPresti CM, Schnobrich DJ, Dversdal RK, Schembri F (2019) A road map for point-of-care ultrasound training in internal medicine residency. Ultrasound J. 11(1):10
5. International federation for emergency medicine (IFEM) (2014) Point-of care ultrasound curriculum guidance [Internet]. https://www.ifem.cc/point-of-care-ultrasound-curriculum-guidances/. Accessed Apr 2020
6. Olgers TJ, Ter Maaten JC (2020) Point-of-care ultrasound curriculum for internal medicine residents: what do you desire? A national survey. BMC Med Educ 20(1):30
7. Gasho CJ, Torralba KD, Chooljian DM, Cohen A, Dinh VA (2019) Impact of a lung ultrasound course for rheumatology specialists (IMPACT-2). Clin Exp Rheumatol 37(3):380–384
8. Zawadka M, Graczyńska A, Janiszewska A, Ostrowski A, Michałowski M, Rykowski M, Andruszkiewicz P (2019) Lessons learned from a study of the integration of a point-of-care ultrasound course into the undergraduate medical school curriculum. Med Sci Monit 2(25):4104–4109
9. Arienti V, Di Giulio R, Cogliati C, Accogli E, Aluigi L, Corazza G, Ultrasound SIMI Study Group (2014) Bedside ultrasonography (US), Echoscopy and US point of care as a new kind of stethoscope for Internal Medicine Departments: the training program of the Italian Internal Medicine Society (SIMI). Intern Emerg Med 9:805–814
10. Dinh VA, Giri PC, Rathinavel I, Nguyen E, Hecht D, Dorotta I, Nguyen HB, Chrissian AA (2015) Impact of a 2-day critical care ultrasound course during fellowship training: a pilot study. Crit Care Res Pract 2015:675041
11. Acuña J, Rubin M, Hahn B, Das D, Kapoor M, Adhikari S, Greenstein J (2020) Point-of-care ultrasound in United States pediatric emergency medicine fellowship programs: the current state of practice and training. Pediatr Emerg Care. https://doi.org/10.1097/PEC.0000000000001955
12. Rhue AL, VanDerveer B (2018) Wilderness first responder: are skills soon forgotten? Wilderness Environ Med 29(1):132–137. https://doi.org/10.1016/j.wem.2017.11.005
13. Kimura BJ, Sliman SM, Waalen J, Amundson SA, Shaw DJ (2016) Retention of ultrasound skills and training in "point-of-care" cardiac ultrasound. J Am Soc Echocardiogr 29(10):992–997
14. Town JA, Bergl PA, Narang A, McConville JF (2016) Internal medicine residents' retention of knowledge and skills in bedside ultrasound. J Grad Med Educ 8(4):553–557
15. Løkkegaard T, Todsen T, Nayahangan LJ, Andersen CA, Jensen MB, Konge L (2020) Point-of-care ultrasound for general practitioners: a systematic needs assessment. Scand J Prim Health Care 38(1):3–11
16. European Core Curriculum for Emergency Medicine (2017). https://eusem.org/images/ebeem/European-Core-Curriculum-for-EM-Version-1.2-April-2017-final-version-1.pdf. Accessed Apr 2020
17. Blumenberg C, Barros AJD (2018) Response rate differences between web and alternative data collection methods for public health research: a systematic review of the literature. Int J Public Health 63(6):765–773
18. Kruger J, Dunning D (1999) Unskilled and unaware of it: how difficulties in recognizing one's own incompetence lead to inflated self-assessments. J Pers Soc Psychol 77(6):1121–1134. https://doi.org/10.1037//0022-3514.77.6.1121

16

Evaluation of a novel handheld point-of-care ultrasound device in an African emergency department

Samuel L. Burleson*, Jonathan F. Swanson, Erin F. Shufflebarger, Douglas W. Wallace, Matthew A. Heimann, James C. Crosby, David C. Pigott, John P. Gullett, Maxwell A. Thompson and Christopher J. Greene

Abstract

Background: Many point-of-care ultrasound devices are now "pocket-sized" or handheld, allowing easy transport during travel and facilitating use in crowded spaces or in austere low-resource settings. Concerns remain about their durability, image quality, and clinical utility in those environments.

Method: Five emergency physicians with training in point-of-care ultrasound employed the Butterfly iQ, a novel handheld ultrasound device, in routine clinical care in a busy, high-acuity African emergency department over a period of 10 weeks. We retrospectively evaluated the performance of the Butterfly iQ from the perspectives of both the clinicians using the device and expert ultrasound faculty reviewing the images.

Results: We found advantages of the Butterfly iQ in a high-acuity African emergency department include its use of a single probe for multiple functions, small size, ease of transport, relatively low cost, and good image quality in most functions. Disadvantages include large probe footprint, lower, though still adequate, cardiac imaging quality, frequent overheating, and reliance on internet-based cloud storage, but these were surmountable. We also report a wide variety of patient presentations, pathology, and procedures to which the device was used.

Conclusion: We conclude the Butterfly iQ is an effective, though imperfect, point-of-care ultrasound device in a low-resource emergency setting. We will continue to employ the device in clinical emergency care and teaching in this setting.

Keywords: Point-of-care ultrasound, Handheld, Butterfly iQ, Resource-limited settings, Emergency, Tropical infectious disease

Introduction

Newly-marketed point-of-care ultrasound (POCUS) devices like the Butterfly iQ (iQ, Butterfly Network, Inc, Guilford, CT, USA) have generated significant excitement over their potential in emergency departments (EDs), critical care units, and resource-limited settings (RLS). Potential benefits of the iQ include small size, lower cost, integration with the user's mobile phone or tablet, and use of silicon-chip based technology obviating the need for multiple transducers. There has been little critical evaluation of the device itself, particularly in RLS. We describe our use of the Butterfly iQ in routine clinical operations in a busy, high-acuity African ED and review its performance and applicability to RLS.

Personnel and setting

Five emergency physicians from the United States worked alongside the ED staff of a busy referral hospital in rural east Africa treating medical and surgical patients of all ages over a period of 10 consecutive weeks in the fall of 2019. All physicians have surpassed accepted POCUS

*Correspondence: slburleson@uabmc.edu
Department of Emergency Medicine, University of Alabama at Birmingham, Old Hillman Building Suite 251, 619 19th St S, Birmingham, AL 35249, USA

training guidelines [1]. Two (SLB and JFS) have completed or are enrolled in a Point-of-care Ultrasound in Resource Limited Settings fellowship [2]. Advanced imaging is available, but access is limited by the need for payment prior to testing; in practice, patients often wait hours or days prior to imaging. Patients were selected by clinicians at the bedside if POCUS was indicated as a part of routine clinical care; therefore, informed consent was not required. Patients were scanned with the Butterfly iQ connected to an Apple iPad (iPad 5th Generation, Apple, Cupertino, CA, USA). Images were later reviewed for quality assurance by ultrasound fellowship-trained faculty. Final diagnoses were determined from a combination of the medical record, discussions with inpatient teams, and expert image review.

Results and discussion

The Butterfly iQ performed well and met clinician needs for a POCUS machine in this single RLS. Its advantages over cart-based machines are magnified, where financial resources, floor space, and reliable power may be scarce. Advantages and disadvantages of the Butterfly iQ are summarized in Table 1.

Advantages

The combination of flexibility and mobility of a single probe with preset modes replacing multiple transducers is the paramount benefit of the device. We successfully employed the iQ in a wide variety of scans and patient presentations (see Table 2, Figs. 1, 2, 3) and procedural guidance (see Table 3).

Image quality, particularly in the abdominal and musculoskeletal modalities, was excellent, though not generally up to the standards of a cart-based system. With few exceptions (see below), image quality in all modalities was adequate to answer the clinical question.

The software application is user-friendly, allowing rapid alternation between preset scanning modes, enabling multiple protocols on the same patient with only a few gestures. Some routine calculation functions (such as gestational age) were not available during our experience with the device. We found the increased screen size of an iPad compared to a mobile phone beneficial for most uses.

The cost of the device (approximately US$2000), plus a required $420 annual subscription fee to the cloud-based image storage) places it within reach of some individual clinicians, and many healthcare institutions, even in RLS. Battery life was adequate, usually enough to last an entire 12-h shift on a full charge, though we did not specifically measure continuous scanning time. When necessary, we were able to charge the device from main power on shift. Small, relatively inexpensive, third party solar-powered chargers could also provide additional charging.

Table 1 Advantages and disadvantages of the butterfly iQ

ADVANTAGES
Single probe replaces multiple traditional transducers, capable of many scan types
Image quality excellent compared to other handhelds
Low cost
User-friendly app
DISADVANTAGES
Cardiac imaging lower quality than other modes
Relatively frequent overheating
Single probe relatively heavy with large footprint, occasionally compressing small structures

Disadvantages

Echocardiography habitually seemed lower quality than other modes. There was an apparent drop in resolution and frame rate, most noticeably associated with the use of color Doppler. Like other pocket-sized devices, the iQ also lacks spectral Doppler. Despite these limitations, we were able to detect significant cardiovascular pathology. All views were generally obtainable, adequate to guide resuscitation, and answer basic clinical questions pertinent to the RLS [3].

Images are stored on a cloud-based server requiring internet access to upload. Until they are uploaded, the images remain in an "outbox", where they can easily be deleted. Without reliable internet access, many images remained in this "outbox" for the duration of our field work, inhibiting our ability to share or review images.

We encountered several challenges related to the device's hardware. The first was periodic overheating, rendering further scanning impossible until the device cooled. Overheating was not appreciably tied to any specific scanning mode or function. We mitigated this by briefly running water over the waterproof end of the device until cooled. We noticed a small rubber seal loosening near the end of the transducer by the closing of our field experience, without any discernible change in function. We found the cord length (125 cm) slightly short, especially when performing POCUS-guided procedures. The probe itself weighs 0.7 lb (0.3 kg), more than twice most other transducers, and its footprint is larger than a phased array probe, which was occasionally problematic when placing ultrasound-guided peripheral IVs and scanning between ribs, respectively. This may have contributed to the decreased quality of some echocardiographic images.

Table 2 Point-of-care ultrasound findings using Butterfly iQ in African Emergency Department

Age/sex	Presentation	US exams	US findings
44 yo M	Afib RVR, Cardiogenic shock	Cardiac	Calcified left atrial thrombus
3 yo M	Abdominal pain, Fussy, Bloody stool	GI	Intussusception
28 yo F	Submandibular swelling	MSK	Submandibular abscess
25 yo M	Dyspnea on exertion, Hx of PCE	Cardiac, Lung	Large PCE without tamponade, Bilateral pleural effusions
Young Adult M	Leg pain	MSK	Mid-shaft femur fracture with displacement
23 yo F	Abdominal pain, Hx of abdominal mass	GI	Dermoid cyst (recurrent)
78 yo M	Early satiety, Rectal mass on exam	GI	Novel dx of diffuse hepatosplenic lesions concerning for malignancy
28 yo M	Necrotic finger	MSK	Abscess vs necrosis
3 mo M	Acute respiratory failure	Cardiac, Lung	Novel dx of Atrial Septal Defect
114 yo M	Dyspnea	Cardiac, Lung	Novel dx of HFrEF
13 yo F	Novel Afib and hypoxia, Hx of RHD	Cardiac	Massive MR, LA dilation, Small PCE (Consistent with known RHD)
14 yo M	Dyspnea, Anasarca on exam, Hx of RHD and malaria	Cardiac	HFrEF, TR with RA dilation, MR (Consistent with known RHD)
24 yo M	Left flank pain	GI	Splenic lesion (Subcapsular hematoma vs Infiltration)
1 yo M	Hypoxia, fever, sepsis	Lung	Bilateral B-lines
1 yo F	Hypoxia, Hx of Ventricular Septal Defect	Cardiac, Lung	RV Dilation and hypertrophy, Persistent VSD, Bilateral B-lines
74 yo F	Respiratory arrest	Cardiac	Dilated/poorly contractile RV, Full IVC
2 mo F	Failure to thrive	CNS	Hydrocephalus
Young Adult M	Leg pain	MSK	Mid-shaft tibia fracture with displacement
Elderly Adult M	Recent DVT, Dyspnea	Cardiac	Right heart strain
20 yo F	2-week post-partum, Peritonitis on exam	GI	Pelvic free fluid
28 yo M	"Hematemesis" found to be hemoptysis, Hypoxia	Cardiac, Lung, GI	Splenic lesion, Bilateral B-lines, Normal LV Ejection Fraction
Elderly Adult M	Dyspnea, Anasarca on exam, Hypoxia	Cardiac, Lung	Dilated RA and RV, TR, Bilateral B-lines, Pleural effusions, Ascites
23 yo F	Suicide attempt by drowing, Third trimester pregnancy	OB	Normal Fetal heart rate and Fetal movement
7 yo M	Abdominal pain, vomiting	GI	SBO from worm burden
25 yo M	Dyspnea and chest pain with near-syncope, Novel Afib with RVR	Cardiac	Thickened Mitral Valve, Dilated LA, Massive MR (Suspected RHD)
5 yo M	Abdominal distention	GI	Enlarged bladder with mild hydronephrosis
3 yo F	Constipation, Reports of "worms in stool"	GI	SBO, No parasites visualized
85 yo M	RUQ abdominal pain and jaundice	GI	Intrahepatic biliary dilation, RUQ Mass
35 yo F	Chest pain, Hx of Tuberculosis	Lung	Loculated pleural effusion
37 yo M	Abdominal pain, Constipation	GI	SBO, Dilated gallbladder
76 yo M	Hypoxia and sepsis	Lung	Subpleural consolidations and B-lines
19 yo F	Hx of tamponade on outpatient echocardiogram	Cardiac	Large PCE, No tamponade
25 yo M	Hypoxia, Novel Afib with RVR	Cardiac	Massive LA dilation and MR, Thickened anterior mitral valve leaflet (Suspected RHD)

Afib, Atrial fibrillation; CNS, Central Nervous System; Dx, Diagnosis; HFrEF, Heart Failure with Reduced Ejection Fraction; GI, Gastrointestinal/Genitourinary; Hx, History; IVC, Inferior Vena Cava; LA, Left Atrium; MR, Mitral Regurgitation; MSK, Musculoskeletal/Soft tissue; OB, Obstetric; PCE, Pericardial Effusion; RA, Right Atrium; RHD, Rheumatic Heart Disease; RUQ, Right Upper Quadrant; RV, Right Ventricle; RVR, Rapid Ventricular Response; SBO, Small Bowel Obstruction; TR, Tricuspid Regurgitation

Limitations

These findings represent a retrospective review of the authors' personal experiences with the Butterfly iQ device during routine clinical work in an African ED in an attempt to evaluate its performance in RLS. Patients were scanned at the discretion of the clinician at the bedside or because of restricted access to other diagnostics, introducing the possibility of selection bias. No patient-oriented outcomes were assessed and no comparisons between devices were available.

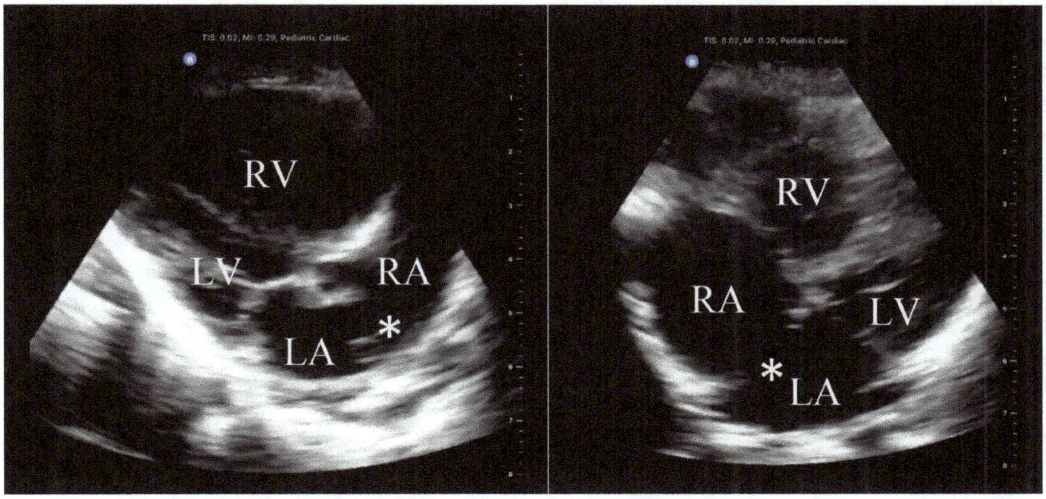

Fig. 1. 3-month-old male presenting with acute respiratory distress. POCUS revealed a dilated right atrium and ventricle with a prominent atrial septal defect, seen in parasternal long view (left) and a slightly modified apical four chamber view (right). LA, Left Atrium, LV, Left Ventricle, RA, Right Atrium, RV, Right Ventricle, *, Atrial Septal Defect

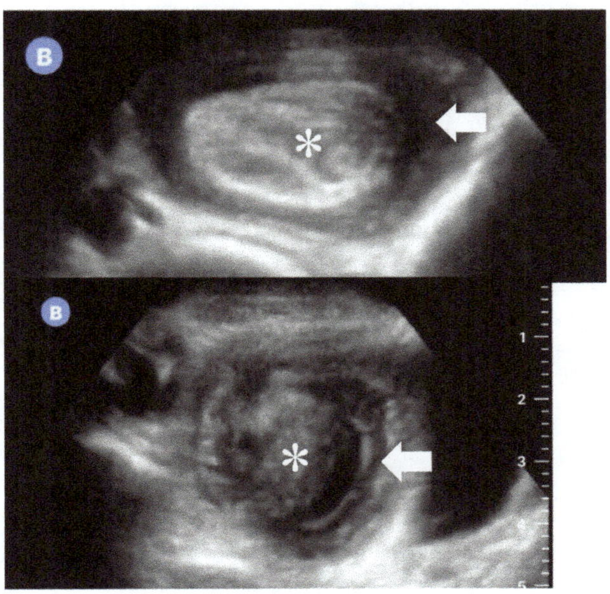

Fig. 2 Abdominal point-of-care ultrasound of a previously healthy 3-year-old male with abdominal pain, nausea, and vomiting diagnosed with intussusception, confirmed and treated by air contrast enema. **a** reveals a stereotypical "target sign", hyperechoic compressed inner loop of bowel (*) telescoping within a hypoechoic, edematous outer loop (arrow). **b** reveals the target sign in another cross sectional plane, with multiple layers of telescoping bowel

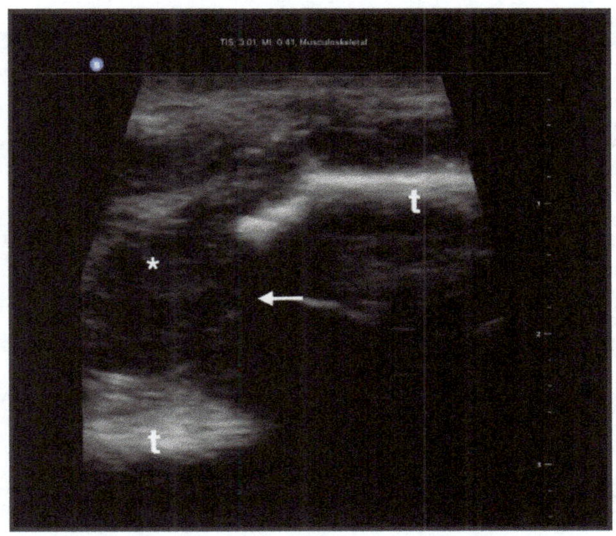

Fig. 3 Musculoskeletal ultrasound of a young male patient with blunt trauma demonstrating two separate sections of tibial cortex (t), with displacement (arrows). Note the associated fracture hematoma visualized (*)

Conclusion

The Butterfly iQ was employed in a wide variety of patient presentations, scanning indications, and procedural guidance in a busy, high acuity RLS ED. Advantages include its use of a single probe for multiple functions, small size, relatively low cost, and good image quality in most functions. Disadvantages include large probe

Table 3 Procedures guided by Butterfly iQ in an African Emergency Department

"Easy IJ"—peripheral IV cannula placed in internal jugular vein for short-term resuscitation [4]
Peripheral IV cannulation
Endotracheal tube placement [5]
Foreign body localization and removal
Paracentesis
Thoracentesis

footprint, lower, though adequate, cardiac imaging quality, frequent overheating, and reliance on internet-based cloud storage, but these were surmountable. We believe the iQ is an effective POCUS device for emergency care in the RLS and we will continue to employ it for patient care and clinical teaching.

Abbreviations
ED: Emergency department; POCUS: Point-of-care ultrasound; RLS: Resource-limited settings.

Acknowledgements
Not applicable.

Authors' contributions
SLB—primary and corresponding author, manuscript conceptualization, image acquisition, image interpretation and review, table and figure visualization, editing and revision. JFS—secondary author, manuscript conceptualization, image acquisition, image interpretation and review, table and figure visualization, editing and revision. EFS—manuscript conceptualization, image acquisition, image interpretation and review, table and figure visualization, editing and revision. DWW—manuscript conceptualization, image acquisition, image interpretation and review, table and figure visualization, editing and revision. MAH—manuscript conceptualization, image interpretation and review, table and figure visualization, editing and revision. JCC—manuscript conceptualization, image interpretation and review, table and figure visualization, editing and revision. DCP—manuscript conceptualization, image interpretation and review, editing and revision. JPG—manuscript conceptualization, image interpretation and review, editing and revision. MAT—manuscript conceptualization, image interpretation and review, editing and revision. CJG—manuscript conceptualization, image acquisition, table and figure visualization, editing and revision. All authors read and approved the final manuscript.

Authors' information
Authors' information was included under section PERSONELL AND SETTING: Five emergency physicians from the United States worked alongside the ED staff of a busy referral hospital in rural east Africa treating medical and surgical patients of all ages over a period of 10 consecutive weeks in the fall of 2019. All physicians have surpassed accepted ultrasound training guidelines [1]. Two (SLB and JFS) have completed or are enrolled in a Point-of-care Ultrasound in Resource Limited Settings fellowship [2]

References

1. Accreditation Council for Graduate Medical Education (2016) Program requirements for graduate medical education in emergency medicine. Revised common program requirements. https://urldefense.proofpoint.com/v2/url?u=https-3A__www.acgme.org_Portals_0_PFAssets_ProgramRequirements_CPRs-5F2017-2D07-2D01.pdf&d=DwIGaQ&c=vh6FgFnduejNhPPD0fl_yRaSfZy8CWbWnIf4XJhSqx8&r=Fh5PU_nOJAk3bM1eZddWH6GpaXEY-HwRMRuAL39fctDlnX_DZuA9PluyOke3kpyc&m=VgMJL2jdkUc8-OiH1iVkdBhkf3nGrnkifYBSKRWdrac&s=CjncrAgZvc4a_PEkxXSdMVJ_WmPgbfF10kjzvm5uDR0&e=. Accessed 27 Nov 2020
2. Burleson SL, Pigott DC, Gullett JP et al (2020) Point-of-care ultrasound in resource-limited settings: the PURLS fellowship. Ultrasound J 12:14
3. Huson MAM, Kaminstein D, Kahn D et al (2019) Cardiac ultrasound in resource-limited settings (CURLS): towards a wider use of basic echo applications in Africa. Ultrasound J 11:34
4. Zitek T, Buby E, Hudson H et al (2018) Ultrasound-guided placement of single-lumen peripheral intravenous catheters in the internal jugular vein. West J Emerg Med 19(5):808–812
5. Gottlieb M, Holladay D, Burns KM et al (2019) Ultrasound for airway management: an evidence-based review for the emergency clinician. Am J Emerg Med. https://doi.org/10.1016/j.ajem.2019/12.019

17

Development and implementation of a point of care ultrasound curriculum at a multi-site institution

Frances M. Russell[1*], Audrey Herbert[1], Robinson M. Ferre[1], Bita Zakeri[2], Valerie Echeverria[3], Dina Peterson[3] and Paul Wallach[4]

Abstract

In 2014, over 60% of medical schools were incorporating point of care ultrasound (POCUS) into their curriculum. Today, over 6 years later, many more schools are teaching POCUS or are in the planning stages of implementing a POCUS curriculum. In 2019, the AAMC reported that 53 schools or over one-third of US medical schools have multi-site campuses for undergraduate medical education. Implementation of a POCUS educational initiative at a multi-site campus presents unique challenges for teaching a uniform curriculum statewide. This article will discuss the POCUS curriculum and implementation process at a large multi-site institution.

Keywords: Point of care ultrasound, Medical education, Medical students, Integrated curriculum, Multi-site campus

Background

Point of care ultrasound (POCUS) is a limited ultrasound examination used by the clinician at the bedside to answer a focused clinical question, guide treatment decisions and/or for procedural guidance [1–4]. POCUS in undergraduate medical education continues to expand with over 60% of medical schools incorporating this training into their curriculum [5, 6]. In 2018, Indiana University School of Medicine began to plan and implement a 4-year longitudinal POCUS curriculum to train medical students. Indiana University School of Medicine is currently the largest medical school in the United States, with over 360 students per year spread across 9 separate campuses throughout the state of Indiana. The size and geographic distance of the campuses presented unique challenges for teaching POCUS statewide. These same challenges are faced by many multi-site schools across the nation. In this manuscript we discuss the POCUS curriculum and implementation process at a large multi-site institution.

Curriculum development and implementation

POCUS, like many other clinical skills, can be broken down into smaller sub-competencies that can be both individually taught and assessed. These have previously been described for POCUS [7, 8] and include: (1) understanding the indications for a POCUS exam; (2) having the ability to operate an ultrasound machine and obtain interpretable images; (3) recognizing basic pathologic conditions and differentiating those from normal; (4) successfully applying the results of a POCUS exam to a patient's clinical care. The purpose of our curriculum was two-fold: (1) to create a scaffolding to augment learning in anatomy and physical exam; (2) to use POCUS as a clinical skill to aid in diagnosis and procedural assistance.

Integrating this curriculum within 4 years of undergraduate medical education curriculum allowed for cognitive scaffolding across theoretical and practical knowledge and skills learned, ultimately enhancing traditional learning and leading to improved diagnostic and procedural skills. Components of the curriculum

*Correspondence: framruss@iu.edu
[1] Department of Emergency Medicine, Indiana University School of Medicine, 720 Eskenazi Ave, Fifth Third Faculty Office Building, 3rd Floor Emergency Medicine Office, Indianapolis, IN 46202, USA
Full list of author information is available at the end of the article

included online modules, proctored hands-on scanning sessions, open lab time with peer teaching and assessments.

Instructional material and modules

To provide didactic instruction, an online POCUS course was developed that consisted of ultrasound modules that corresponded to instructional material being taught at different time points within the undergraduate medical curriculum. The initial phase of POCUS implementation included sixteen unique modules made available to students prior to hands-on instruction, see Fig. 1.

These modules were developed to augment existing educational objectives, as well as to give students the POCUS foundation and skills necessary to enhance their clinical practice. Modules were divided into diagnostic, procedural and symptom-based categories. Diagnostic modules were divided into beginner and advanced sections. The beginner level of each module focused on anatomic structures, image acquisition and interpretation; the advanced level focused on pathology, interpretation, clinical integration and treatment. The different levels of learning in each module were intentionally designed to increase cognitive scaffolding across the curriculum, leading to deeper levels of understanding of anatomy, pathology and treatment. In the first year of curriculum integration, assessment of 147 students found that 73% watched the online didactics prior to the hands-on scanning session for anatomy, while 27% did not complete the pre-lab assignments.

Hands-on instruction

Proctored hands-on POCUS instruction was integrated into the curriculum throughout multiple classes including anatomy, physical examination skills, clerkships and emergency medicine. During anatomy and physical examination courses, for first and second year students, POCUS labs were required. Depending on the resources available at each campus these labs were held either five times over the year with the content mirroring what the students were learning during dissection or were combined into a single lab with training for the same amount of time.

Survey data collected from 100 first year medical students after anatomy hands-on POCUS instruction, found that 71% agreed that the pre-lab modules helped prepare them to manipulate the US equipment, while 11% disagreed. Eighty-seven percent reported increased confidence with identifying the gallbladder and performing a cardiac exam after the lab, while 1% felt it worsened their ability. The majority of students commented that they "would have liked more time" in the curriculum to learn ultrasound. Survey data collected from 108s year students after their physical examination hands-on POCUS instruction, found that 91% agreed that the pre-lab modules helped prepare them to manipulate the US equipment, while 2% disagreed. Ninety-eight percent reported increased confidence with performing a FAST and cardiac exam after the lab. Two percent were neutral and none felt that the lab worsened their ability.

During clerkships and emergency medicine rotations for third and fourth year students, hands-on instruction was required during orientation and available throughout the rotation depending on the site. During hands-on labs students performed peer-to-peer scanning or used a standardized patient.

Introduction:
Physics, Knobology, Orientation

Diagnostic:
Aorta, Breast, Cardiac and IVC, Extended FAST (trauma ultrasound), First trimester obstetric, Gallbladder, Kidneys and bladder volume, Lung, Ocular, and Soft tissue

Procedural:
Nerve blocks, Paracentesis, Thoracentesis and Vascular access (central and peripheral)

Symptom based/resuscitation:
Rapid ultrasound for hypotension (RUSH protocol), and Ultrasound in shortness of breath

Fig. 1 POCUS Modules

Open scanning labs

Open scanning labs were optional and offered to students as an additional opportunity to gain hands-on experience and to further review the module content. Open labs were promoted through the school's electronic newsletter and intranet site. For first and second year medical students labs were held every other week at each campus and scheduled to coincide with free-time built into the students' curricular program. These sessions were proctored by a registered diagnostic medical sonographer or a sonography student to ensure expert guidance. For third and fourth year medical students labs were held once a month and were not proctored.

Assessments

We started assessments during the second year of implementation. Within the anatomy course we added post-lab knowledge assessment questions to the already existing end of block examinations. These assessments included true/false and multiple choice questions, and covered anatomic structures on POCUS images and image acquisition. Assessments have yet to be added to the physical examination course and clerkships; however, we plan on adding assessments in an objective structure clinical examination (OSCE) format and using simulation for identification of pathology and incorporation into clinical practice.

Feedback

Feedback was imperative for successful implementation of this educational initiative. We regularly collected feedback from both students and faculty to continually adjust and improve the experience for both. Feedback was mainly collected through post-lab surveys and directly from students (representative of years 1–3) who sat on the POCUS committee. Faculty feedback regarding the design of the curriculum, online modules and training sessions was critical to the development and integration POCUS into the existing curriculum.

Equipment

Physical space and POCUS equipment were key components in planning a longitudinal POCUS experience across all 9 campuses. Diagnostic POCUS machines are expensive and physical space to house them can be challenging to find. Ancillary equipment (e.g., ultrasound gel, tables for models to lay on, cleaning solution, towels for draping, etc.) required for hands-on scanning labs was also an important consideration in budgeting and planning.

After exploring different types of POCUS equipment, it was evident that handheld POCUS equipment offered several advantages over larger cart-based imaging systems. Handheld POCUS equipment could be purchased at a fraction of the cost and secure storage of these devices required little space. Handheld equipment could also be checked out to individual users for several days at a time, thus allowing equipment to be used outside of dedicated lab time.

Taking into consideration quality, cost and diversity of the handheld devices equal numbers of Butterfly iQ (Butterfly Network, Inc, Guilford, CT, USA) and Philips Lumify (Philips North America Corp, Andover, MA, USA) devices were purchased. Having two different machines provided variation in POCUS educational tools for learners. Butterfly iQ uses CMET technology, which enables a single probe the ability to image both superficial and deep structures. We purchased Lumify phased array probes to image cardiac, lung and abdomen.

Simulators

Simulators were bought with the idea of teaching procedural guidance, introducing students to pathology on POCUS and learning clinical integration. For this reason Blue Phantom (CAE, Inc, Montreal, Quebec, Canada) and SonoSim LiveScan (SonoSim, Inc, Santa Monica, CA) were purchased for all campuses. During the Anesthesia clerkship a hands-on ultrasound guided vascular access lab was taught using the vascular models. These branched vessel ultrasound phantoms served as low fidelity simulators and were reusable.

SonoSim LiveScan was incorporated into the physical examination course hands-on lab for second year students in a case based format to illustrate pathology and for students to get comfortable incorporating POCUS into clinical practice.

Location and check out procedure for equipment

Selection of an optimal space to both store equipment and train learners across all 9 campuses in an equitable manner was important. We chose the simulation center, medical library and hospital space designated for teaching. The space used varied by campus based on availability, size and accessibility for students. Handheld POCUS devices and tablets were securely stored in locked cabinets at each site along with other necessary supplies such as gel and cleaning solution.

In addition to scheduled POCUS events, faculty and students could check-out equipment to practice scanning. A reservation software program was used to reserve and track equipment and track the length of check-out time. Detailed instructions for checking out equipment were disseminated through the school using a newsletter and intranet site.

Coordination with stakeholders

To implement a longitudinal POCUS curriculum at a multi-site campus, key sponsors, educators and course directors were initially identified across the state. Under the direction of the Executive Associate Dean for Educational Affairs a POCUS committee was created to coordinate and communicate with key stakeholders. Members of this committee included faculty of diagnostic radiology, ultrasound-trained emergency medicine faculty, radiology faculty, medical students from each phase of education and a program manager.

The POCUS committee developed, piloted and subsequently oversaw a phased implementation of the 4-year curriculum. To incorporate the POCUS modules within the existing courses, the committee worked collaboratively with course directors and local and regional deans to develop a plan for deployment of the curriculum within the targeted courses at all sites. Communication at multiple levels was crucial in synchronizing the integration of POCUS across the state.

In addition, a point of care ultrasound advisory committee was developed at the onset, and members consisted of phase Deans, multidisciplinary ultrasound trained faculty, and simulation center leadership. The initial focus of this group was to coordinate implementation strategies across the state, disseminate information widely, give feedback and collaborate with key stakeholders. The committee was successful in creating a space to network and collaborate with invested faculty from across multiple departments. However, the committee became less active through the implementation process. The plan, as the curriculum is further improved and expanded, is that the advisory committee will stay involved.

Finding local champions

Local champions, with expertise in POCUS and teaching, spearheaded training and implementation of the curriculum on each campus. We identified regional campus champions through regional deans' recommendation and through individuals who nominated themselves. Student enthusiasm for this initiative, availability of resources, along with support of the regional campus deans presented an inviting opportunity for faculty to get involved. These faculty worked directly with the central POCUS planning team. Regional champions locally guided faculty and student training, phased implementation of POCUS modules within the curriculum and ensured an equitable student learning experience across all campuses.

Faculty education

Lack of faculty skill and confidence in performing and teaching POCUS remains a large barrier to implementation of a longitudinal curriculum and holds true especially at a multisite campus, where instruction is bound geographically [5, 6]. We held multiple continuing medical education (CME) accredited training sessions for faculty in an effort to increase POCUS utilization and medical student teaching by varied faculty across the school. These sessions were promoted over email and offered during different days and times of the week to increase the number of opportunities for participants to attend. Almost 80 faculty across multiple specialties completed a 6-h POCUS CME training workshop. These workshops included didactics and hands-on instruction covering multiple exam types. A primary goal of these workshops was to increase confidence and knowledge with POCUS and give faculty the tools to teach POCUS to medical students. Data analysis of 78 faculty participants found that a majority of the faculty were novice to ultrasound (68%). By assessing confidence, knowledge and skill we found that after a short training faculty had increased confidence with using and teaching POCUS ($p<0.01$), showed improved knowledge from 50 to 86% ($p<0.01$) and were able to correctly identify anatomic structures with ultrasound with good image quality [9].

Interprofessional

While faculty training was being implemented, senior sonography students with an interest in POCUS, ultrasound fellows and fourth year medical students who had previously completed a 1-month elective in POCUS served as a critical resource for medical student training. Sonography students served as proctors during required and independent hands-on labs.

Ultrasound fellows and fourth year medical students, likewise, served as instructors during required hands-on labs. Lab facilitator guides were created, which included objectives of the lab, required images to obtain and tips for acquiring images. These, in addition to the modules, were available online and reviewed by proctors prior to lab.

Placement of POCUS within the curriculum

Sixteen modules were included in the initial POCUS curriculum. The content of these modules were compared to the existing curriculum to decide, where each module would best fit. Anatomy and physical examination courses were identified as two subject areas, where POCUS would augment the curriculum. POCUS modules were divided into beginner and advanced. Beginner modules included anatomy and image acquisition and these were incorporated into the anatomy course. For these modules we focused on content that would subsequently be used in clinical POCUS exams. For example, dedicated modules that focused on anatomic structures identifiable on cardiac ultrasound were developed. Students were able to use POCUS to visualize anatomic structures in real-time, using POCUS views that would later be incorporated into the clinical evaluation of patients. This served to not only supplement existing curriculum, but to also serve as a foundation for future POCUS education see Fig. 2.

During the clinical phase of the curriculum, placement of POCUS modules were paired to the respective clerkship, where they were most applicable. For example, first trimester obstetric ultrasound was chosen for implementation in the obstetrics and gynecology clerkship, extended focus assessment of sonography in trauma was implemented in the surgery clerkship, etc. As many faculty in these specialties already use targeted POCUS in their practice, existing faculty skill and knowledge base could, therefore, be capitalized.

Piloting curriculum

To evaluate the feasibility of implementation and achievement of educational objectives, we piloted the POCUS curriculum at one regional campus in the anatomy course. Three sessions were held throughout the

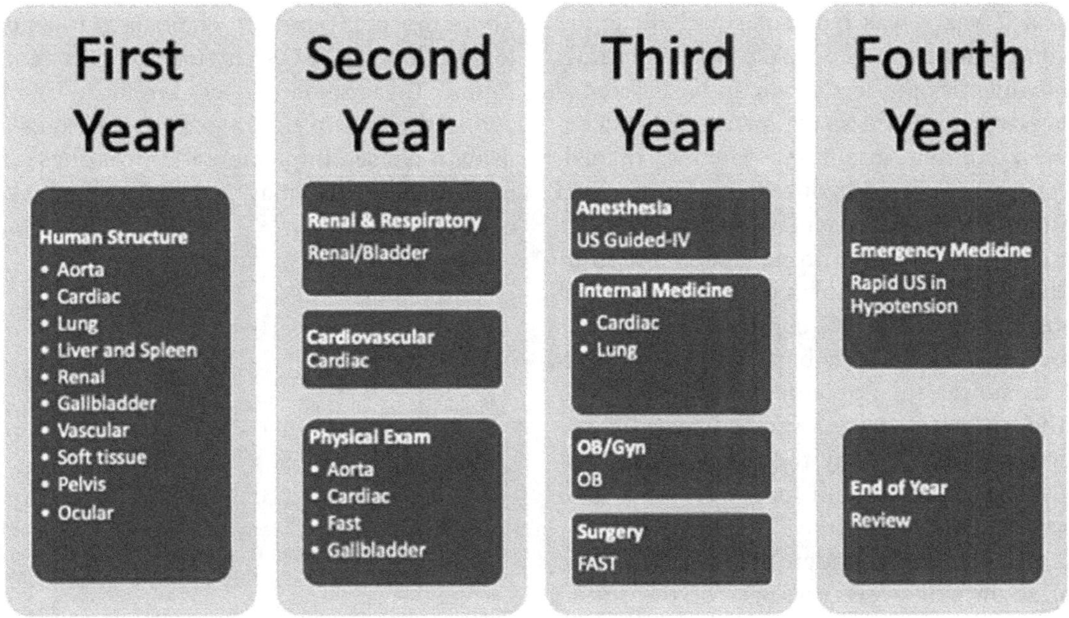

Fig. 2 Undergraduate medical education curriculum showing where POCUS modules were implemented, specifically in which year of schooling and in what course

year using asynchronous viewing of online modules and hands-on instruction to deliver content. Students were then surveyed regarding implementation of POCUS within anatomy. Survey data of 40 students after course implementation found that 100% of students indicated that ultrasound enhanced their understanding of anatomy, and found adding ultrasound to anatomy lab to be beneficial to their learning. We found the piloted curriculum to be feasible and well received by both faculty and students. The following year it was implemented across all nine campuses.

Phased implementation

Due to resource limitations, including time in current curriculum and lack of trained faculty, POCUS was implemented using a phased approach. We started by integrating POCUS into anatomy, clerkships and emergency medicine. These areas were targeted as they required the least amount of training and resources, or already had a POCUS component. In addition, independent scanning labs were offered throughout the year. The following year we expanded to the physical examination and pathophysiology courses. We also added in knowledge assessments to the anatomy course. Using a phased approach we were able to ensure an equivalent POCUS experience for students across all campuses. Additionally, it allowed more faculty to gain more exposure to POCUS without the curriculum becoming overwhelming.

Student consent form

Consent was required from a student if they volunteered to serve as an ultrasound model at any time. An electronic consent form was developed specifically for this use. All students were asked to accept or decline participation as a model for other students or learners in an educational setting. The form was placed within the Medical Student Administration System, which is a student portal. All first-year students were instructed to complete the consent form during their anatomy course. POCUS hands-on lab facilitators verified consent completion prior to any hands-on scanning. Students could change consent status at any time.

Development of an US Website

The POCUS website was created with the intent to have all information stored in one central location that could be easily disseminating in a timely fashion to all faculty, staff and medical students. The website houses modules, lab facilitator guides, equipment check-out procedures, open lab times and consent forms.

Amendments and future directions

Implementing a POCUS curriculum across a large multi-site medical school has been successful, in large part because of support from the executive leadership, collaboration with key stakeholders and the universal positive reception from medical students. Each of these three elements have been and remain critical for success. Competition for curricular space and time within the first 2 years was particularly challenging. Our staged implementation approach with centrally created online didactics put less strain on basic science faculty and created time and space for them to incorporate this new content into their courses. Indeed, due to the logistical constraints of a multi-site medical school, the initial aims of curricular integration were focused on creating material, training faculty and finding time within the existing curriculum. Creation of didactic content by the POCUS committee and finding local experts to assist with hands-on instruction proved vital to successful implementation. However, we believe, the ultimate success and longevity of the curriculum will be measured by the uptake and ownership from course directors and local educators, and not the central POCUS committee.

By design, assessment of student's POCUS knowledge and hands-on skill were not part of the initial implementation of the curriculum. Incorporating knowledge-based assessment into pre-existing testing strategies, such as pre-existing block exams, has and will continue to be important for integration. Skill-based assessments are being planned for clinical rotations with the plan to incorporate hands-on POCUS assessment into pre-existing OSCEs that occur at the end of third year. While standardized patients do not have pathology, students will be required to perform the appropriate POCUS exam, identifying to examiners the anatomy and location of the pathologic findings germane to the case. They will then be given images of pathology for the case, asked to interpret the images and apply them to the patient in the exam scenario. For pre-clinical years, this coming academic year we will begin skill-based assessment as students submit images for review, which they will upload to our learning management system and graded using a simple rubric.

Finally, while not focused on the individual student, we plan to introduce competitive gamification of POCUS during the fourth year, similar to what has previously been described [10]. Subject material would be comprehensive from all 4 years of POCUS instruction. Teams of students would compete at stations designed to assess knowledge and or specific skill.

While national curricular standards do not exist for POCUS integration, professional organizations like Society of Ultrasound in Medical Education (SUSME) allow for sharing of ideas and resources for schools looking to begin a POCUS curriculum. Content sharing through MedED Portal and Canvas Commons are additional ways we hope to share our experience and content.

Conclusion

There are many unique challenges to implementing a longitudinal POCUS curriculum at a multi-site institution. These same barriers are faced by many schools across the country. This report describes an approach using a phased implementation that has been found to be successful, and may serve as a reference for POCUS curriculum design.

Acknowledgements
None.

Authors' contributions
FMR, AH, RMF, BZ were responsible for concept. FMR takes responsibility for paper as a whole. All authors read and approved the final manuscript.

Author details
[1] Department of Emergency Medicine, Indiana University School of Medicine, 720 Eskenazi Ave, Fifth Third Faculty Office Building, 3rd Floor Emergency Medicine Office, Indianapolis, IN 46202, USA. [2] Education and Continuing Medical Education, Indiana University School of Medicine, Indianapolis, IN, USA. [3] Indiana University School of Medicine, Indianapolis, IN, USA. [4] Department of Internal Medicine, Office of the Dean, Indiana University School of Medicine, Indianapolis, IN, USA.

References

1. Moore CL, Copel JA (2011) Point-of-care ultrasonography. N Engl J Med 364(8):749–757
2. Smith-Bindman R, Aubin C, Bailitz J, Bengiamin B, Camargo C, Corbo J, Dean AJ, Goldstein RB, Griffey RT, Jay GD, Kang TL, Kriesel DR, Ma OJ, Mallin M, Manson W, Melnikow J, Miglioretti DL, Miller SK, Mills LD, Miner JR, Moghadassi M, Noble VE, Press GM, Stoller ML, Valencia VE, Wang J, Wang RC, Cummings SR (2014) Ultrasonography versus computed tomography for suspected nephrolithiasis. N Engl J Med 371:1100–1110
3. Jones AE, Tayal VS, Sullivan DM, Kline JA (2004) Randomized, controlled trial of immediate versus delayed goal-directed ultrasound to identify the cause of nontraumatic hypotension in emergency department patients. Crit Care Med 32(8):1703–1708
4. Melniker L, Leibner E, McKenney MG, Lopez P, Briggs WM, Mancuso CA (2006) Randomized controlled clinical trial of point-of-care, limited ultrasonography for trauma in the emergency department: the first sonography outcomes assessment program trial. Ann Emerg Med 48(3):227–235
5. Rempell JS, Saldana F, DiSalvo D (2016) Pilot point-of-care ultrasound curriculum at harvard medical school: early experience. West J Emerg 17(6):734–740
6. David P, Bahner DP, Goldman E, Way D, Royall NA, Liu YT (2014) The state of ultrasound Education in U.S. medical schools: results of a national survey. Acad Med 89(12):1681–1686
7. Damewood SC, Leo M, Bailitz J, Gottlieb M, Liu R, Hoffmann B, Gaspari RJ (2020) Tools for measuring clinical ultrasound competency: recommendations from the ultrasound competency work group. AEM Educ Train 4(Suppl 1):S106–S112
8. (2017) Ultrasound guidelines: emergency, point-of-care and clinical ultrasound guidelines in medicine. Ann Emerg Med 69(5):e27–e54
9. Russell FM, Herbert A, Zakeri B, Blaha M, Ferre RM, Sarmiento EJ, Wallach PW (2020) Training the trainer: faculty from across multiple specialties show improved confidence, knowledge and skill in point of care ultrasound after a short intervention. Cureus 12(12):e11821
10. Lewiss RE, Hayden GE, Murray A, Liu YT, Panebianco N, Liteplo AS (2014) SonoGames: an innovative approach to emergency medicine resident ultrasound education. J Ultrasound Med 33(10):1843–1849

18

The role of point-of-care ultrasound in the diagnosis of pericardial effusion: a single academic center retrospective study

Matthew G. Hanson[1] and Barry Chan[2*]

Abstract

Background: Symptomatic pericardial effusion (PCE) presents with non-specific features and are often missed on the initial physical exam, chest X-ray (CXR), and electrocardiogram (ECG). In extreme cases, misdiagnosis can evolve into decompensated cardiac tamponade, a life-threatening obstructive shock. The purpose of this study is to evaluate the impact of point-of-care ultrasound (POCUS) on the diagnosis and therapeutic intervention of clinically significant PCE.

Methods: In a retrospective chart review, we looked at all patients between 2002 and 2018 at a major Canadian academic hospital who had a pericardiocentesis for clinically significant PCE. We extracted the rate of presenting complaints, physical exam findings, X-ray findings, ECG findings, time-to-diagnosis, and time-to-pericardiocentesis and how these were impacted by POCUS.

Results: The most common presenting symptom was dyspnea (64%) and the average systolic blood pressure (SBP) was 120 mmHg. 86% of people presenting had an effusion > 1 cm, and 89% were circumferential on departmental echocardiogram (ECHO) with 64% having evidence of right atrial systolic collapse and 58% with early diastolic right ventricular collapse. The average time-to-diagnosis with POCUS was 5.9 h compared to > 12 h with other imaging including departmental ECHO. Those who had the PCE identified by POCUS had an average time-to-pericardiocentesis of 28.1 h compared to > 48 h with other diagnostic modalities.

Conclusion: POCUS expedites the diagnosis of symptomatic PCE given its non-specific clinical findings which, in turn, may accelerate the time-to-intervention.

Keywords: Pericardial effusion, Point-of-care ultrasound, Diagnosis

Introduction

Pericardial effusion (PCE) is a fluid collection in the pericardial sac which can result in life-threatening cardiac tamponade. Cardiac tamponade occurs when the intrapericardial pressure compresses the cardiac chambers resulting in impaired diastolic filling for which the right heart is most susceptible [1, 2]. The fibrous pericardial sac has limited compliance; therefore, tamponade can be precipitated when small volume of fluid accumulates quickly [3, 4]. Alternatively, subacute accumulation can stretch the pericardium, increasing its compliance, such that higher PCE volume is required to result in tamponade [1, 2, 5]. The pericardial sac generally contains 50 mL of fluid, and effusion size is classified based on the pericardial separation distance during diastole with small effusion being < 10 mm (50–100 mL), moderate effusion as 10–20 mm (100–500 mL), and large effusion > 20 mm (> 500 mL) [4, 6, 7].

Often patients with symptomatic PCE or tamponade present with non-specific symptoms and signs such as

*Correspondence: barrytschan@gmail.com
[2] Division of General Internal Medicine, Department of Medicine, Queen's University, Kingston, ON, Canada
Full list of author information is available at the end of the article

dyspnea, peripheral edema, tachycardia, and elevated jugular venous pressure (JVP) [2, 5]. As such, bedside diagnosis is challenging given the non-specific symptomatology and variable exam findings [3, 5]. Classically, Beck's Triad, comprising hypotension, increased JVP, and quiet/distant heart sounds, has been taught to screen for tamponade at the bedside [2, 8, 9]. However, the triad does not reliably predict the presence of tamponade or significant PCE in over 40% of cases [5]. Other clinical features classically described for PCE or tamponade include tachypnea, tachycardia, and pulsus paradoxus are non-specific [2]. For example, pulsus paradoxus may be present in patients with significant respiratory distress (asthma or chronic obstructive pulmonary disease exacerbation), or any mechanism that exaggerates the interventricular dependence. Conversely, pulsus paradoxus can be absent in patients with left ventricular hypertrophy, hypovolemia or atrial septal defects even in the presence of clinically significant PCE [2, 10, 11]. Some studies have looked at adjuncts to the physical exam including electrocardiogram (ECG) analysis, using chest X-ray (CXR), or point-of-care ultrasound (POCUS) to aid the diagnosis of PCE or cardiac tamponade [5, 8, 10, 12–14]. ECG and CXR lack diagnostic sensitivity, whereas POCUS has been shown to be sensitive, specific, and potentially reduces the time-to-intervention [1, 10, 12].

Echocardiography (ECHO) remains as the gold standard imaging modality to verify the presence of a PCE by demonstrating fluid collection in the pericardial space and interrogating for features of tamponade physiology such as systolic right atrial (RA) collapse, early diastolic right ventricle (RV) collapse, respiratory variations of transvalvular flow [1, 3, 4, 7].

To determine the rate of reported symptoms, physical exam findings, ECG and CXR abnormalities, we looked at all patients who underwent pericardiocentesis between 2002 and 2018 at a Canadian tertiary care hospital. Furthermore, we looked at ECHO findings, the length of time-to-diagnosis and time-to-pericardiocentesis, and how these were affected by POCUS.

Methods

Study design

This chart review was performed from 2002–2018 on patients who underwent pericardiocentesis at Kingston Health Sciences Centre, a tertiary care hospital in Kingston, Ontario, Canada. Ethical consent was obtained from the Queen's University Health Sciences & Affiliated Teaching Hospitals Research Ethics Board. Patient electronic medical records were searched for the terms "pericardiocentesis + pericardial tamponade", "pericardiocentesis + cardiac tamponade", and "pericardiocentesis + pericardial effusion".

Patient records were reviewed for the presenting symptomatology, physical examination findings, CXR and ECG reports, POCUS use, time-to-diagnosis, and time-to-pericardiocentesis where available. Demographic data including age, gender, past medical history, and medications were, also, obtained where available.

In terms of POCUS resource at our institution, the prevalence of trained POCUS users in 2002 is unknown though its use was limited to Emergency Medicine. By 2018, 100% of the Emergency Physicians were POCUS users with the majority trained via the Emergency Department ECHO (EDE) 1 program; and 30% of General Internal Medicine were POCUS users with training ranging from part of their subspecialty fellowship program to proprietary training courses such as the Canadian Point of Care Ultrasound Society (CPOCUS). With regard to POCUS machinery, the first mention of the use of POCUS in our study was 2007, at the time, there was a total of 3 POCUS machines all of which were situated in the emergency room. As of 2018, there were 9 machines (1 for Cardiology, 2 for Critical Care, 3 for Emergency Medicine, 3 for General Internal Medicine).

As there is no POCUS archiving and reporting system locally, the beside sonographic findings and interpretation were extracted from written documentation (paper chart or electronic medical record). The CXR and ECG interpretations were derived from the finalized reports of the respective radiologist and cardiologist.

The time-to-diagnosis interval was computed from the time of presentation to the earliest mention of the presence of a PCE for a respective diagnostic modality. The time-to-pericardiocentesis interval was computed from the time of presentation to the earliest mention of the procedure being commenced or underway. Patients requiring more than one pericardiocentesis during a given visit only had the first procedure considered for the study. The differences in the means of the presenting hemodynamic profiles between the groups that was first diagnosed via POCUS and departmental ECHO were analyzed with the Welch's t-test with the threshold p-value adjusted through the Bonferroni correction.

Data are reported as an overall average of all charts and include those where data were unavailable in the denominator unless otherwise specified. Statistical analysis was performed with Statistical Package for Social Sciences (SPSS) Version 26.

Results

Baseline characteristics

The search algorithm returned 342 unique charts

In all comers receiving pericardiocentesis, the average age was 63.3 ± 14 years and males were slightly more common than females (56 vs 44%, respectively). The most common comorbid conditions were hypertension (37%) and malignancy (27%) (Table 1). 79 were procedurally related PCE (23%) with ablation for atrial fibrillation/flutter being the most common cause.

Upon review of all the charts available via the search terms which included "Pericardiocentesis", the procedures were all performed as inpatient.

Most common presentation complaint, physical exam, ECG, CXR findings

The most common presenting complaint was dyspnea which was present in 66% of patients; and 41% had elevated JVP.

Most patients had compensated initial hemodynamics where 43% had a normal heart rate and only 9.6% were hypotensive with SBP ≤ 90 mmHg.

Table 1 Baseline characteristics ($n = 342$)

Age (years)	63.3 ± 14.1
Gender	*n* (%)
Male	193 (56)
Female	149 (44)
Cardiovascular risk factors	
Hypertension	127 (37)
Diabetes	65 (19)
Coronary artery disease	59 (17)
Atrial fibrillation/flutter	63 (18)
Inflammatory conditions	
Rheumatologic conditions	25 (7)
Pericarditis	10 (3)
Malignancy	91 (27)
Recent cardiac procedure	31 (9)
Hemodynamics on presentation	
Systolic blood pressure (mmHg)	121 ± 27
Diastolic blood pressure (mmHg)	72 ± 14
Systolic blood pressure ≤ 90 mmHg (*n*) (%)	33 (9.6)
Heart rate (beats per minute)	94 ± 22
On oral anticoagulation	
Warfarin	26 (8)
Direct oral anticoagulant	5 (1)
Other cardiac medications	
ACE inhibitor/angiotensin receptor blocker	88 (26)
Alpha-blocker	18 (5)
Beta-blocker	77 (23)
Dihydropyridine calcium channel blocker	37 (11)
Non-dihydropyridine calcium channel blocker	22 (6)
Diuretics	81 (24)
Anti-arrhythmics	29 (8)
Vasodilators	9 (3)

47% had tachycardia on ECG at the time of presentation; and 54% had cardiomegaly on CXR. The remainder of other clinical features, ECG, and radiographic findings are tabulated in Table 2.

Modality of initial diagnosis, time-to-diagnosis, and time-to-intervention

For non-procedurally related PCE, 35.5% were identified by departmental ECHO, 23.3% via POCUS, and 19.8% through other imaging modalities for which computed tomography (CT) scan was most common.

The time-to-diagnosis with POCUS and departmental ECHO were on average 5.9 h and 45.1 h, respectively. Time-to-pericardiocentesis was 28.1 h in the POCUS group in comparison to 49 h for the departmental ECHO group (Table 3). After adjustment with the Bonferroni correction (p-value threshold < 0.0167 is considered to indicate statistical significance), there was no statistical difference between the presenting hemodynamic profile between the two groups (Table 4).

Echocardiography

Of all patients who received a pericardiocentesis and had a measured effusion pocket, 67% had a PCE ≥ 2 cm, 17% were 1–2 cm, and 3.5% with < 1 cm. 89% had circumferential effusion (Table 5). 64% had evidence of systolic

Table 2 Presenting symptoms, physical exam, electrocardiogram, and chest X-ray findings ($n = 342$)

	Yes *n* (%)	No *n* (%)	Not available *n* (%)
Presenting symptoms			
Dyspnea	227 (66)	52 (15)	63 (18)
Orthopnea	51 (15)	151 (44)	140 (41)
Chest pain	108 (32)	151 (44)	83 (24)
Presyncope	45 (13)	184 (54)	113 (33)
Syncope	20 (6)	208 (61)	114 (33)
Peripheral edema	41 (12)	189 (55)	112 (33)
Physical exam			
Respiratory distress	67 (20)	183 (54)	220 (64)
Pulsus paradoxus (> 10 mmHg)	123 (36)	168 (49)	51 (15)
Muffled heart sound	10 (3)	271 (79)	61 (18)
Elevated jugular venous pulse	140 (41)	188 (55)	14 (4)
Electrocardiogram			
Sinus tachycardia	161 (47)	153 (45)	28 (8)
Low voltage	123 (36)	168 (49)	51 (15)
Alternans	10 (3)	271 (79)	61 (18)
Chest X-ray			
Cardiomegaly	184 (54)	55 (16)	103 (30)
Pulmonary edema	15 (4)	227 (66)	100 (29)

Table 3 Diagnostic modality, time-to-diagnosis, and time-to-intervention (non-procedure related $n = 263$)

Initial diagnostic modality (n)	Time-to-diagnosis in hours (n)	Time-to-pericardiocentesis in hours (n)
Departmental ECHO (93)	45.1(35)	49.0 (67)
POCUS (61)	5.9 (47)	28.1 (55)
Other[a] (53)	12.0 (30)	56.1 (45)
Not available (56)	–	–

[a] Other imaging includes CT ($n = 49$), abdominal ultrasound ($n = 1$), cardiac MRI ($n = 1$), and ventilation/perfusion (VQ) scan ($n = 1$), intraoperative transesophageal ECHO ($n = 1$)

right atrial (RA) collapse, and 58% had early diastolic right ventricular (RV) collapse.

Discussion

PCE is challenging to diagnose clinically. Larose et al. noted 80% of 50 cardiac tamponade who necessitated pericardiocentesis received either the wrong diagnosis (36%) or not considered as part of the differential diagnosis (44%) [15]. The most common symptom is dyspnea is non-specific for clinically significant PCE. Furthermore, many of the classically taught physical exam findings do not accurately rule in or out PCE. In comparison to a meta-analysis by Jacob et al. to our review, 54% (33–74%) vs 41% had elevated JVP, 22% (11–34%) vs 15% with muffled heart sounds, and hypotension in 28% (14–39%) vs 10%, respectively [5]. The difference in the rates of hypotension could be explained by patient population selection. In the meta-analysis, the study with the highest hypotension rate (39%), iatrogenic PCE accounted for 31% of the cases whereas our study was 23%. Trauma and surgically related PCE tend to develop acute tamponade in comparison to medical etiologies. In addition, majority of the studies took place in the 1980s (1963–1997) and comparing to a more contemporary review [16] only 15% patients presenting to the emergency department with non-traumatic causes of cardiac tamponade were hypotensive on arrival which was similar with our findings. Gandhi et al. also, noted there was less hypotensive

Table 4 Comparison of hemodynamics on presentation of the POCUS and departmental ECHO groups with the Welch's *t*-test

	POCUS ($n = 75$)	Departmental ECHO ($n = 126$)	Mean difference	p-value[a]
Mean systolic blood pressure (mmHg)	112 (95% CI 107–117)	121 (95% CI 116–126)	8.3 (95% CI 1.2–15.5)	0.022
Mean diastolic blood pressure (mmHg)	73 (95% CI 69–77)	73 95% CI 70–76)	0.63 (95% CI −3.6–4.9)	0.77
Mean heart rate (beats per minute)	99 (95% CI 94–104)	94 (95% CI 82–106)	−5.4 (95% CI −11–0.3)	0.63

[a] With the Bonferroni adjustment, a p-value of < 0.0167 is considered to indicate statistical significance

Table 5 Departmental echocardiographic findings

	All ($N = 342$)			Non-procedural etiology ($N = 263$)			Iatrogenic/procedural etiology ($N = 79$)		
	Yes	No	Not available	Yes	No	Not available	Yes	No	Not available
Right atrial collapse	219 (64%)	68 (20%)	55 (16%)	187 (71%)	47 (18%)	29 (11%)	32 (41%)	21 (27%)	26 (33%)
Right ventricle collapse	199 (58%)	89 (26%)	54 (16%)	164 (62%)	7 (27%)	28 (11%)	35 (44%)	18 (23%)	26 (33%)
Left atrial collapse	10 (3%)	275 (80%)	57 (17%)	8 (3%)	225 (86%)	30 (11%)	2 (3%)	50 (63%)	27 (34%)
Left ventricle collapse	4 (1%)	282 (83%)	56 (16%)	2 (1%)	231 (89%)	30 (11%)	2 (3%)	51 (65%)	26 (33%)
Significant respiratory variation	98 (29%)	41 (12%)	203 (59%)	86 (33%)	33 (13%)	144 (55%)	12 (15%)	8 (10%)	59 (75%)
Mechanical alternans	8 (2%)	36 (11%)	298 (87%)	8 (3%)	32 (12%)	223 (85%)	0 (0%)	4 (5%)	75 (95%)
Effusion location									
Circumferential	307 (90%)			255 (97%)			52 (66%)		
Regional	19 (6%)			6 (2%)			13 (16%)		
Not available	16 (4%)			2 (1%)			14 (18%)		
Deepest effusion pocket (measured during diastole)									
< 1 cm	13 (4%)			5 (2%)			8 (10%)		
1–2 cm	57 (17%)			41 (16%)			16 (20%)		
> 2 cm	228 (67%)			204 (78%)			24 (30%)		
Not available	33 (10%)			11 (4%)			22 (28%)		
Pericardial clot	11 (3%)			2 (1%)			9 (11%)		

presentation (32% vs 15%) comparing cardiac tamponade cohorts from 1998–1991 to 2002–2005 [19]. This could be explained by an increased index of suspicion for the condition over the past decade [19] and access to echocardiography to assist in the diagnosis [20].

In our study, many were hemodynamically compensated on presentation with fewer than 10% being hypotensive despite 84% of all cases had moderate-to-large effusions with > 50% having RA and/or RV collapse. This is in keeping with previous studies that demonstrated normotension or even hypertension in patients with subacute or chronic PCE accumulation resulting in cardiac tamponade [16–18]. These echocardiographic-to-clinical discrepancies illustrate the hemodynamic spectrum spanning from subclinical to clinically overt yet compensated to outright decompensatory shock [11, 18].

Given the insidious nature of PCE, evaluation with POCUS could reduce the time-to-diagnosis which had truncated by 39 h in our study. In terms of time-to-pericardiocentesis, our data demonstrated the POCUS group received the intervention 21 h earlier than the departmental ECHO group. A smaller retrospective study by Alert et al. found a similar signal whereby the POCUS arm received pericardiocentesis 59 h earlier than the control [12]. However, this trend towards diagnostic and interventional efficiency should be interpreted with caution. Intuitively, POCUS would readily allow significant PCE to be identified, therefore leading to earlier diagnosis and intervention if indicated. Conversely, those who are sicker may more likely receive POCUS interrogation by the concerned physician—a selection bias. In our study, however, there was no significant hemodynamic difference between the two groups on presentation. Perhaps this could be explained by an increase use of POCUS as training programs foster the skillset into their curriculums. As of 2012, 100% of Fellow of the Royal College of Physicians of Canada–Emergency Medicine residency programs (FRCPC-EM) and 88% of the Certification in the College of Family Physicians Emergency Medicine (CCFP-EM) residency programs have formally incorporated POCUS as part of their curriculums [21]. A recent national in 2016 amongst Canadian emergency physicians demonstrated an overall increase in POCUS usage compared to 2007 [22]. Critical Care and General Internal Medicine are, also, recommending POCUS training which will foster its clinical utilization [23, 24].

This study has several limitations. First of all, it takes place at a single university hospital, therefore the results may not extrapolate to other systems where the etiological prevalence differs especially in trauma centers.

Secondly, this is a retrospective study spanning from 2002 to 2018 whereby many charts were only partially converted to the electronic version for review and, also, given the lack of systematic history and physical exam findings data documentation, and POCUS archiving system, the dataset is subjected to significant registry bias as certain elements may not have been recorded or explicitly sought. Furthermore, some of the cases were transferred from peripheral hospitals whereby the presenting complaints, vitals, and initial diagnostic tests were not available. Uncaptured PCE that was discovered by POCUS that warranted a pericardiocentesis will affect the time-to-diagnosis and time-to-pericardiocentesis aggregate estimation as well. Nevertheless, as discussed above, the rates determined from our limited study are congruent with to a large meta-analysis [5]. Also, the POCUS group's time-to-diagnosis was on average 39 h less than the group diagnosed via departmental echocardiography. This time margin is quite wide unlikely explainable by exclusion of undocumented POCUS alone.

This study did not include two groups: (a) those who died from cardiac tamponade as they would not have received pericardiocentesis and (b) those who were diagnosed with a PCE and discharged without a pericardiocentesis. As such, their respective time-to-diagnosis intervals are not incorporated into the calculation. However, given both groups did not receive pericardiocentesis, its exclusion will not affect the time-to-pericardiocentesis estimation. Also, the intent of the study is to investigate only those with clinically significant PCE who warranted pericardiocentesis on the same admission.

The estimation of the time-to-diagnosis and time-to-pericardiocentesis is dependent on timestamps from the time of initial presentation to the date and time when the procedure being performed is recorded. As such, the time frame will not be precise to the minute. Consequently, the interval is reported in hours instead which will be less error prone. However, a prospective study is necessitated to verify the value of POCUS upon these definitive endpoints and with current POCUS archiving systems the analysis can be more rigorous.

Conclusion

Clinically significant PCE presents with non-specific findings whereby a high degree of clinical suspicion is necessitated. However, POCUS is a readily available bedside diagnostic tool that can quickly rule in the diagnosis. Whether it may expedite definitive intervention, further studies would be required.

Abbreviations

DBP: Diastolic blood pressure; ECHO: Echocardiogram; ECG: Electrocardiogram; CXR: Chest X-ray; JVP: Jugular venous pulse; LA: Left atrium; LV: Left ventricle; PCE: Pericardial effusion; POCUS: Point-of-care ultrasound; RA: Right atrium; RV: Right ventricle; SBP: Systolic blood pressure; VQ: Ventilation perfusion.

Acknowledgements
Many thanks to Dr. Christopher Smith, Division Head of General Internal Medicine at Queen's University, who has been supportive with this research endeavour.

Authors' contributions
There was no funding provided for this article. Data collection was done by BC, data analysis and manuscript preparation were done by MGH and BC. All authors read and approved the final manuscript.

Author details
[1] Division of Cardiology, Department of Medicine, Queen's University, Kingston, ON, Canada. [2] Division of General Internal Medicine, Department of Medicine, Queen's University, Kingston, ON, Canada.

References

1. Vakamudi S, Ho N, Cremer PC (2017) Pericardial effusions: causes, diagnosis, and management. Prog Cardiovasc Dis 59(4):380–388. https://doi.org/10.1016/j.pcad.2016.12.009
2. Roy CL, Minor MA, Brookhart MA (2007) Does this patient with a pericardial effusion have cardiac tamponade? JAMA 297(16):1810–1818. https://doi.org/10.1001/jama.297.16.1810
3. Ceriani E, Cogliati C (2016) Update on bedside ultrasound diagnosis of pericardial effusion. Intern Emerg Med 11(3):477–480. https://doi.org/10.1007/s11739-015-1372-8
4. Hoit BD (2017) Pericardial effusion and cardiac tamponade in the new millennium. Curr Cardio Rep 19(7):57. https://doi.org/10.1007/s11886-017-0867-5
5. Jacob S, Sebastian JC, Cherian PK, Abraham A, John SK (2009) Pericardial effusion impending tamponade: a look beyond Beck's triad. Am J Emerg Med 27(2):216–219. https://doi.org/10.1016/j.ajem.2008.01.056
6. Azarbal A, LeWinter MM (2017) Pericardial effusion (2017). Cardiol Clin. 35(4):515–524. https://doi.org/10.1016/j.ccl.2017.07.005
7. Alerhand S, Carter JM (2019) What echocardiographic findings suggest a pericardial effusion is causing tamponade? Am J Emerg Med 37(2):321–326. https://doi.org/10.1016/j.ajem.2018.11.004
8. Liu RB, Donroe JH, McNamara RL, Forman HP, Moore CL (2017) The practice and implications of finding fluid during point-of-care ultrasonography: a review. JAMA Intern Med 177(12):1818–1825. https://doi.org/10.1001/jamainternmed.2017.5048
9. Beck CS (1935) Two cardiac compression triads. JAMA 104(9):714–716. https://doi.org/10.1001/jama.1935.02760090018005
10. Argula RG, Negi SI, Banchs J, Yusuf SW (2015) Clinical investigations role of a 12-lead electrocardiogram in the diagnosis of cardiac tamponade as diagnosed by transthoracic echocardiography in patients with malignant pericardial effusion. Clin Cardio 28(3):139–144. https://doi.org/10.1002/clc.22370
11. Argulian E, Messerli F (2013) Misconceptions and facts about pericardial effusion and tamponade. Am J Med 126(1):858–861. https://doi.org/10.1016/j.amjmed.2013.03.022
12. Alpert EA, Amit U, Guranda L, Mahagna R, Grossman SA, Bentancur A (2017) Emergency depart point-of-care ultrasonography improves time to pericardiocentesis for clinically significant effusions. Clin Exp Emerg Med. 4(3):128–132. https://doi.org/10.15441/ceem.16.169
13. Nagdev A, Stone MB (2011) Point-of-care ultrasound evaluation of pericardial effusions: does this patient have cardiac tamponade? Resuscitation 82(6):671–673. https://doi.org/10.1016/j.resuscitation.2011.02.004
14. Mathur AP, Saini A, Lucas BP et al (2013) Diagnostic accuracy retrospectively of electrocardiographic findings and cancer history for tamponade in patients determined to have pericardial effusion by transthoracic echocardiogram. Am J Cardiol 111(7):1062–1066. https://doi.org/10.1016/j.amjcard.2012.11.064
15. Larose E, Ducharme A, Mercier LA et al (2000) Prolonged distress and clinical deterioration before pericardial drainage in patients with cardiac tamponade. Can J Cardiol 16:331–336 (**PMID: 10744796**)
16. Kapoor T, Locurto M, Farina GA et al (2012) Hypotension is uncommon in patients presenting to the emergency department with non-traumatic cardiac tamponade. J Emerg Med 42(2):220–226. https://doi.org/10.1016/j.jemermed.2010.05.071
17. Brown J, MacKinnon D, King A et al (1992) Elevated arterial blood pressure in cardiac tamponade. N Engl J Med 327(7):463–466. https://doi.org/10.1056/nejm199208133270704
18. Reddy PS, Curtiss EI, Uretsky BF (1990) Spectrum of hemodynamic changes in cardiac tamponade. Am J Cardiol 66(20):1487–1491. https://doi.org/10.1016/0002-9149(90)90540-h
19. Gandhi S, Scheneider A, Mohiuddin S et al (2008) Has the clinical presentation and clinician's index of suspicion of cardiac tamponade changed over the past decade. Echocardiography 25(3):237–241. https://doi.org/10.1111/j.1540-8175.2007.00592.x
20. Levine MJ, Lorell BH, Diver DJ et al (1991) Implications of echocardiographically assisted diagnosis of pericardial tamponade in contemporary medical patients: detection before hemodynamic embarrassment. J Am Coll Cardiol 17(1):59–65. https://doi.org/10.1016/0735-1097(91)90704-d
21. Kim DJ, Theoret J, Liao MM et al (2012) The current state of ultrasound training in Canadian emergency medicine programs: perspectives from program directors. Acad Emerg Med 19(9):e1073–e1078. https://doi.org/10.1111/j.1553-2712.2012.01430.x
22. Leschyna M, Hatam E, Britton S et al (2019) Current state of point-of-care ultrasound usage in Canadian emergency departments. Cureus 11(3):e4246. https://doi.org/10.7759/cureus.4246
23. Arntfield RT, Millington SJ, Ainsworth CD et al (2014) Canadian recommendations for critical care ultrasound training and competency. Can Respir J 21(6):341–345. https://doi.org/10.1155/2014/216591
24. Ma IWY, Arishenkoff S, Wiseman J et al (2017) Internal medicine point-of-care ultrasound curriculum: consensus recommendations from the Canadian Internal Medicine Ultrasound (CIMUS) group. J Gen Intern Med 32:1052–1057. https://doi.org/10.1007/s11606-017-4071-5

Comparison of in-person versus tele-ultrasound point-of-care ultrasound training during the COVID-19 pandemic

Nilam J. Soni[1,2,17*], Jeremy S. Boyd[3,4], Gregory Mints[5], Kevin C. Proud[1,2], Trevor P. Jensen[6], Gigi Liu[7], Benji K. Mathews[8], Christopher K. Schott[9,10], Linda Kurian[11], Charles M. LoPresti[12,13], Phil Andrus[14], Robert Nathanson[1,2], Natalie Smith[1,2], Elizabeth K. Haro[1,2], Michael J. Mader[1,2], Jacqueline Pugh[2], Marcos I. Restrepo[1,2] and Brian P. Lucas[15,16]

Abstract

Background: Lack of training is currently the most common barrier to implementation of point-of-care ultrasound (POCUS) use in clinical practice, and in-person POCUS continuing medical education (CME) courses have been paramount in improving this training gap. Due to travel restrictions and physical distancing requirements during the COVID-19 pandemic, most in-person POCUS training courses were cancelled. Though tele-ultrasound technology has existed for several years, use of tele-ultrasound technology to deliver hands-on training during a POCUS CME course has not been previously described.

Methods: We conducted a retrospective observational study comparing educational outcomes, course evaluations, and learner and faculty feedback from in-person versus tele-ultrasound POCUS courses. The same POCUS educational curriculum was delivered to learners by the two course formats. Data from the most recent pre-pandemic in-person course were compared to tele-ultrasound courses during the COVID-19 pandemic.

Results: Pre- and post-course knowledge test scores of learners from the in-person ($n=88$) and tele-ultrasound course ($n=52$) were compared. Though mean pre-course knowledge test scores were higher among learners of the tele-ultrasound versus in-person course (78% vs. 71%; $p=0.001$), there was no significant difference in the post-course test scores between learners of the two course formats (89% vs. 87%; $p=0.069$). Both learners and faculty rated the tele-ultrasound course highly (4.6–5.0 on a 5-point scale) for effectiveness of virtual lectures, tele-ultrasound hands-on scanning sessions, and course administration. Faculty generally expressed less satisfaction with their ability to engage with learners, troubleshoot image acquisition, and provide feedback during the tele-ultrasound course but felt learners completed the tele-ultrasound course with a better basic POCUS skillset.

Conclusions: Compared to a traditional in-person course, tele-ultrasound POCUS CME courses appeared to be as effective for improving POCUS knowledge post-course and fulfilling learning objectives. Our findings can serve as a roadmap for educators seeking guidance on development of a tele-ultrasound POCUS training course whose demand will likely persist beyond the COVID-19 pandemic.

Background

Competency in point-of-care ultrasound (POCUS) requires basic knowledge of ultrasound technology, skills in image acquisition and interpretation, and ability to integrate findings into clinical decision-making.

*Correspondence: sonin@uthscsa.edu
[1] South Texas Veterans Health Care System, San Antonio, TX, USA
Full list of author information is available at the end of the article

Historically, practicing clinicians have gained POCUS skills by attending in-person continuing medical education (CME) courses, and these courses have been shown to be effective [1].

Due to travel restrictions and physical distancing requirements during the COVID-19 pandemic, most in-person POCUS training courses were cancelled, although the demand for POCUS training may have increased given the utility of POCUS in COVID-19 [2]. Many traditional lecture-based CME courses were converted to virtual courses relatively easily during the pandemic, but a major challenge in creating a virtual POCUS CME course is the need for hands-on training with live and simulation models, which is the primary reason many learners attend an in-person POCUS course. Tele-ultrasound technology has been used to perform remote scanning of patients [3, 4], especially in resource-limited settings [5, 6], but few studies have described its use for virtual hands-on training of clinicians [7–11]. Furthermore, no prior studies have described use of tele-ultrasound technology for hands-on POCUS training as part of an accredited CME course for practicing clinicians.

We converted an established in-person POCUS CME course to a tele-ultrasound course during the COVID-19 pandemic. The goal of the tele-ultrasound POCUS CME course was to provide the same educational experience, including hands-on training, using a virtual format. We compared the change in POCUS knowledge of learners, fulfillment of course objectives, and faculty and learner feedback of the in-person versus tele-ultrasound POCUS CME courses.

Methods

We conducted a retrospective observational study comparing an established in-person POCUS course in February 2020 (pre-pandemic) versus new tele-ultrasound POCUS courses in July 2020 and February 2021 during the COVID-19 pandemic. The same POCUS educational curriculum was used for the in-person and tele-ultrasound courses, although the format of delivering educational content differed. All learners and faculty were considered for inclusion and only excluded if their pre- or post-course datasets were incomplete. The University of Texas Health San Antonio Investigational Review Board deemed this retrospective educational study to be exempt from formal review.

In-person course

We held in-person POCUS courses every 6–12 months from 2013 until the COVID-19 pandemic in early 2020. These 2-day courses combined focused lectures, image review sessions, and hands-on scanning sessions (Additional file 1: Table S1). Both live models and simulators were used. A learner-to-faculty ratio of 3:1 or 2:1 was maintained for all hands-on training. Data from the most recent in-person course in February 2020 were used for comparison to the tele-ultrasound courses.

Tele-ultrasound course

To meet the ongoing demand of POCUS training during the COVID-19 pandemic, we converted our traditional 2-day in-person course into a 4-week tele-ultrasound course. While the number of CME hours from didactics and hands-on training stayed the same (16.25 h) (Additional file 1: Table S2), the curriculum was spread over 4 weeks for two reasons. First, learners and faculty needed additional time to become comfortable using the tele-ultrasound software. Second, our course coordinators were online to connect faculty and learners, initiate the hands-on scanning sessions, and troubleshoot any problems that arose during the session. Thus, we scheduled individual hands-on scanning sessions at different times, rather than all learners and faculty scanning simultaneously. The learner-to-faculty ratio was 2:1 or 1:1 for all hands-on scanning sessions. Hands-on scanning objectives of the in-person and tele-ultrasound courses were similar (Additional file 1: Tables S3 and S4).

We utilized tele-ultrasound software (Reacts by Philips & Innovative Imaging Technologies, Montreal, Canada). This software allowed simultaneous visualization of a learner's hand position and ultrasound screen (Fig. 1).

We piloted our tele-ultrasound course with 12 learners at four remote critical access hospitals in southeastern Alaska in July 2020, followed by a larger course with 43 learners from 14 different states in the United States and abroad in February 2021. Twenty-six experienced POCUS faculty specializing in internal medicine, hospital medicine, critical care, and emergency medicine from 15 different U.S. institutions provided virtual hands-on POCUS instruction by tele-ultrasound. Faculty and learners were scheduled for 2-h hands-on scanning sessions that allowed for 60–90 min of actual scanning. Live models were relatives of learners, course participants, or volunteer staff or patients.

Learners completed pre- and post-course knowledge tests (Additional file 1: File S1), CME course evaluations (Additional file 1: File S2), tele-ultrasound course evaluations (Additional file 1: File S3), and participated in a live post-course debriefing. The knowledge test included 30 questions focusing on fundamentals of ultrasonography, image interpretation, and integration of POCUS findings in clinical decision-making. After both the in-person and tele-ultrasound POCUS courses, learners completed a standard CME course evaluation that gathered both quantitative and qualitative feedback. Learners evaluated fulfillment of course objectives and quality of

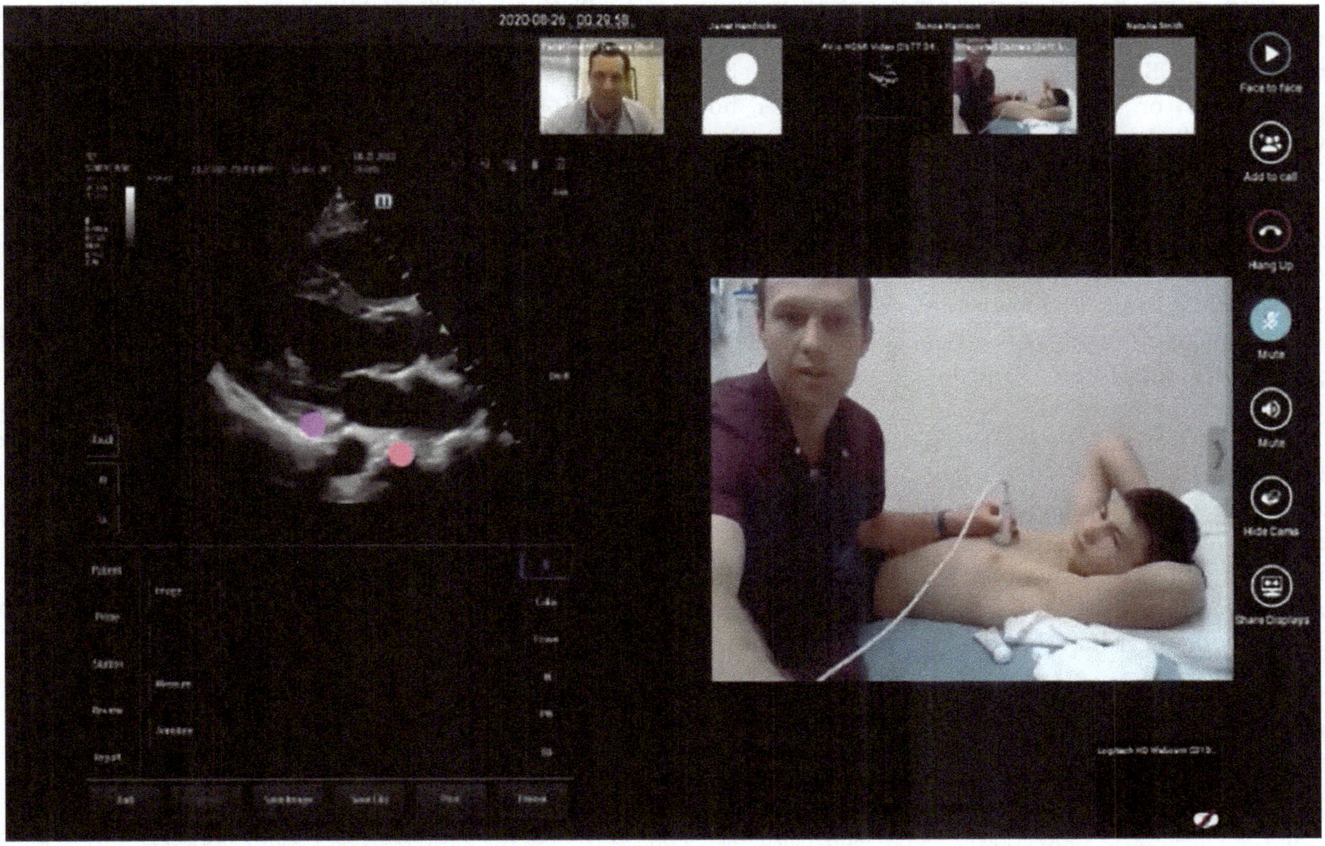

Fig. 1 Tele-ultrasound hands-on scanning session. Live hands-on scanning sessions were conducted using tele-ultrasound software (Reacts by Philips & Innovative Imaging Technologies). The platform allowed simultaneous visualization of the learner's hands position (right) and ultrasound screen (left) which allowed faculty to guide learners in image acquisition. Both faculty and learners could point to structures on the ultrasound screen using different colored pointers (left)

lectures and hands-on scanning sessions by rating their agreement with standardized statements on a scale of 1–5 (1 = "not at all" or "low agreement"; 5 = "excellent" or "high agreement"). We gathered qualitative feedback from learners of the in-person and tele-ultrasound courses in three domains: (1) teaching effectiveness of faculty for hands-on sessions; (2) new knowledge or practice strategies gained; and (3) practice changes implemented after attending the course. Qualitative data were collected from learners using free text boxes in the CME course evaluation and tele-ultrasound course evaluation, and during live post-course debriefing sessions. Faculty evaluated the tele-ultrasound course by completing the same tele-ultrasound course evaluation as learners that included faculty-specific questions and during a live post-course debriefing session for faculty.

Mean knowledge test scores and differences in scores were compared using the Mann–Whitney test. Paired t-tests were used to test the hypothesis of an increase in knowledge test scores from pre- to post-course for each course format. Proportions of learners rating "excellent" on course evaluations were compared for each objective using the Z-test for proportions. A p-value of < 0.05 was considered statistically significant. Qualitative data from learners and faculty were reviewed and discussed by two co-authors (NJS, EKH) and recurring themes were compiled.

Results

Eighty-eight learners from the in-person course and 52 from the tele-ultrasound course completed all pre- and post-course assessments. The vast majority of learners were novices with no or minimal experience using POCUS and did not or infrequently used POCUS (few times per year). Twenty-six faculty participated in the tele-ultrasound course, and 54% of the same faculty taught both the in-person and tele-ultrasound courses. Learner and faculty characteristics are displayed in Additional file 1: Table S5.

The mean pre-course knowledge test scores were higher for learners in the tele-ultrasound versus in-person course (78% vs. 71%; $p = 0.001$), but the post-course scores of learners in the tele-ultrasound course improved to a similar level as those in-person course (89% vs. 87%;

$p=0.069$), although with a lower net overall improvement. Thus, learners demonstrated a significant improvement in POCUS knowledge after participating in either the in-person or tele-ultrasound course. Further, both courses fulfilled course objectives similarly based on CME course evaluations (Table 1).

Both learners and faculty of the tele-ultrasound POCUS course completed a separate course evaluation assessing the tele-ultrasound course format (Additional file 1: Tables S6 and S7). Overall, learners rated the tele-ultrasound course highly (4.6–5.0 on a 5-point scale) for lectures, tele-ultrasound hands-on scanning sessions, and course administration.

Similar to learners, the majority of faculty rated the effectiveness of the tele-ultrasound course administration and hands-on sessions highly; however, the virtual lectures were felt to be less effective by faculty than learners (3.7 vs. 4.8). Compared to learners, faculty generally expressed less satisfaction with the tele-ultrasound scanning sessions regarding their ability to engage learners, troubleshoot image acquisition, and provide feedback. Faculty did not express differences in difficulty of teaching specific cardiac or non-cardiac applications using tele-ultrasound, but difficulty visualizing the learner's probe position was a common complaint.

We highlight some of the key points gathered from the qualitative feedback. First, regarding teaching effectiveness of faculty during hands-on sessions, some learners of the in-person course disliked faculty taking control of the ultrasound transducer without letting the learner troubleshoot his/her own image. Second, learners in both the in-person and tele-ultrasound courses reported increased confidence in their ability to utilize POCUS in patient care post-course. Third, similar practice changes were anticipated by learners after participating in either the in-person or tele-ultrasound course, the most common being increased frequency of POCUS use in patient care. Additional advantages and disadvantages of the tele-ultrasound course from the perspectives of learners and faculty are presented in Table 2.

Table 1 Comparison of knowledge test scores and fulfillment of course objectives by the in-person vs. tele-ultrasound POCUS courses

	In-person (n = 88)	Tele-ultrasound (n = 52)	p-value
Knowledge test scores			
Pre-course (%)			
Mean	71	78	0.001
Median [IQR]	73 [60–83]	83 [71–85]	
Range	34–98	49–95	
Post-course (%)			
Mean	87	89	0.069
Median [IQR]	88 [83–91]	90 [85–93]	
Range	49–98	54–100	
Differences (%)			
Mean	16	11	0.017
Median [IQR]	12 [7–22]	7 [2–18]	
Range	(− 7)–51	(− 12)–39	
p-value	< 0.0001	< 0.0001	
Fulfillment of course objectives[a]			
Fundamental principles of ultrasound technology and basic operation of a portable ultrasound machine	4.7	4.7	0.81
Techniques to perform focused diagnostic ultrasound examinations at the bedside, including imaging of the heart, lungs, abdomen, and lower extremity veins	4.8	4.8	0.53
Techniques to guide performance of bedside procedures with ultrasound guidance, including central venous catheterization, thoracentesis, paracentesis, and lumbar puncture	4.5	4.4	0.32
Indications, basic protocols, and limitations of bedside ultrasound imaging	4.7	4.6	0.65
Practice interpretation of normal and abnormal ultrasound images	4.7	4.7	0.81
Mentored scanning with experienced faculty to learn hands-on imaging techniques	4.7	4.7	0.70

[a] Mean scores per 5-point scale (1 = not at all; 2 = minimal; 3 = neutral; 4 = good; 5 = excellent) with *p*-values calculated for proportion giving an excellent rating

Table 2 Summary of learner and faculty feedback of the tele-ultrasound courses

	Learners	Faculty
Lectures		
Advantages	More convenient and comfortable Recorded lectures good for review Small group size is less intimidating	Flexible scheduling
Disadvantages	Easier to get distracted	Difficult to engage learners
Hands-on scanning		
Advantages	Time for self-directed practice in between scanning sessions Personalized teaching Opportunity to troubleshoot scanning without faculty intervening physically Flexible scheduling of sessions	More satisfying teaching 1–2 learners Less exhausting phys cally Time to convey learner needs between faculty Flexible scheduling of sessions
Disadvantages	Reliable internet signal required Tele-ultrasound software can glitch Learners could benefit from peer observation	Learner fatigue during 1–2 h hands-on sessions Inability to demonstrate skills Struggling learners difficult to guide No control over learners' setting (lighting, room and model positioning, space limitations, etc.)
Procedure training		
Advantages	None	None
Disadvantages	Limited number of simulation models can be sent to learner	Inability to demonstrate technique on simulation model
General		
Advantages	No travel required Lower total training costs	Lower risk of COVID-19 exposure Faculty honoraria equitably paid based on involvement in course
Disadvantages	Multi-week course is time consuming Time zones differences can cause scheduling errors	Strong administrative support is imperative for course coordination Extended course duration compared to 2-day in-person course

Discussion

For many learners, the primary reason to attend an in-person POCUS CME course is the opportunity to practice hands-on scanning on live models and ultrasound-guided procedures on simulators under the guidance of expert faculty. We have demonstrated that hands-on scanning is feasible using tele-ultrasound technology, and a tele-ultrasound POCUS CME course can improve learners' post-course knowledge to a similar level as an in-person course. We have also identified important advantages and disadvantages of the two course formats and considerations for course directors seeking to develop a tele-ultrasound POCUS CME course.

Learners' POCUS knowledge improved significantly after participating in either the in-person or tele-ultrasound POCUS course. This finding has important implications for future dissemination of POCUS training since lack of training is the number one barrier to POCUS implementation [12–14]. Historically, POCUS training has been obtained primarily through in-person courses, but the limited availability and required travel of in-person courses are important limitations. Avoiding travel, reducing time away from work and personal responsibilities, and reducing total training costs were unique advantages of the tele-ultrasound course format.

Additional advantages and disadvantages of a tele-ultrasound POCUS course surfaced from qualitative feedback gathered. Most important, faculty felt learners completed the tele-ultrasound course with a better basic POCUS skillset than the traditional in-person course, which may be attributed to the longer course duration (4 weeks vs. 2 days), lower learner-to-faculty ratio (1 or 2:1 vs. 2 or 3:1), and greater comfort and convenience for learners scanning in their home environment. Learners commented that the multi-week format of the tele-ultrasound courses allowed them more time to absorb the course material and practice scanning in between hands-on sessions. Further, the total number of hours spent scanning by faculty was higher with the tele-ultrasound courses because the learner-to-faculty ratios were lower; however, faculty did not lose time traveling as they would for an in-person course which was an important advantage to some faculty. Finally, learners preferred to troubleshoot their own images without faculty intervening physically by taking control of the transducer. This was an advantage per learners, but a disadvantage per faculty who often preferred to take physical control of the transducer to intervene or demonstrate image acquisition.

For course directors interested in developing a tele-ultrasound POCUS course, we highlight three important considerations: selection of videoconferencing and tele-ultrasound software, selection of learners and faculty, and course coordination.

First, several general videoconferencing platforms exist (e.g., Zoom, Skype, Cisco WebEx, GoToMeeting, Microsoft Teams, BlueJeans Meetings, Google Hangouts Meet, and Jabber). Essential features for a virtual POCUS course include high-quality transmission of ultrasound images without a lag or choppiness, sufficient online storage for recording lectures, and ease of use for both learners and faculty with features (chat, screensharing, etc.). Regarding tele-ultrasound platforms, both ultrasound-specific and general videoconferencing software can be used. Two examples of ultrasound-specific software are Reacts (Philips/Innovative Imaging Technologies, Montreal, Canada) and Butterfly Teleguidance (Butterfly Network, Guilford, CT, USA). A unique advantage of these tele-ultrasound platforms is simultaneous camera and ultrasound image transmission using a cellular or internet signal, allowing faculty to coach learners in image acquisition while simultaneously seeing the learner's hand position and ultrasound image. Reacts can be used with most major brands of ultrasound machines, whereas Butterfly Teleguidance is available only with Butterfly ultrasound devices. Some tele-ultrasound software allow faculty to remotely adjust ultrasound machine settings to optimize the image, which can be an important feature if learners are struggling with knobology. General videoconferencing software may be used for tele-ultrasound using remote desktops or screensharing, or by pointing the videoconferencing camera directly on the ultrasound screen, but variable degrees of image degradation occur with the latter option.

Second, success of hands-on scanning sessions using tele-ultrasound is dependent on both the learners and faculty. Learners must have reliable access to an ultrasound device compatible with the selected tele-ultrasound software; a reliable internet signal with sufficient bandwidth to simultaneously transmit ultrasound and video images; and availability of a live model for hands-on scanning. Experienced faculty that have previously demonstrated mastery in guiding learners in image acquisition *without* touching the transducer should be selected for the tele-ultrasound hands-on scanning sessions. All faculty must use standard terminology for transducer manipulation (slide, tilt, rotate, rock) to avoid confusing learners that scan with multiple faculty. Less experienced faculty can learn from more experienced faculty by shadowing during a live tele-ultrasound session.

Third, compared to an in-person course, substantially more educational staff time is needed to coordinate a tele-ultrasound POCUS CME course. Unique tasks included screening and selecting learners and faculty as mentioned above; organizing, packing, and shipping loaned tele-ultrasound equipment to learners; scheduling 2-h tele-ultrasound sessions between learners and faculty; and connecting learners and faculty online during scanning sessions.

Regarding costs, the tele-ultrasound course budget was similar to the in-person course. However, funds were spent differently in the tele-ultrasound course: more funds were spent on educational staff time for course coordination, faculty honoraria for scanning sessions, and purchasing and shipping of tele-ultrasound equipment, while funds were saved on faculty travel and venue expenditures, such as catering and room rental. For learners, there were significant cost savings by avoiding travel.

We recognize our findings have limitations and require confirmation. Though many faculty and learners felt better hands-on scanning skills were achieved by learners upon completion of the tele-ultrasound course, it was not feasible to test learners' hands-on skills pre- and post-course. Additionally, although both courses had the same number of CME credit hours, the duration of the tele-ultrasound course was 4 weeks while the in-person course was 2 days. Next steps include piloting a 2-day tele-ultrasound course to test the feasibility and logistics of having multiple learners and faculty scanning simultaneously using tele-ultrasound compared to a traditional in-person 2-day course.

In conclusion, we have demonstrated that a virtual POCUS CME course with hands-on scanning sessions using tele-ultrasound is feasible. Both the traditional in-person and tele-ultrasound POCUS courses fulfilled learning objectives and significantly improved learners' post-course knowledge to a similar level. By improving learners' access to expert faculty for mentored scanning, tele-ultrasound can help bridge the gap in POCUS training in the coming years.

Abbreviations

CME: Continuing medical education; POCUS: Point-of-care ultrasound.

Supplementary Information

Additional file 1: **Table S1.** Two-day In-person POCUS Course Agenda. **Table S2.** Four-week Tele-ultrasound POCUS Course Agenda. **Table S3.** In-person Course Scanning Session Objectives. **Table S4.** Tele-ultrasound Course Scanning Session Objectives. **File S1.** Pre- and Post-course Knowledge Test. **File S2.** CME Course Evaluation. **File S3.** Tele-ultrasound Course Evaluation. **Table S5.** Characteristics of Learners and Faculty. **Table S6.** Tele-ultrasound Course Evaluations by Learners and Faculty. **Table S7.** Faculty Evaluation of the Tele-ultrasound Course.

Acknowledgements
None.

Authors' contributions
NJS, JSB, GM, KCP, TPJ, GL, BKM, CKS, LK, CML, PA, RN, NS, EKH, MM, JP, MIR, and BPL contributed substantially to the study design, data analysis and interpretation, and writing of the manuscript. NJS has full access to all of the data in the study and takes responsibility for the integrity of the data and the accuracy of the data analysis. All authors read and approved the final manuscript.

Author details
[1]South Texas Veterans Health Care System, San Antonio, TX, USA. [2]Department of Medicine, UT Health San Antonio, San Antonio, TX, USA. [3]Department of Emergency Medicine, Veterans Affairs - Tennessee Valley Healthcare System, Nashville, TN, USA. [4]Department of Emergency Medicine, Vanderbilt University Medical Center, Nashville, TN, USA. [5]Division of Hospital Medicine, Weill Cornell Medicine, New York, NY, USA. [6]Division of Hospital Medicine, University of California San Francisco Medical Center at Parnassus, San Francisco, CA, USA. [7]Division of General Internal Medicine, Department of Medicine, Johns Hopkins School of Medicine, Baltimore, MD, USA. [8]Department of Hospital Medicine, Regions Hospital, HealthPartners, St. Paul, MN, USA. [9]Department of Critical Care Medicine, Veterans Affairs of Pittsburgh Health Care System, Pittsburgh, PA, USA. [10]Departments of Critical Care Medicine and Emergency Medicine, University of Pittsburgh Medical Center, University of Pittsburgh, Pittsburgh, PA, USA. [11]Division of Hospital Medicine, Donald and Barbara Zucker School of Medicine at Hofstra/Northwell, Hempstead, NY, USA. [12]Louis Stokes Cleveland Veterans Affairs Medical Center, Cleveland, OH, USA. [13]Case Western Reserve University School of Medicine, Cleveland, OH, USA. [14]Department of Emergency Medicine, Donald and Barbara Zucker School of Medicine at Hofstra/Northwell, Hempstead, NY, USA. [15]White River Junction VA Medical Center, White River Junction, VT, USA. [16]Department of Medicine, Dartmouth Geisel School of Medicine, Hanover, NH, USA. [17]University of Texas Health San Antonio, South Texas Veterans Health Care System, 7703 Floyd Curl Drive, MC 7982, San Antonio, TX 78229, USA.

References

1. Greenstein YY, Littauer R, Narasimhan M, Mayo PH, Koenig SJ (2016) Effectiveness of a critical care ultrasonography course. Chest 151(1):34-40
2. Mathews BK, Koenig S, Kurian L et al (2020) Clinical progress note: point-of-care ultrasound applications in COVID-19. J Hosp Med 15(6):353–355
3. Gibson LE, Low SA, Bittner EA, Chang MG (2020) Ultrasound teleguidance to reduce healthcare worker exposure to coronavirus disease 2019. Crit Care Explor 2(6):e0146
4. Olivieri PP, Verceles AC, Hurley JM, Zubrow MT, Jeudy J, McCurdy MT (2020) A pilot study of ultrasonography-naïve operators' ability to use tele-ultrasonography to assess the heart and lung. J Intensive Care Med 35(7):672–678
5. Britton N, Miller MA, Safadi S, Siegel A, Levine AR, McCurdy MT (2019) Tele-ultrasound in resource-limited settings: a systematic review. Front Public Health 7:244
6. Rabie NZ, Sandlin AT, Barber KA et al (2017) Teleultrasound: how accurate are we? J Ultrasound Med 36(11):2329–2335
7. Arntfield RT (2015) The utility of remote supervision with feedback as a method to deliver high-volume critical care ultrasound training. J Crit Care 30(2):441.e441-441.e446
8. Schroeder AN, Hall MM, Kruse RC (2020) Sports ultrasound training during a pandemic: developing a "hands-on" skill through distance learning. Am J Phys Med Rehabil 99(9):860–862
9. Dreyfuss A, Martin DA, Farro A et al (2020) A novel multimodal approach to point-of-care ultrasound education in low-resource settings. West J Emerg Med 21(4):1017–1021
10. Ramsingh D, Ma M, Le DQ et al (2019) Feasibility evaluation of commercially available video conferencing devices to technically direct untrained nonmedical personnel to perform a rapid trauma ultrasound examination. Diagnostics 9(4):188. https://doi.org/10.3390/diagnostics9040188
11. Salerno A, Tupchong K, Verceles AC, McCurdy MT (2020) Point-of-care teleultrasound: a systematic review. Telemed J E Health 26(11):1314–1321
12. Wong J, Montague S, Wallace P et al (2020) Barriers to learning and using point-of-care ultrasound: a survey of practicing internists in six North American institutions. Ultrasound J 12(1):19
13. Sanders JL, Noble VE, Raja AS, Sullivan AF, Camargo CA Jr (2015) Access to and use of point-of-care ultrasound in the emergency department. West J Emerg Med 16(5):747–752
14. Stowell JR, Kessler R, Lewiss RE et al (2017) Critical care ultrasound: a national survey across specialties. J Clin Ultrasound 46(3):167-177.

20

A retrospective evaluation of point of care ultrasound for acute cholecystitis in a tertiary academic hospital setting

David P. Evans*, Jordan Tozer, Lindsay Taylor, Michael J. Vitto and Michael Joyce

Abstract

Background: In 2008 the Council of Emergency Medicine Residency Directors delineated consensus recommendations for training in biliary ultrasound for the "detection of biliary pathology".

Objectives: While studies have looked at the accuracy of emergency provider performed clinical ultrasound (ECUS), we sought to evaluated if ECUS could be diagnostic for acute cholecystitis and thus obviate the need for follow-up imaging.

Method: We reviewed all ECUS performed between 2012 and 2017 that had a matching radiology performed ultrasound (RADUS) and a discharge diagnosis. 332 studies were identified. The sensitivity and specificity of both ECUS and RADUS were compared to the patient's discharge diagnosis. The agreement between the ECUS and RADUS was assessed using an unweighted Cohen's Kappa. The time from patient arrival to diagnosis by ECUS and RADUS was also compared.

Results: Using discharge diagnosis as the gold standard ECUS was 67% (56–78%) sensitive, 88% (84–92%) specific, NPV 90% (87–95%), PPV 60% (50–71%), +LR 5.6 (3.9–8.2), −LR 0.37 (0.27–0.52) for acute cholecystitis. RADUS was 76% (66–87%) sensitive, 97% (95–99%) specific, NPV 95% (092–97%), PPV 86% (76–95%), +LR 25.6 (12.8–51.4), and −LR 0.24 (0.15–0.38). ECUS was able to detect gallstones with 93% (89–96%) sensitivity and 94% (90–98%) specificity leading to a NPV 90% (85–95%), PPV of 95% (92–98%), +LR 14.5 (7.7–27.4), −LR 0.08 (0.05–0.13). The unweighted kappa between ECUS and RADUS was 0.57. The median time between obtaining ECUS vs. RADUS diagnosis was 124 min.

Conclusions: ECUS can be beneficial in ruling out acute cholecystitis, but lacks the test characteristics to be diagnostic for acute cholecystitis.

Keywords: Biliary ultrasound, Medical education, Cholecystitis

Introduction

Background

Cholecystitis afflicts over 20 million people in the United States [1]. Amongst people with biliary disease approximately 1–4% develop biliary colic annually [2–5]. Of these symptomatic patients, 20% will go on to develop a potentially life-threatening complication such as acute cholecystitis [6]. This comes at a direct annual cost to the U.S. health care system of 6.3 billion dollars [7]. Unfortunately, historical and physical exam findings lack the ability to identify acute cholecystitis in the clinical setting [8]. Given this, clinicians in the emergency department (ED) routinely order radiology-performed ultrasound (RADUS) of the gallbladder to "rule out" acute cholecystitis. RADUS is typically performed by an ultrasound technician and interpreted by a radiologist. This approach leads to inherit lag times in radiology-based

*Correspondence: david.evans@vcuhealth.org
Department of Emergency Medicine, Virginia Commonwealth School of Medicine, Main Hospital 2nd floor, room 606, Suite 600, 1250 East Marshal St, PO BOX 980401, Richmond, VA 23298-0401, USA

imaging that prolong ED wait times causing throughput delays and contributing to overcrowding [9, 10]. Due to these issues, emergency physicians have begun to explore the use of clinician-performed ultrasound (ECUS) to evaluate patients for possible biliary disease [11–13]. This led to the 2008 Council of Emergency Medicine Residency Directors consensus recommendations for training in biliary ultrasound for the "detection of biliary pathology" [14]. Following these recommendations it became commonplace at our institution for resident physicians to perform a ECUS of the gallbladder for any patient presenting with right upper quadrant or epigastric pain. It is also common at our institution for an attending physician working in the triage area to order formal right upper quadrant scans through radiology, while the patient is in triage.

Importance

Following these recommendations, academic emergency departments began to teach clinical ultrasound to all residents, requiring a basic competency prior to graduation. In the decade, since these recommendations were made, few studies have looked at the accuracy of emergency physician performed clinical ultrasound (ECUS) and none have evaluated if ECUS could be diagnostic for biliary pathology and thus obviate the need for follow-up imaging [15, 16].

Goals of this investigation

The goal of this investigation was to perform a retrospective chart review study evaluating ECUS test characteristics for acute cholecystitis as compared to the patients discharge diagnosis. Secondary objectives were to evaluate how ECUS correlated to RADUS, the time difference to obtaining ECUS vs. RADUS, the use of cholescintigraphy in the ED, and lastly to evaluate how different clinical ultrasound test characteristics for acute cholecystitis performed.

Materials and methods

Study design

This was a retrospective review of historical data retrieved from the ultrasound archiving system (Qpath, Telexy, Canada) of a large urban teaching hospital from January 1, 2012 to January 1, 2017. All studies were performed on Sonosite Xport machines (Fujifilm Sonosite, Bethell, WA). The study was approved by our Institutional Review Board.

Setting and selection of participants

All emergency physician-performed focused gallbladder studies completed during the eligible period that had a matching radiology-interpreted study and formal discharge diagnosis were included. Patients that underwent HIDA scan for inconclusive radiology-performed ultrasound were included in the data. The time from the initial patient encounter by ED physician to diagnosis by ECUS, RADUS and HIDA was recorded and compared.

Primary data analysis

Detecting pathology

The protocol for all ECUS studies of the gallbladder at our institution consisted of a 4 second clip of the gallbladder both in long and short access, as well as image of the common bile duct. The gallbladder wall is to be measured on the short axis, where it abuts the liver anteriorly with a normal measurement of less than 0.34 cm. The common bile duct is verified with color Doppler and its inner diameter measured in the longitudinal axis with a normal measurement of less than 0.7 cm. Abnormal findings would include gallstones, wall thickening, pericystic fluid, sonographic murphy's sign or enlargement of the common bile duct. The ECUS studies were grouped into the following diagnostic categories: no pathology, cholelithiasis, cholelithiasis with cholecystitis, acalculous cholecystitis, choledocolithiasis, polyps, and other based solely on the ED physician's final interpretation. The sensitivity, specificity, positive likelihood and negative likelihood ratios for both ECUS and RADUS were compared using the patient's discharge diagnosis for the same above categories. The discharge diagnosis was obtained from the patient's discharge summary. All chart reviews were conducted by DE. Data was collected and stored in Excel (Microsoft, Redmond, WA). All statistical testing was performed with Stata (version 12.1; StataCorp, College Station, Tx).

Test for agreement

The agreement between the ECUS diagnosis and the RADUS diagnosis was assessed using an unweighted Cohen's Kappa. An initial test for agreement used all diagnosis categories and a second test for agreement combined the diagnoses of acalculous cholecystitis, choledocolithiasis, and polyps into the other category, as they had low representations in the data. Cohen's Kappa was calculated again for the agreement between the two new sets of diagnoses.

Time analysis

The time between the initial physician encounter to ECUS diagnosis, RADUS diagnosis, and HIDA diagnosis, was calculated for each patient. Eleven patients were omitted from this analysis, because they received a RADUS study prior to being seen by an emergency physician. Eighty-eight additional patients had missing values for their times and were omitted from the analysis. For

Table 1 EUS vs. RADUS for acute cholecystitis

	EUS (955 CI)	RADUS (95% CI)
Sensitivity	67% (56–78%)	76% (66–87%)
Specificity	88% (84–92%)	97% (95–99%)
NPV	90% (87–95%)	95% (92–97%)
PPV	60% (50–71%)	86% (76–95%)
+LR	5.6 (3.9–8.2)	25.6 (12.8–51.4)
−LR	0.37 (0.27–0.52)	0.24 (0.15–0.38)

Table 2 EUS ability to detect gallstones

Sensitivity	93% (89–96%)
Specificity	94% (90–98%)
NPV	90% (85–95%)
PPV	95% (92–98%)
+LR	14.5 (7.7–27.4)
−LR	0.08 (0.05–0.13)

the patients that received a HIDA scan, the time from initial encounter to the HIDA scan diagnosis was calculated. The median times to ECUS diagnosis, RADUS diagnosis, and HIDA diagnosis were calculated and compared.

Results

Of the 3121 total ECUS studies of the gallbladder performed during the study period 332 were identified that met inclusion criteria. Of these, 189 patients were diagnosed with cholelithiasis and 47 were diagnosed with cholecystitis by ECUS, while 131 patients were diagnosed with cholelithiasis and 56 were diagnosed with cholecystitis by RADUS.

When compared to the discharge diagnosis of acute cholecystitis, RADUS was more sensitive (76% vs. 67%) and specific (97% vs. 88%), with better predictive value compared to ECUS (Table 1). When looking at the discharge diagnosis of cholelithiasis ECUS was 92.7% sensitive and 93.6% specific compared to RADUS, which was 95.4% sensitive and 84.1% specific (Table 2). The unweighted kappa between ECUS and RADUS was 0.57.

Of the 332 subjects, 83 had surgery with available pathology for review. Of the patients who went to the operating room, 53 were diagnosed with cholecystitis, 25 with cholelithiasis, and 5 with gallstone pancreatitis. Of the 53 patients diagnosed with cholecystitis, 30 (56.6%) were diagnosed on ECUS as having cholecystitis and 22 (41.5%) were diagnosed with gallstones without signs of cholecystitis. In comparison, 37 (70%) were diagnosed on RADUS as having cholecystitis and 13 (24%) were diagnosed with gallstones without signs of cholecystitis.

Acalculous cholecystitis was diagnosed by ECUS in 16 patients and by RADUS in 9 patients. Of the 332 patients studied; however, only one received a discharge diagnosis of acalculous cholecystitis.

In our study population, ECUS deemed 103 patients to have no significant gallbladder pathology. Of these, 12 patients were diagnosed with cholelithiasis on RADUS, one of which had a subsequent HIDA scan that showed no pathology. None of the 103 patients with a negative ECUS were diagnosed with acute cholecystitis and none returned to the study institution in the 6 months after their ED visit with a diagnosis of acute cholecystitis.

Therefore, dichotomizing biliary ultrasound into pathology vs. no pathology ECUS was 93.6% (90–97.1%) sensitive and 67.6% (60–75.2%) specific with positive LR of 2.89 (2.27–3.66) and negative likelihood ratio of 0.09 (0.05–0.17). Conversely, RADUS was 96.3% (93.6–98.9) sensitive and 73.9% (66.7–81.1) specific with a positive LR of 3.69 (2.8–4.88) and negative LR of 0.04 (0.02–0.10).

The median time between acquisition of the ECUS and RADUS was 124 min, while the median time between ECUS and HIDA scan was 800 min.

Discussion

Biliary disease places a significant burden on the United States healthcare system with up to 20% of the more than 20 million with disease developing potentially life-threatening complications. Knowing that medical history and physical exam cannot reliably identify biliary disease, a rapid but accurate screening test is desirable. This is beneficial for multiple reasons, including early identification of complications, as well as ED throughput. Avoiding the need for further imaging could decrease time to disposition, and improve patient outcomes through earlier identification of significant complications and thus earlier intervention. When compared to RADUS, we found that ECUS was slightly less sensitive (67% vs. 76%) and specific (88% vs. 97%) for acute cholecystitis when using discharge diagnosis as the gold standard.

In the 17 patients who received HIDA scan none had a change in their diagnosis. The average delay in diagnosis between HIDA and ECUS was over 13 h. This result is consistent with previous studies showing no benefit to HIDA scan in the ED [17].

After dichotomization of patients into those with pathology and those with no significant sonographic findings by ECUS, the sensitivity of ECUS for determining presence of disease was 93.6% (90–97.1%). None of the 103 patients with negative ECUS had a diagnosis of acute cholecystitis or returned to the study institution within 6 months with acute cholecystitis. This makes ultrasound a valuable screening tool in the hands of the emergency physician, and can allow for earlier discharge of well appearing patients if there is no concern for alternate etiology.

In a patient in which the emergency physician has a high pretest probability for acute cholecystitis, the positive likelihood ratio of 5.6 (3.9–8.2) for ECUS can be considered diagnostic and the emergency physician could possibly forego further imaging prior to surgical consult. Given its lower specificity in detecting pathology in general, it could be argued that ECUS lacks the test characteristics to be diagnostic if the clinical picture is unclear; therefore, a confirmatory radiology study may be considered at the discretion of the emergency physician.

Many EDs around the country are experiencing significant boarding and throughput issues. Previous studies have shown that pelvic ECUS was 66 min faster than RADUS, which lead to a 120-min shorter LOS [18, 19]. At our institution, ECUS lead to a 124-min decrease in time to result compared to RADUS. This finding is in agreement with previous literature that indicates that there could potentially be even more time saved in time to disposition.

Finally, it is prudent to consider the possible financial implication of ECUS in addition to the improved throughput time. Previous work has shown that ECUS programs as a whole, including procedural use, have increased ED revenue by $35,500 with a potential for a $107,700 revenue increase with improved utilization and documentation [20]. This does not take into account the reduction in expenses of formal RADUS. To our knowledge, no study has investigated the potential cost savings of a negative biliary ECUS that does not require a more expensive follow-up RADUS.

This study relied on image acquisition and interpretation by emergency physicians with variable levels of training in performing ECUS. It has been demonstrated in several previous studies that interpretation accuracy improves with increasing number of biliary studies [21], with no improvement over 50 studies [22]. In our study, the attending physician assigned to each case reviewed and attested to the ECUS interpretation prior to it becoming final, per department policy. These physicians were credentialed in ultrasound per the ACEP guidelines, having completed a minimum of 25 prior biliary studies.

Another limitation to consider is the median time to receive the RADUS interpretation may be longer depending on the indication for scan. For example, if a "right upper quadrant" RADUS was ordered this would increase the time the technician would spend obtaining the imaging when compared to a specific "biliary" RADUS. Furthermore, compared to a clinical ultrasound exam fewer views are required to adequately diagnose biliary pathology when compared to a more comprehensive right upper quadrant RADUS.

Like many busy EDs, our emergency department has a physician in triage that may order RADUS studies before the ECUS can be performed. This led to 11 studies being performed by RADUS prior to the treating physician seeing the patient. While these studies were excluded, because no ECUS was performed, accounting for these studies could have shortened the time difference noted between ECUS and RADUS.

The gold standard we used was the diagnosis given to the patient at discharge. While we believe this to be a meaningful patient-oriented outcome, recorded discharge diagnoses are subject to inherit human recording error. To mitigate any discharge diagnosis error that may have occurred, each patient was followed for 6 months by chart review to ensure there was no return to the study institution for repeat assessment. It is conceivable that a follow-up visit occurred elsewhere.

Finally, it should be noted that the retrospective nature of this study opens it to selection bias. The patients who had clear diagnosis made on ECUS could have not received a formal RADUS. Therefore, patients with unclear diagnoses or physically difficult to perform ultrasounds may have been more likely to receive both a ECUS and a RADUS of the gallbladder.

Conclusions

ECUS is a valuable screening tool in the hands of the emergency physician, which can improve time to diagnosis and potential disposition, in patients in whom biliary colic is suspected. ECUS also has the potential to decreases time to intervention when there is high clinical suspicion of acute cholecystitis. If ECUS is equivocal for a patient in whom the emergency physician has suspicion for biliary pathology, then a confirmatory RADUS should be obtained.

Abbreviations

ECUS: Emergency provider performed clinical ultrasound; RADUS: Radiology performed ultrasound; HIDA: Hepatobiliary iminodiacetic acid scan; NPV: Negative predictive value; PPV: Positive predictive value; +LR: Positive likelihood ratio; −LR: Negative likelihood ratio; ACEP: American College of Emergency Medicine; ED: Emergency department; LOS: Length of stay.

Acknowledgements

The study has been presented at the following meetings: (1) "A Prospective Evaluation of Emergency Department Performed Ultrasound for Biliary Disease in an Academic Setting." Society of Academic Emergency Medicine, 2018 Annual Meeting. Indianapolis IN; May 16th, 2018. (2) "A Prospective Evaluation of Emergency Department Performed Ultrasound for Biliary Disease in an Academic Setting." American Institute of Ultrasound in Medicine, 2018 Annual Meeting. New York City NY; March 26th, 2018.

Authors' contributions

DPE conceived the study and designed the trial. DPE, JT, LT supervised the conduct of the trial and data collection. MJ and LT provided statistical advice on study design and analyzed the data; DPE chaired the data oversight committee. DPE, LT, JT, MJ, and MV drafted the manuscript, and all authors contributed substantially to its revision. DPE takes responsibility for the paper as a whole. All authors read and approved the final manuscript.

References

1. Everhart JE, Khare M, Hill M, Maurer KR (1999) Prevalence and ethnic differences in gallbladder disease in the United States. Gastroenterology 117:632–639
2. Attili AF, De Santis A, Capri R (1995) The natural history of gallstones: the GREPCO experience. The GREPCO Group. Hepatology 21:655–660
3. Wenckert A, Robertson B (1966) The natural course of gallstone disease: eleven year review of 781 nonoperated cases. Gastroenterology 50:376–381
4. Gracie WA, Ransohoff DF (1982) The natural history of silent gallstones: the innocent gallstone is not a myth. N Engl J Med 307:798–800
5. Barbara L, Sama C, Morselli Labate AM (1987) A population study on the prevalence of gallstone disease: the Sirmione sstudy. Hepatology 7:913–917
6. Friedman GS, Raviola CA, Fireman B (1989) Prognosis of gallstones with mild or no symptoms: 25 years of follow-up in a health maintenance organization. J Clin Epidemiol 42:127–136
7. American Gastroenterological Association (2001) The burden of gastrointestinal diseases. American Gastroenterological Association, Bethesda
8. Trowbridge RL, Rutkowski NK, Shojania KG (2003) Does this patient have acute cholecystitis? JAMA 289(1):80–86
9. Blaivas M, Harwood RA, Lambert MJ (1999) Decreasing length of stay with emergency ultrasound examination of the gallbladder. Acad Emerg Med 6:1020–1023
10. Kell MR, Aherne NJ, Coffey C, Power CP, Kirwan WO, Redmond HP (2002) Emergency surgeon-performed hepatobiliary ultrasonography. Br J Surg 89:1402–1404
11. American College of Emergency Physicians (2009) Emergency ultrasound guidelines. Ann Emerg Med 53:550–570
12. Mateer J, Plummer D, Heller M et al (1994) Model curriculum for physician training in emergency ultrasound. Ann Emerg Med 23:95–102
13. Bektas F, Eken C, Soyuncu S et al (2009) Contribution of goal-directed ultrasonography to clinical decision-making for emergency physicians. Emerg Med J 26:169–172
14. Akhtar S, Theodore D, Gaspari R et al (2009) Resident training in emergency ultrasound: consensus recommendations from 2008 council of emergency medicine residency directors conference. Acad Emerg Med 16(Suppl 2):S32–S36
15. Summers SM, Scruggs W, Menchine MD et al (2010) A prospective evaluation of emergency department bedside ultrasonography for the detection of acute cholecystitis. Ann Emerg Med 56(2):114–122
16. Torres-Macho J, Antón-Santos JM, García-Gutierrez I (2012) Initial accuracy of bedside ultrasound performed by emergency physicians for multiple indications after a short training period. Am J Emerg Med 30(9):1943–1949
17. Blaivas M, Adhikari S (2007) Diagnostic utility of cholescintigraphy in emergency department patients with suspected acute cholecystitis: comparison with bedside RUQ ultrasonography. J Emerg Med 33(1):47–52
18. Wilson SP, Connolly K, Lahham S et al (2016) Point-of-care ultrasound versus radiology department pelvic ultrasound on emergency department length of stay. World J Emerg Med 7(3):178–182
19. Burgher SW, Tandy TK, Dawdy MR (1998) Transvaginal ultrasonography by emergency physicians decreases patient time in the emergency department. Acad Emerg Med 5(8):802–807
20. Soremekun OA et al (2009) Financial impact of emergency department ultrasound: current and potential revenue. Acad Emerg Med 16(7):674–680
21. Gaspari RJ, Dickman E, Blehar D (2009) Learning curve of bedside ultrasound of the gallbladder. J Emerg Med 37(1):51–56
22. Jang TB, Ruggeri W, Dyne P, Kaji AH (2010) The learning curve of resident physicians using emergency ultrasonography for cholelithiasis and cholecystitis. Acad Emerg Med 17(11):1247–1252

21

Clinical applications of the venous excess ultrasound (VExUS) score: conceptual review and case series

Philippe Rola[1]*, Francisco Miralles-Aguiar[2], Eduardo Argaiz[3], William Beaubien-Souligny[4], Korbin Haycock[5], Timur Karimov[6], Vi Am Dinh[7] and Rory Spiegel[8]

Abstract

The importance of functional right ventricular failure and resultant splanchnic venous congestion has long been under-appreciated and is difficult to assess by traditional physical examination and standard diagnostic imaging. The recent development of the venous excess ultrasound score (VExUS) and growth of point-of-care ultrasound in the last decade has made for a potentially very useful clinical tool. We review the rationale for its use in several pathologies and illustrate with several clinical cases where VExUS was pivotal in clinical management.

Keywords: Point-of-care ultrasound, VExUS score, Congestive nephropathy, Venous congestion, Congestive heart failure

Background

The venous side of the circulation has long played second fiddle to the arterial side, who has enjoyed much of the medical fanfare both in acute and chronic disease. The arterial blood pressure, its tracing and its variation have been the subject of much study and are deeply ingrained in the day-to-day and even minute-to-minute of medical culture.

Of course, while arterial blood pressure is indeed critically important, the venous side may be just as critical as its more popular counterpart, and its physiological impact on organ function is vastly more important than commonly thought.

While the approach we discuss here is undoubtedly new, the physiology is not. As early as 1931, Winton noted that the impact of raising venous pressure was greater than an equal decrease in arterial pressure in terms of urine output [1].

This is not entirely surprising when one realizes that the true perfusion pressure of an organ is in fact not mean arterial pressure (MAP) minus central venous pressure (CVP), but rather precapillary arteriolar pressure minus postcapillary venular pressure. In the former equation, the MAP is generally above 90, while in the latter, the inflow pressure can be in the 35–40 mmHg range (Fig. 1) [2]. Hence, the pressure gradient is much narrower, and the impact of raising venous pressure is much greater than commonly thought.

Ultrasound markers of venous congestion are not new either. Portal vein pulsatility has been described about 30 years ago in the setting of heart failure [3] although it was never incorporated in the comprehensive echocardiographic assessment.

The development of point-of-care ultrasound (POCUS) has brought together acute care clinicians and pathology with a powerful tool able to assess physiology at the bedside. The group of Denault and Beaubien-Souligny have been particularly instrumental in showing the strong link between portal vein pulsatility and acute kidney injury in the subgroup of cardiac surgical patients [4–6].

*Correspondence: philipperola@gmail.com
[1] ICU Chief of Service, Santa Cabrini Hospital, Montreal, QC, Canada
Full list of author information is available at the end of the article

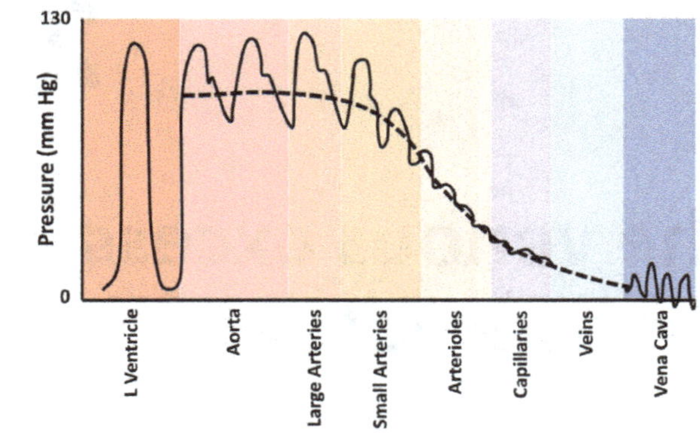

Fig. 1 Pressure at different points in the circulatory system. Note the precapillary arteriolar pressure is substantially lower than the large arterial pressures

Recently, our group developed the venous excess ultrasound (VExUS) score, which incorporates hepatic venous, intrarenal venous Doppler and inferior vena cava (IVC) assessment to portal vein Doppler, and found the presence of a severe score to be very specific for the prediction of acute kidney injury following cardiac surgery, even more so than portal vein pulsatility alone [7].

In this case series, we will describe cases where the use of POCUS and more specifically, VExUS, was useful in identifying pathophysiology and assisting in clinical decision-making.

Case presentations

Case 1

A 75-year-old male was admitted with worsening dyspnea, anasarca and acute renal failure. The critical care outreach service was consulted for placement of a catheter to drain ascites for symptomatic relief. He was known for alcoholic cirrhosis and severe congestive heart failure with an ejection fraction of 20%. He had been getting frequent—almost weekly—paracentesis in the past 6 months to control his dyspnea. His admission creatinine was 121 mmol/L and rose in a sawtooth pattern over 2 weeks to 285 mmol/L, prompting alternating increases and decreases in his furosemide dose. In the next days, his renal function continued to deteriorate, furosemide was held and attempts were made to manage this cardiorenal syndrome using albumin infusions in an effort to improve a "low-flow state". He was deemed to be in end-stage cardiorenal syndrome and the ascites management was meant to be a palliative therapy.

On examination the patient was in mild respiratory distress on nasal prongs, his blood pressure was 126/85, his heart rate 72 and his respiratory rate 24. His abdomen was distended and tense, he had marked anasarca involving both legs. His sensorium was clear, his extremities were warm and without mottling. There were chronic venous stasis changes in his lower legs.

His POCUS examination revealed a large, dilated and fixed IVC measuring over 30 mm in both axes and along the whole intrahepatic course (Fig. 2a), his portal vein showed 100% pulsatility with reversal of flow (Fig. 2b), his hepatic vein Doppler showed reversal of flow of the S wave (Fig. 2a). These findings correspond to a VExUS grade 3 venous congestion. He had massive ascites and a severe dilated cardiomyopathy with an ejection fraction of 20%. He was admitted to the stepdown intensive care unit for drainage and further management.

Over the next days, continuous drainage of ascites was done until a total of 12 L had been removed. Intravenous furosemide was restarted at a higher dose until a net balance of negative 1000 cc per 8 h shift was obtained. Progressively, the pulsatility of the portal vein decreased until it was approximately 30%. The IVC regained respiratory

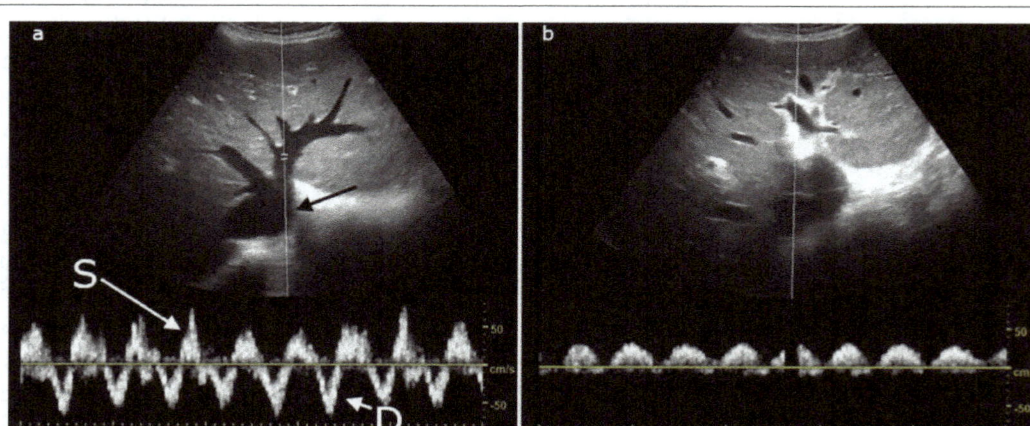

Fig. 2 Case 1: **a** IVC short axis view (black arrow) and hepatic vein Doppler showing the D wave (short white arrow) and reversal of the S wave (long white arrow). **b** Portal vein Doppler showing > 100% pulsatility with some flow reversal

variation and measured approximately 25–28 mm in both axes along most of its intrahepatic course. After an initial rise following admission to the intensive care unit (310 mmol/L/3.51 mg/dL), the creatinine decreased until it was normal (85 mmol/L/0.96 mg/dL).

The patient was discharged home with follow-up to the advanced CHF clinic.

In this case, the patient's congestive cardiorenal syndrome was thought to be due to reduced effective circulating volume state due to poor left ventricular function, despite the lack of other clinical markers of poor perfusion. Essentially, a lack of forward flow was blamed for the renal failure, rather than poor perfusion due to congestive factors. This is a common error, and physical examination can be very challenging. The use of VExUS allowed the recognition of the venous congestive role in the patient's problem. With aggressive fluid removal, the decongestion of the venous circulation via diuretics and ascites drainage allowed for improvement in renal perfusion pressure and function. It is important to note that while abdominal decompression may have helped by relieving direct pressure on the kidney, this alone did not resolve the portal vein pulsatility which remained significant after several liters having been drained, which instantly normalized intra-abdominal pressure clinically. Unfortunately this was not measured pre- and post-drainage, which would have been interesting.

This case also illustrates the difficulty of properly assessing venous congestion in the setting of cardiac and hepatic disease, as well as differentiating the subtypes of cardiorenal syndrome, and how POCUS with VExUS scoring can identify pathological congestion and guide therapy. The presence of a dilated IVC is not sufficient to demonstrate clinically important congestion, as the IVC may be chronically dilated with varying degrees of actual venous congestion. The commonly seen delay in changes in serum creatinine (as its serum value does not reflect renal function in real time) with interventions can make management challenging (whether attempting to increase or decrease intravascular volume), whereas with bedside physiological evidence of the presence or absence of venous congestion, more congruent therapeutic decisions may be made.

Case 2

A 45-year-old male presented to the emergency department with worsening right upper quadrant abdominal pain after being referred for suspected acute cholecystitis diagnosed by ultrasound 2 weeks ago at another hospital. He arrived at the county emergency department with an ultrasound report indicating gallbladder wall edema and pericholecystic fluid, suspicious for acute cholecystitis. Because the report did not include images and was 2 weeks old, a repeat abdominal ultrasound and labs were ordered by an advanced care provider after consultation with the supervising physician.

The patient denied any past medical history and denied peripheral edema, dyspnea on exertion, or orthopnea. Vital signs were unremarkable and physical exam was significant for right upper abdominal tenderness to palpation, but no pedal edema, abnormal heart sounds, or crackles in the lung fields were appreciated in the noisy emergency department.

Laboratory results were significant for WBC of 14K, and mild elevations in AST and ALT. Creatine was 124 mmol/L (1.4 mg/dL). Ultrasound was interpreted by the radiologist as gallbladder wall thickening, pericholecystic fluid, without gallstones suspicious for acalculous cholecystitis (Fig. 3a). Surgical consultation was initiated by the advanced care provider and the surgery service evaluated the patient and planned to take him to surgery for a cholecystectomy later in the afternoon.

The supervising emergency physician was updated on the case and decided to review the ultrasound images. It was noted that the IVC and hepatic vein were plethoric and the portal vein Doppler was biphasic. Due to these findings, elevated venous pressure was suspected. A Focused Cardiac Ultrasound (FoCUS) and POCUS abdominal exam were therefore performed by the physician.

Abdominal POCUS was significant for a plethoric IVC without respiratory variation. Hepatic vein Doppler showed high amplitude A waves with S < D forward flow waves (Fig. 3b). There was a triphasic portal vein Doppler pattern (Fig. 3c), and biphasic interrupted intrarenal venous flow (Fig. 3d). These findings correspond to a VExUS grade 2 venous congestion, however there are severe flow abnormalities in the portal system. Furthermore, a more comprehensive bedside echocardiography exam showed biventricular dilation with a left ventricular ejection fraction of < 10%, restrictive left ventricular filling pattern, significant functional mitral regurgitation, and pulmonary hypertension. Left ventricular outflow tract velocity time integral (LVOT VTI) interrogation revealed a stroke volume of only 18 mL and cardiac output of 1.4 L/min.

The surgical service was contacted and after further discussion it was decided to cancel plans for surgery. The patient was discharged home for outpatient follow-up with cardiology and a furosemide prescription.

As shown in this case, the effects of venous congestion can mimic other pathological entities. In this particular instance, elevated venous pressures due to previously undiagnosed congestive heart failure led to impaired venous drainage of the portal system and congestion of the gallbladder wall which was initially mistaken as acute

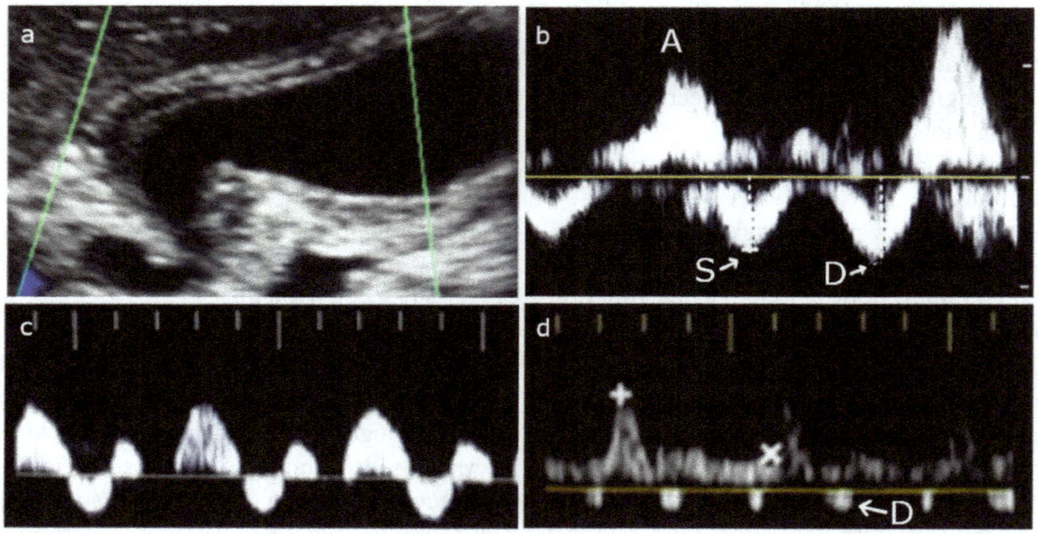

Fig. 3 Case 2: **a** gallbladder showing signs of acalculous cholecystitis. **b** Hepatic vein Doppler with high amplitude A waves with S < D forward flow waves. **c** Triphasic portal vein Doppler **d** biphasic interrupted intrarenal venous flow

cholecystitis. When the ultrasound was reviewed, recognition of the plethoric IVC and abnormal Doppler findings of the portal vein combined with the lack of other findings suggestive of cholecystitis led to the both the diagnosis of congestive heart failure and prevented an unnecessary surgical procedure.

Case 3

An 81-year-old male patient with moderate pulmonary hypertension and severe mitral insufficiency underwent mitral valve replacement with a bioprosthetic valve.

In the first 24 h, the patient needed transfusion of three units of blood, 800 mL of plasma and also pooled platelets. His fluid balance was positive by 2910 mL.

On physical examination, he weighed 90 kg, the heart rate was 73 bpm and arterial blood pressure was 138/56 mmHg. Oxygen saturation was 98% on high-flow nasal cannula (HFNC) with inspired oxygen at 40%. A pulmonary artery catheter showed moderate right ventricular (RV) dysfunction with pulmonary artery pressure 50/23 mmHg, central venous pressure (CVP) of 15 cm/H_2O on noradrenaline 0.1 mcg/kg/min + dobutamine 10 mcg/kg/min. He was in mild respiratory distress and pulmonary auscultation revealed crackles in the lower third of both lung fields. In addition, there was mild edema in the lower limbs and pulses were normal. The hemoglobin was 9.5 mg/dL, creatinine 256 umol/L (2.9 mg/dL) and urea 18 (mmol/L 110 mg/dL).

His POCUS examination revealed an EF of 65% with impaired relaxation; moderate right ventricular dysfunction with tricuspid annular plane systolic excursion (TAPSE) of 13 mm. His VExUS score showed a dilated and fixed IVC measuring over 25 mm in both axes and his portal vein showed 65% pulsatility (Fig. 4a). Hepatic vein Doppler showed reversal of flow of the S wave (Fig. 4b) and renal Doppler showed discontinuous monophasic flow with only a diastolic phase (Fig. 4c). These findings correspond to a VExUS grade 3 venous congestion.

Intravenous furosemide was started at high dose until a net balance of negative 1200 cc per 24 h was obtained. The patient was then on noradrenaline 0.05 mcg/kg/min, dobutamine 5 mcg/kg/min with a HR of 87 bpm, BP of 127/45, PAP 48/19 mm/Hg, and a CVP of 10 mmHg. The Hb was 10.2 mg/dL.

Progressively, the pulsatility of the portal vein decreased until it was 34.7% (Fig. 4d) and renal Doppler improved to discontinuous biphasic flow with systolic and diastolic phases (Fig. 4e). The IVC regained respiratory variation and measured approximately 22 mm in both axes. After the initial rise, the creatinine decreased to 194 mmol/L (2.2 mg/dL) and the urea improved to 32 mmol/L (90 mg/dL).

On the third day, furosemide infusion was continued targeting a higher negative fluid balance. A negative balance of 3200 cc per 24 h was achieved and dobutamine was further decreased to 3 mcg/kg/min.

At this point the blood pressure was 130/70, heart rate 75 bpm, and CVP was 2 mmHg. POCUS examination showed an IVC measuring approximately 15 mm in both axes with a respiratory variation greater than 50%. The portal vein showed 20% pulsatility (Fig. 4f) and the hepatic vein Doppler improved to normal with S > D flow (Fig. 4g). Creatinine levels continued to decline to 132 mmol/L (1.5 mg/dL) and the urea to 21 mmol/L

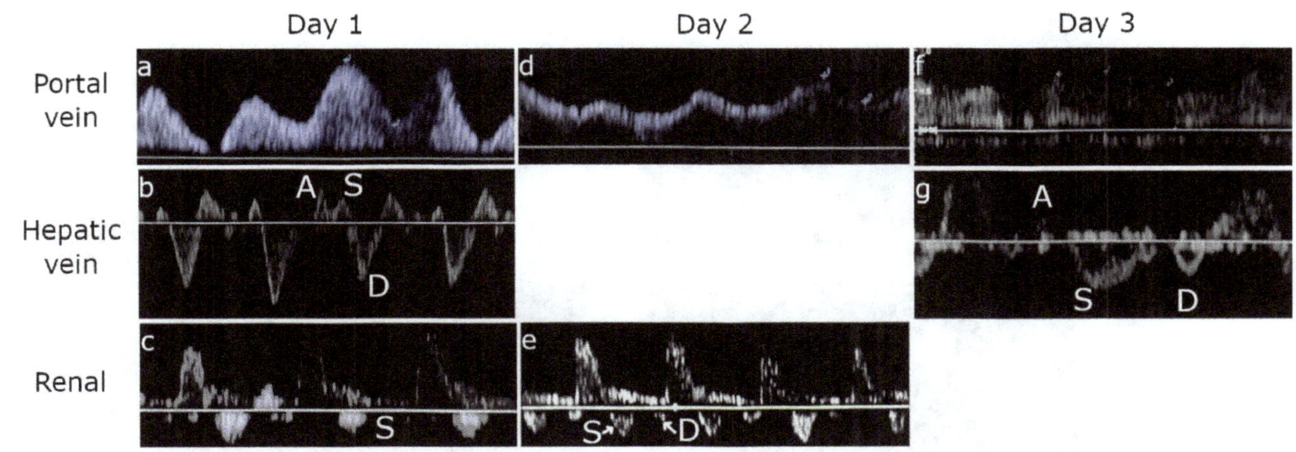

Fig. 4 Case 3: Doppler profiles of portal vein, hepatic vein, and intrarenal vasculature at days 1, 2 and 3

(60 mg/dL) and further improved to normal levels by the 4th day, and the patient was discharged to the cardiac surgery ward.

The pre-existence of pulmonary hypertension in this patient complicated the interpretation of the significance of the elevated CVP and dilated IVC. The chronicity of this condition leads to the question of the degree of previous compensated congestion versus the contribution of more acute elevations in venous pressures. VExUS allowed the assessment of venous congestion and its contribution to the patient's hemodynamic derangement. Despite inotropic support, the RV was significantly volume overloaded leading to decreased venous return in the face of acutely elevated right atrial pressures. This in turn led to a decreased perfusion gradient of the kidneys and likely further renal fluid retention. Diuresis thus allowed venous decongestion and improved renal perfusion in addition to offloading the RV, returning it to the steeper part of the Frank–Starling curve.

Case 4

A 57-year-old patient with group 1 pulmonary hypertension had been recently seen at an ambulatory clinic with an increase in the serum creatinine to 235 mmol/L (2.66 mg/dL) (baseline 96 mmol/L/1.09 mg/dL). Because of this, bumetanide and spironolactone were suspended.

Three weeks later the patient presented to the ED for worsening lower extremity edema and ascites. Physical exam was notable for Grade II ascites and lower extremity edema. Vital signs were HR 52, BP 94/62 mmHg, and O2 saturation of 98%. The creatinine was 311 mmol/L (3.52 mg/dL) and the potassium was 6.7 meq/L. VExUS assessment showed an IVC of 30 mm with no inspiratory collapse, hepatic vein with systolic flow reversal, a portal vein with greater than 100% pulsatility, and discontinuous monophasic intrarenal venous flow (Fig. 5a). POCUS showed normal LV systolic function, a dilated RV, and severe tricuspid regurgitation. B-type natriuretic peptide (BNP) was 1404 pg/mL. Given the severe venous congestion and hyperkalemia, the patient was treated with furosemide 200 mg IV. However, despite this treatment the patient produced no urine. A high-flow catheter was placed and hemodialysis was started with ultrafiltration of 2.5 L. Immediately after ultrafiltration, VExUS scan was repeated showing improvement in venous congestion. The IVC was persistently plethoric (30 mm), the hepatic vein improving to S < D, the portal vein pulsatility decreasing to 45%, and intrarenal venous Doppler became an interrupted biphasic pattern (Fig. 5b). Moments later the patient spontaneously produced 800 mL of urine. A furosemide infusion (200 mg/day) + spironolactone 50 mg BID was started and eventually achieved a negative fluid balance of 15.5 L. Serum creatinine improved to 151 mmol/L (1.71 mg/dL) and the patient was discharged home with oral bumetanide and spironolactone.

This case again demonstrates the value of VExUS in differentiating inadequate from excessive diuretic therapy. Initially, because of the rise in creatinine, the patient was mistakenly determined (without VExUS exam) to be over aggressively diuresed. Cessation of diuretic therapy then led to further renal dysfunction and clinical decompensation. The use of VExUS not only implicated venous congestion as the major culprit in the patient's deterioration, but served as a guide to both the initiation of ultrafiltration dialysis when furosemide failed, and served to guide titration of the ultrafiltration therapy.

Case 5

A 28-year-old gravida 5, para 2 female at 32 weeks of a twin pregnancy presented with vaginal bleeding and contractions. The patient had an emergent C-section

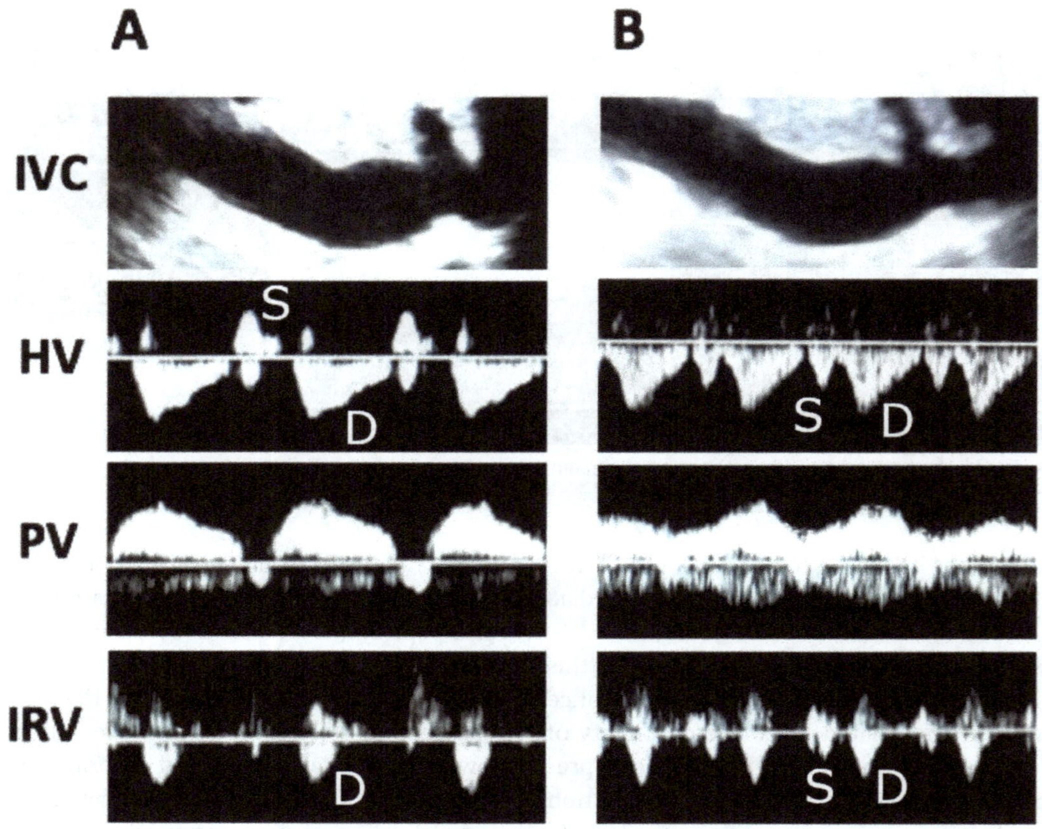

Fig. 5 Case 4: **a** initial congestive Doppler profiles. **b** Doppler profiles after hemodialysis with ultrafiltration of 2.5 L

performed and went into disseminated intravascular coagulation (DIC) requiring massive blood transfusion protocol (> 10 Units). On arrival to the ICU the patient was anuric, hypotensive and on high doses of phenylephrine, norepinephrine, and vasopressin. Her lactate was 11.3mMol/L and Hgb was 6.7 g/dL. The patient's therapy was being partially guided by a continuous cardiac output monitor which showed a stroke volume variation of 23%, so she also received over 6 L of IV fluid, as she was considered "volume responsive".

On physical exam the patient was intubated tachycardic with SpO2 of 94% on 80% FiO2 and PEEP of 10 cm H2O.

POCUS showed a dilated IVC, a retrograde S wave on hepatic Doppler, and 100% pulsatile portal vein. In addition, the cardiac ultrasound showed an enlarged right ventricle with a D-sign shape and severe tricuspid regurgitation. The patient had diffuse B-lines in both lung fields and on lower extremity ultrasound, a mobile clot was seen in the left common femoral vein (Fig. 6a–f). The overall VExUS pattern was Grade 3 signifying severe venous congestion.

A CT pulmonary angiogram was obtained showing bilateral small subsegmental pulmonary emboli. Since the patient was anuric, nephrology was consulted for emergent ultrafiltration and 5 L of fluid was taken off within 24 h. Anticoagulation was contraindicated because of the recent C-section and active DIC. An IVC filter was placed for the mobile DVT.

Over the next 2 days the patient's lactate normalized and vasopressor requirements improved. The patient was eventually extubated 3 days later and discharged after 17 days total of hospitalization.

In this case, the use of VExUS demonstrated that the patient's refractory shocked state was related to volume overload as well as the already recognized RV dysfunction. Without the use of VExUS the RV dysfunction may have been only attributed to the pulmonary emboli.

The continuous cardiac output monitor provided the clinicians erroneous data with regard to the patient's volume status, likely due to the severe RV dysfunction and subsequent interventricular dependence hemodynamic factors.

The use of VExUS demonstrated significant venous congestion and led to an active fluid offloading strategy rather than continued attempts to use ventricular preloading to resolve the hypotension and shock. This strategy was further supported by the echocardiographic "D-sign" showing that the RV dilation from volume overload was encroaching on LV diastolic

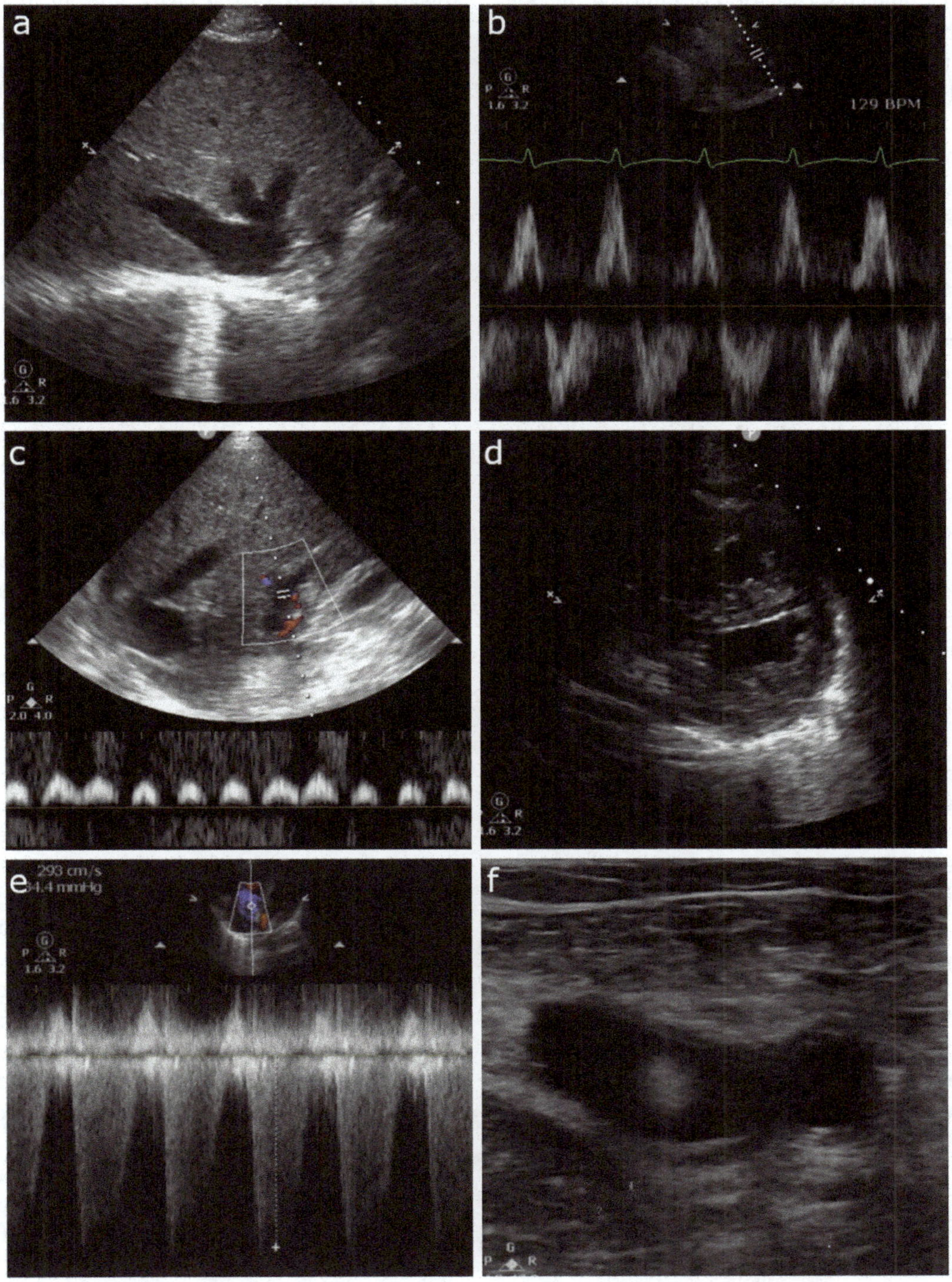

Fig. 6 Case 5: **a** dilated IVC. **b** Hepatic vein Doppler with retrograde S wave. **c** Portal vein Doppler with 100% pulsatility. **d** PSAX view of the heart with D-shaped left-ventricle. **e** CW Doppler at the tricuspid valve showing tricuspid regurgitation. **d** Mobile clot seen in the left femoral vein

filling. With removal of the excess volume, the dysfunctional septal shift resolved, thus increasing left ventricular filling and cardiac output.

Venous congestion and the VExUS grading system: pathological basis, pitfalls and limitations

Systemic venous congestion can be evaluated and

quantified by Doppler interrogation of multiple splanchnic organs. The VExUS grading system utilizes Doppler evaluation of the hepatic vein, portal vein and intrarenal venous vein. In the presence of a plethoric inferior vena cava, each of these veins are evaluated and assigned to either being normal, mild congestion, or severe congestion. VExUS grade 0 is with no sign of congestion in any organ, VExUS grade 1 is with only mild congestive findings, VExUS grade 2 is with severe findings in only one organ, and VExUS grade 3 is with severe congestive findings in at least 2 of 3 organ systems (Fig. 7).

Hepatic vein Doppler patterns are the result of interactions between venous return-driven by the mean systemic filling pressure (Pmsf) and the right atria and right ventricle. Pmsf is generated by the elastic recoil of the sum total of the venous system. The venous system is highly compliant and acts as a large blood reservoir that can be recruited in times of hypovolemia via an increase in venous tone. Blood volume that occupies the venous compartment without distending the walls of the veins is called unstressed volume, and exerts no influence on venous return. However, any additional volume that distends the walls of the venous system will generate a pressure due to elastic recoil of the veins. The pressure resulting from this recoil, known as the Pmsf, serves as the driving force that generates venous return to the right ventricle. Forces impeding venous return are the resistance of the venous system and the right atrial pressure that exists due to imperfect efficiency of the right ventricle. During the cardiac cycle, when right atrial pressure exceeds Pmfs, the blood flow will be away from the heart and conversely, flow will be towards the heart when Pmfs exceeds right atrial pressure. Therefore, normal hepatic Doppler waveforms are characterized by an initial above the baseline wave associated with right atrial contraction, followed by below the baseline flow during systole (due to right atrial relaxation, movement of the tricuspid annulus toward the apex of the heart, and an increase in atrial volume capacity as the ventricles decrease their volume within the non-compliant pericardium), and finally a below the baseline flow wave during diastole as the right atrium becomes a passive conduit for blood to enter the relaxing right ventricle. These waves are known as the A, S, and D waves, respectively, and correspond to the well-known A wave, X descent, and Y descent of the jugular venous pulse. Generally, as average right atrial pressures rise, the A wave becomes more prominent and the S wave will decrease in amplitude relative to the D wave until there is a systolic reversal of flow and fusion with the A wave.

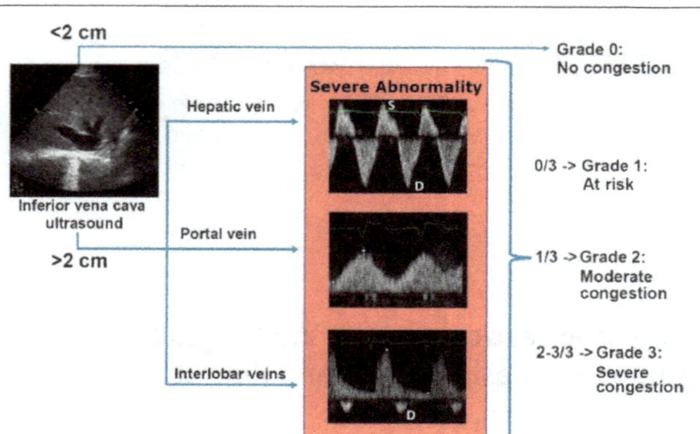

Fig. 7 Doppler profiles showing severe congestive patterns

Under normal circumstances, the venous compartment is highly compliant with high capacitance, and therefore, with increasing distance from the heart, the venous pulse is dampened so that in the smaller veins, flow becomes undulating and phasic in nature. However, in states of right ventricular failure or intravascular volume overload, the venous compartment becomes congested and the limits of venous compliance are reached. Under these circumstances, the normal dampening of the venous pulse due to the compliant nature of the smaller veins is lost, and the pulsations are transmitted back into the smaller veins.

The portal vein is separated from the rest of the systemic venous circulation by the hepatic sinusoids that it empties into. The hepatic sinusoids then drain into the hepatic veins that finally drain into the IVC. Due to this distance from the heart, normal portal venous flow is undulating and phasic in nature and blood travels in a hepatopetal direction at about 20 cm/s. As venous congestion rises, the hepatic vein's retrograde flow generated by atrial contraction is transmitted up through the hepatic sinusoids and into the portal vein where it gives rise to impedance to the portal hepatopetal flow. This causes the normal undulating flow to become progressively pulsatile and this phenomenon is compounded when there is systolic reversal of venous return to the heart. Eventually, the pulsatility becomes significant enough to cause a biphasic or back-and-forth pattern of portal flow.

Intrarenal venous Doppler waveform obtained from the interlobar or arcuate vessels is usually considered adequate when both arterial (above the baseline) and venous (below the baseline) flow signals are seen clearly for two or more cardiac cycles.

The intrarenal venous Doppler signal is normally a continuous monophasic flow below the baseline. With increasing venous congestion, the venous flow becomes pulsatile, then progresses to an interrupted biphasic flow which correlates to the S and the D waves of the hepatic vein's flow.

Similar to the hepatic vein pattern, as venous congestion further worsens, the S wave becomes smaller and the D wave is more pronounced until the S wave disappears entirely, leaving only a monophasic D wave.

The intrarenal venous Doppler waveform is considered abnormal when there is discontinuous venous flow with either a systolic/diastolic (discontinuous biphasic) pattern or a diastolic only pattern (discontinuous monophasic).

The assessments presented in this case series are not without important caveats. The IVC can be compressed by increased intra-abdominal pressure independently of right atrial pressure [8]. In chronic pulmonary hypertension, it can experience significant size remodeling [9]. The hepatic vein might not show significant alterations even in severe tricuspid regurgitation if right atrial compliance is preserved [10]. The portal vein can display a pulsatile flow in thin healthy subjects without venous congestion [11], this is also the case in patients with arteriovenous malformations [12]. In patients with stiff liver parenchyma as in cirrhosis or non-alcoholic fatty liver disease, transmission of pressure from the right atrium through the liver sinusoid is dampened and this may lead to a non-pulsatile portal vein even in the presence of severe venous congestion [13, 14]. The intrarenal venous doppler is technically difficult to obtain which can lead to suboptimal recordings [15]. It is also possible that parenchymal renal disease could alter intre-renal doppler venous waveforms [15]. Given these limitations, it is important to avoid interpretation of any of these exams in isolation. Performing a protocolized exam including IVC, HV, PV and IRVD will increase the overall accuracy of the evaluation. In support of this idea, the protocolized combination of scans, summarized by the VExUS grading system, showed increased predictive value for AKI in cardiac surgery patients [7].

Discussion

These cases illustrate how assessing venous splanchnic congestion can be of critical importance in a wide variety of clinical scenarios. The vague and somewhat unclear concept of "volume status" remains a challenge for clinicians in general due to the limitations of physical examination. Indeed, in many patients, identifying the presence of venous congestion associated with potential end-organ dysfunction may not be possible without invasive monitoring or ultrasound assessments. But beyond the definition of euvolemia, the more practical questions center around when to give or when to remove fluid. While VExUS will not likely provide much information on the need for fluid, it may provide stop points to fluid resuscitation and identify patients who are likely to tolerate and benefit from fluid removal. While the focus in fluid resuscitation has long been cardiac output or forward flow, the literature suggests strongly that venous congestion, as determined by CVP or by venous Doppler indices, will at a certain point offset the benefits of increasing said forward flow [4–7, 16]. In fact, Vellinga et al., in studying the microcirculation, showed that a CVP above 12 actually resulted in a decreased tissue perfusion, and was associated with sluggish capillary flow which they termed "microcirculatory tamponade" [17].

This knowledge should prompt the clinician to be keenly aware of the double-edged nature of fluids and to use available tools at the bedside to tailor fluid resuscitation or removal to avoid pathological markers of venous congestion.

Conclusion

As time passes, positive experiences of first-line clinicians using venous congestion indices as a guide to the management of intravascular volume accumulates in several different clinical settings. While there remains a lack of properly controlled interventional studies regarding the effectiveness of a strategy based on such an approach, there are good reasons to believe that using an approach incorporating POCUS would have clear advantages compared to current practice characterized by high variability among healthcare providers. The VExUS as a window on the venous pathophysiology, might be a key to achieving precise fluid management.

The rapid evolution of knowledge about the VExUS assessment should be of interest to all first-line clinicians involved in daily decision-making about fluid balance management. Moreover, it adds to the growing body of evidence that a modern clinician should be proficient in POCUS to ensure optimal care to their patients.

Acknowledgements
Not applicable.

Authors' contributions
PR, FMA, EA and KH each contributed a case. WBS, RS contributed to discussion and general review. TK contributed to discussion, general review, editing and figure generation. All authors read and approved the final manuscript.

Author details
[1]ICU Chief of Service, Santa Cabrini Hospital, Montreal, QC, Canada. [2]Anasthesia & Surgery Critical Care Service, Hospital Universitario Puerta del Mar, Cádiz, Spain. [3]Instituto Nacional de Ciencias Medicas y Nutricion Salvador, Zubiran, Tlalpan, Mexico City, Mexico. [4]Division of Nephrology, Centre Hospitalier de L'Université de Montréal, Montreal, Canada. [5]Department of Emergency Medicine, Riverside University Health Systems Medical Center, Moreno Valley, CA, USA. [6]Intensive Care, Hôpital Honoré Mercier, Ste-Hyacinthe, QC, Canada. [7]Department of Emergency Medicine and Department of Internal Medicine, Division of Pulmonary and Critical Care Medicine, Loma Linda University Health, Loma Linda, CA, USA. [8]Department of Critical Care, Georgetown University Medstar Washington Hospital Center, Washington, DC, USA.

References

1. Winton FR (1931) The influence of venous pressure on the isolated mammalian kidney. J Physiol 72(1):49–61. https://doi.org/10.1113/jphysiol.1931.sp002761
2. Boron WF, Boulpaep EL (2009) Medical physiology: a cellular and molecular approach, 2nd edn. Saunders/Elsevier, Philadelphia
3. Catalano D, Caruso G, DiFazzio S, Carpinteri G, Scalisi N, Trovato GM (1998) Portal vein pulsatility ratio and heart failure. J Clin Ultrasound 26(1):27–31. https://doi.org/10.1002/(sici)1097-0096(199801)26:1%3c27::aid-jcu6%3e3.0.co;2-l
4. Beaubien-Souligny W, Benkreira A, Robillard P et al (2018) Alterations in portal vein flow and intrarenal venous flow are associated with acute kidney injury after cardiac surgery: a prospective observational cohort study. J Am Heart Assoc 7(19):e009961. https://doi.org/10.1161/JAHA.118.009961
5. Eljaiek R, Cavayas YA, Rodrigue E et al (2019) High postoperative portal venous flow pulsatility indicates right ventricular dysfunction and predicts complications in cardiac surgery patients. Br J Anaesth 122(2):206–214. https://doi.org/10.1016/j.bja.2018.09.028
6. Beaubien-Souligny W, Eljaiek R, Fortier A et al (2018) The Association between pulsatile portal flow and acute kidney injury after cardiac surgery: a retrospective cohort study. J Cardiothorac Vasc Anesth 32(4):1780–1787. https://doi.org/10.1053/j.jvca.2017.11.030
7. Beaubien-Souligny W, Rola P, Haycock K et al (2020) Quantifying systemic congestion with Point-Of-Care ultrasound: development of the venous excess ultrasound grading system. Ultrasound J 12(1):16. https://doi.org/10.1186/s13089-020-00163-w
8. Wachsberg RH (2000) Narrowing of the upper abdominal inferior vena cava in patients with elevated intraabdominal pressure: sonographic observations. J Ultrasound Med 19(3):217–222. https://doi.org/10.7863/jum.2000.19.3.217
9. Via G, Tavazzi G, Price S (2016) Ten situations where inferior vena cava ultrasound may fail to accurately predict fluid responsiveness: a physiologically based point of view. Intensive Care Med 42(7):1164–1167. https://doi.org/10.1007/s00134-016-4357-9 (**Epub 2016 Apr 23**)
10. Pennestrí F, Loperfido F, Salvatori MP, Mongiardo R, Ferrazza A, Guccione P, Manzoli U (1984) Assessment of tricuspid regurgitation by pulsed Doppler ultrasonography of the hepatic veins. Am J Cardiol 54(3):363–368. https://doi.org/10.1016/0002-9149(84)90198-x
11. Gallix BP, Taourel P, Dauzat M, Bruel JM, Lafortune M (1997) Flow pulsatility in the portal venous system: a study of Doppler sonography in healthy adults. AJR Am J Roentgenol 169(1):141–144. https://doi.org/10.2214/ajr.169.1.9207514
12. Wachsberg RH, Needleman L, Wilson DJ (1995) Portal vein pulsatility in normal and cirrhotic adults without cardiac disease. J Clin Ultrasound 23(1):3–15. https://doi.org/10.1002/jcu.1870230103
13. Loperfido F, Lombardo A, Amico CM, Vigna C, Testa M, Rossi E, Costalunga A, Pennestri F, Biasucci LM (1993) Doppler analysis of portal vein flow in tricuspid regurgitation. J Heart Valve Dis 2(2):174–182
14. Baikpour M, Ozturk A, Dhyani M, Mercaldo ND, Pierce TT, Grajo JR, Samir AE (2020) Portal venous pulsatility index: a novel biomarker for diagnosis of high-risk nonalcoholic fatty liver disease. AJR Am J Roentgenol 214(4):786–791. https://doi.org/10.2214/AJR.19.21963 (**Epub 2020 Jan 15**)
15. Jeong SH, Jung DC, Kim SH, Kim SH (2011) Renal venous Doppler ultrasonography in normal subjects and patients with diabetic nephropathy: value of venous impedance index measurements. J Clin Ultrasound 39(9):512–518. https://doi.org/10.1002/jcu.20835 (**Epub 2011 May 4**)
16. Spiegel R, Teeter W, Sullivan S, Tupchong K, Mohammed N, Sutherland M, Leibner E, Rola P, Galvagno SM Jr, Murthi SB (2020) The use of venous Doppler to predict adverse kidney events in a general ICU cohort. Crit Care 24(1):615. https://doi.org/10.1186/s13054-020-03330-6
17. Vellinga NA, Ince C, Boerma EC (2013) Elevated central venous pressure is associated with impairment of microcirculatory blood flow in sepsis: a hypothesis generating post hoc analysis. BMC Anesthesiol 7(13):17. https://doi.org/10.1186/1471-2253-13-17

22

Offshore telementored ultrasound: a quality assessment study

Victoria Vatsvåg[1,2*], Kjetil Todnem[3], Torvind Næsheim[4,5], John Cathcart[1], Daniel Kerr[1] and Nils Petter Oveland[2,6]

Abstract

Background: Telementored ultrasound (US) connects experts to novices through various types of communication and network technologies with the overall aim to bridge the medical imaging gap between patients' diagnostic needs and on-site user experience. The recurrent theme in previous research on remote telementored US is the limited access to US machines and experienced users. This study was conducted to determine whether telementored US was feasible in a remote offshore setting. The aim was to assess if an onshore US expert can guide an offshore nurse through focused US scanning protocols by connecting an US machine to existing videoconference units at the offshore hospitals and to evaluate the diagnostic quality of the images and cineloops procured.

Results: The diagnostic quality of cineloops was scored on a five-point scale. The percentage of cineloops suitable for interpretation (score 3 ≥) for the FATE and e-FAST protocols was 96.4 and 79.1. Lung sliding and seashore sign could be identified in all volunteers. The scan time for the FAST protocol (n = four scanning positions), FATE protocol (n = six scanning positions) and both lungs (n = two scanning positions) was 1 min 20 s, 4 min 15 s and 32 s, respectively.

Conclusion: A novice US user can be guided by a remote expert through focused US protocols within an acceptable time frame and with good diagnostic quality using existing communication and network systems found onboard offshore oil rigs.

Keywords: Ultrasound, Telementored ultrasound, PoCUS, Offshore, Remote

Background

Historically, practising medicine has always been a combination of skills for diagnosis and commencing treatment based on patients' signs and symptoms [1, 2]. As one would expect, doing so in an austere environment is even more challenging where the clinical scenarios and patterns of illness and injury vary widely, and the access to medical equipment and qualified healthcare personnel are limited or even lacking [3]. Norway is an important supplier of oil and gas to the global market and employs approximately 21,000 people running between 80 and 90 oil installations [4]. These platforms and ships are spread along the Norwegian continental shelf and have limited medical and logistic support. Operating in such remote locations and challenging climatic environments requires a well-functioning health service [5]. Today, this remote medical practice is run by offshore nurses in hospital units onboard the installations and search-and-rescue (SAR) personnel working as part of medical evacuation (medevac) teams onboard helicopters [6]. The nurses, often working alone, are trained to carry out focused clinical examinations, perform certain medical tests, including recording vitals and electrocardiograms (ECGs), and provide simple blood and urine tests (e.g., haemoglobin, CRP, glucose). The nurse also has the opportunity to consult with a physician onshore, either by phone or videoconference [7]. However, this remote offshore healthcare service is in many cases insufficient for determining

*Correspondence: victoria.vatsvag@uis.no
[1] School Health Sciences, Ulster University, Co., Antrim, UK
Full list of author information is available at the end of the article

a final diagnosis [8, 9]. Whereas patients hospitalized onshore are referred for further medical imaging, such as X-ray, computerized tomography (CT), magnetic resonance imaging (MRI) or ultrasound (US), to determine their diagnosis [1, 10], this equipment has not, to date, been available for offshore workers. The result is an extended use of medevacs with SAR helicopters to bring the patients off the platforms and admit them to onshore hospitals. This process is a costly affair and not without risks, especially in challenging weather conditions [6]. It can take several hours from alerting the SAR team until the patient reaches definitive care, or in the worst-case scenario, no evacuation is possible due to restricted flying conditions [7]. Therefore, there is a need for extended medical practice with provision of more advanced diagnostic and management advice via telecommunication (i.e., telemedicine [11, 12]). A solution could be to connect US machines to the already installed videoconference units (medical units) found onboard most oil installations [13]. The development of lightweight, battery-powered, and easily transportable devices has made US in the field (i.e., outside hospitals) possible in contrast to bulkier and power-demanding X-ray machines and CT and MRI scanners [14]. Continued improvement in both US and telecommunication technology may open opportunities for improved clinical decision-making [12, 15]. US imaging can be obtained instantly and correlated to the patient's presenting signs and symptoms and repeated if the condition changes [16]. Combining the offshore nurses' physical examination with a focused goal-directed US scan [i.e., point-of-care ultrasound (PoCUS)] can confirm and refute life-threatening diagnoses, thereby assisting the onshore physicians in the initial evaluation and management of critically ill and injured patients [16, 17]. However, the acquisition and interpretation of PoCUS examinations are highly user-dependent [17, 18]. The operator experience amongst offshore nurses and SAR personnel thus appears to be a limitation to widespread use. We believe that this limitation can be compensated through real-time assistance using videoconferencing to link novice operators to geographically separate US experts to enable remote guidance of PoCUS examinations, an activity recognized as telementored US, tele-US or remote telementored US (RTMUS) [17, 19]. This utility of US has been evident in various extreme expeditions, such as to Mount Everest [20]. In the last decade, experience with remote applications for PoCUS has continued to increase, and research has been carried out in a variety of locations, such as rural areas in third world countries and even in space (International Space Station) [21–24]. However, telementored US between offshore nurses and an onshore on-call physician service has never been tested and evaluated. Thus, our study describes the initial experiences from a telementored US trial sending real-time video and US images from an offshore installation.

Objectives

The objectives of this research are as follows:

- Test if the telecommunication technologies and networks available at an offshore oil installation support real-time streaming of US cineloops and images.
- Test if an onshore physician is able to instruct and guide an offshore novice user in performing predefined PoCUS protocols of the lungs, heart and abdomen.
- Analyse the US cineloops and images procured by novice users to determine if the quality is sufficient to extract useful clinical information.

Methods

Study design and setting

This study was a quality assessment study conducted in 2012 at the Statfjord C rig at the Statfjord oil field covering 580 km^2 in the United Kingdom—Norwegian boundary of the North Sea. Statfjord C has a capacity of 345 persons on board served by one single hospital unit. The hospital is manned by one nurse, working 14-day rotations, in collaboration with onshore physicians working on-call 24-7 to assist in diagnosis and treatment decisions [13]. In most cases, the communication is via telephone (i.e., audio communication), but there is the option of using a preinstalled videoconference unit to enable video and audio from the hospital bay (i.e., the patient's bed area) to be transmitted to remotely located computers (with preinstalled communication software) [12]. The US machine was directly connected to the medical unit and transmitted the US image and roof camera video to an onshore computer via an internet connection. The technical setup is illustrated in Fig. 1 and described in detail under "Equipment".

Ethical considerations

This study was exempt from formal ethical approval according to mail correspondence with the regional committees for medical and health research ethics (REK) in Norway. The study protocol was reported to the Norwegian Centre for Research Data (NSD), and considerable efforts were made to protect the interests of the participants. Participation was voluntary; we analysed the data anonymously, informed the participants about the study in writing, and notified them of their right to withdraw consent at any time. A written agreement including the invitation and participation without compensation was

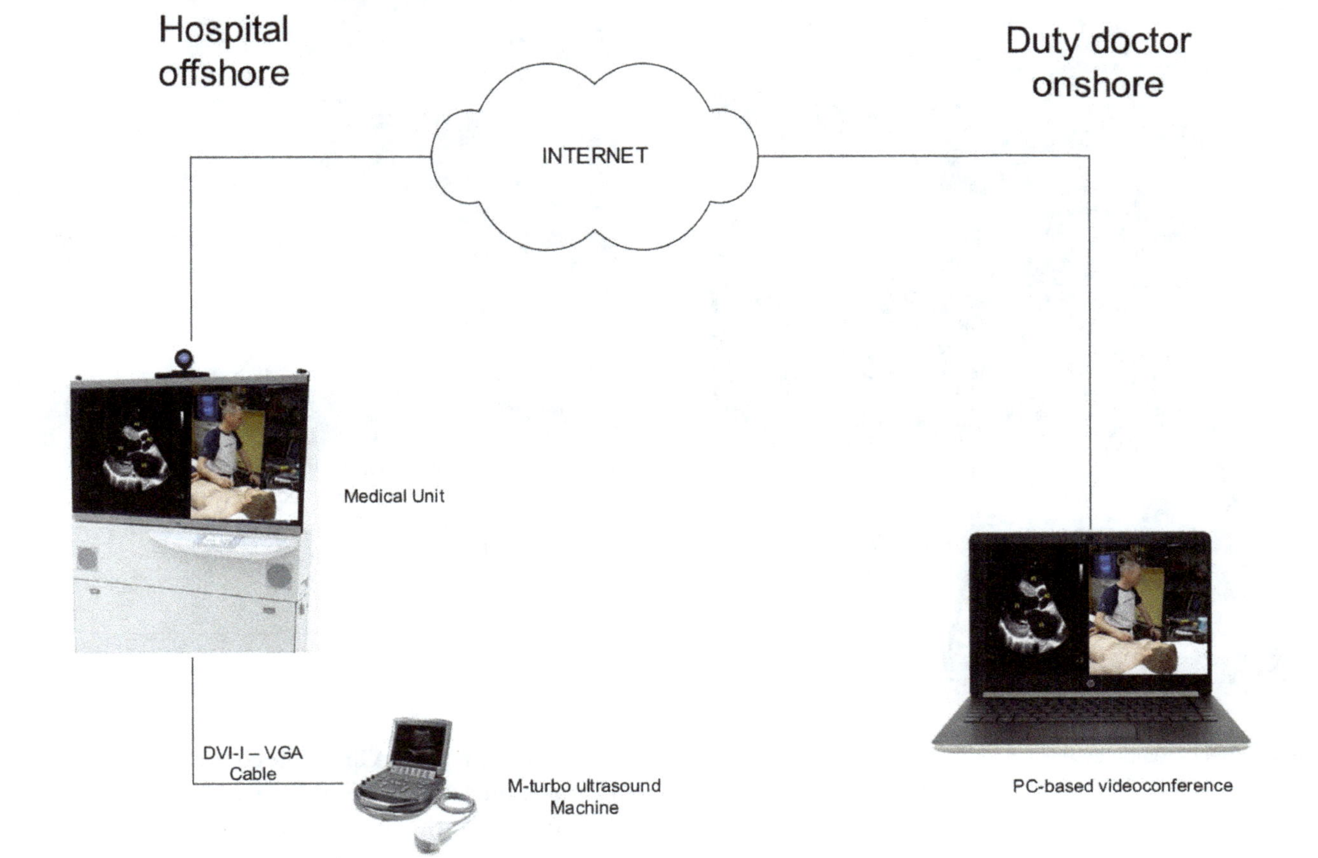

Fig. 1 Technical setup

signed by all parties. In the case that pathology was found during the US scan, the participant was referred to his/her primary care physician. Furthermore, we also encouraged the participants to contact the researchers if they had any concerns or questions.

Equipment

An M-Turbo US machine (FUJIFILM SonoSite Inc, Bothell, WA, USA) with three bandwidth phased-array (P21x probe 5-1 MHz), curved-array (C60xi probe 5–2 MHz) and linear-array (L25x probe 13-6 MHz) transducers (FUJIFILM SonoSite Inc, Bothell, WA, USA) was connected to the videoconference unit (Cisco TelePresence C90, Cisco Systems Inc., San Jose, CA, USA) via a video graphics array (VGA) cable. The M-Turbo machine does not have a VGA outlet and was solved using a small docking station with a digital visual interface integrated (DVI-I) to VGA converter. The videoconference unit is called Medical unit and will be referred as such in the remaining text and figure legends. The VGA cable relays analogue component video signals and data from the US machine to the Medical unit, which together with the main and roof cameras (Cisco P60, Cisco Systems Inc., San Jose, CA, USA), allow real-time communication of audio–video signals between the oil installation to a Medical unit or remote computer with Cisco Jabber communication software (Cisco Systems Inc., San Jose, CA, USA) in the duty doctor's office (Fig. 1). As a default, a 50%–50% split screen solution showing both the US image and video of the patient on the hospital bed was used (Fig. 2). The sharing of the US stream and the bidirectional sharing of audio and video were transferred live through an encrypted video stream. As shown in Fig. 1, the duo-video was transmitted to the duty doctor's Medical unit (Fig. 2) through the corporate network at Statfjord C. All communication equipments, including servers and routers, are readily available and can be bought off the shelf. Todnem et al. [12] have described the use of medical units as an integrated part of the health service on offshore oil installations on the Norwegian continental shelf.

Participants

The participants ($n=37$) in the study were volunteer offshore workers that, based on availability, consented

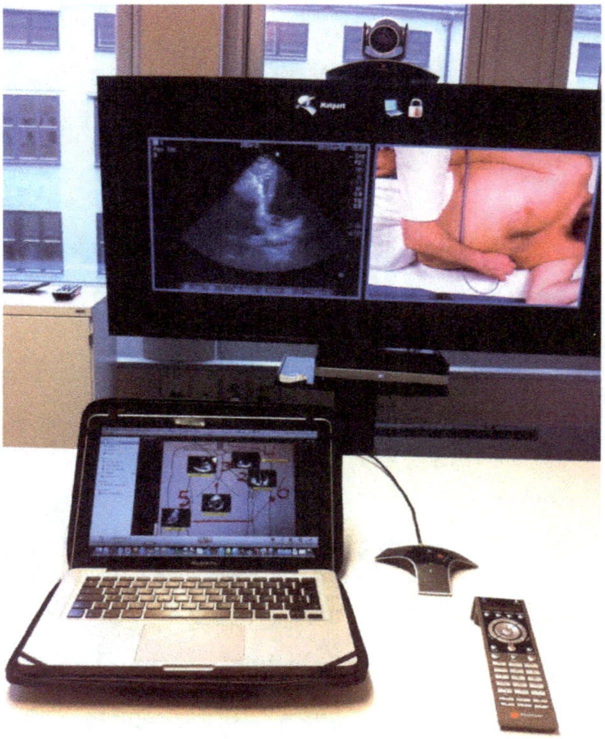

Fig. 2 Onshore computer showing the split screen with both the ultrasound image and roof camera video. Photo: Nils Petter Oveland

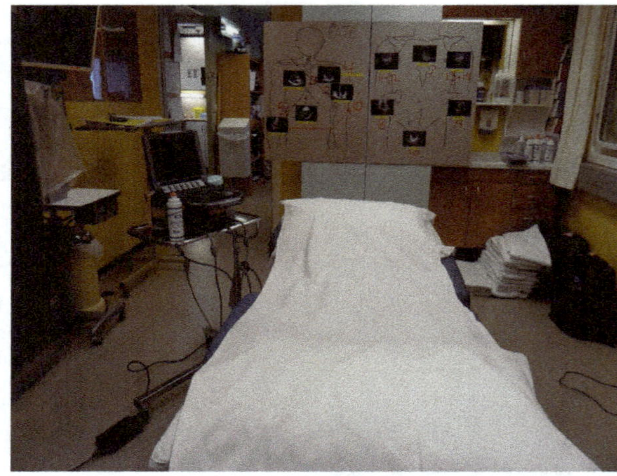

Fig. 3 Scanning positions. Offshore hospital bed with M-Turbo ultrasound machine and wall-mounted scanning cards for Focused Assessed Transthoracic Echo (FATE) and extended Focused Assessment with Sonography for Trauma (e-FAST). Ultrasound video clips and images were recorded from all 14 positions. Photo: Nils Petter Oveland

to serve as US scanning models. No volunteers were rejected from participating and the final number of 37 participants was based on the maximum capacity of a 2-day study period offshore at Statfjord C. All US scanning were performed by the offshore nurse on call ($n = 1$) and remotely guided by an onshore physician ($n = 1$) using videoconference communication as described. The nurse (i.e., novice user) had no previous US scanning experience, and the onshore physician (i.e., expert user) had more than 10-year clinical experience in PoCUS.

Data acquisition

The nurse received an initial ½ h practical demo (i.e., knobology) of the M-Turbo US machine, including how to insert patient data and save US images and cineloops. This was done offshore and the demo was given by the research supervisor. The remotely located onshore physician then guided the nurse through two defined scanning protocols: Focused Assessed Transthoracic Echo (FATE) of the heart and pleural space [25] and extended Focused Assessment with Sonography for Trauma (e-FAST) of the abdominal, pleural and pericardial space and bilateral lung scans [26]. The FATE, FAST, e-FAST and lung protocols are extensively described in the literature [27–29]. The nurse was guided through the examination as described in the FATE protocol and obtained a 6-s cineloop from each position. For each volunteer ($n = 37$), cineloops using the phased-array cardiac probe were recorded at each of the following positions: (1) subcostal 4-chamber view, (2) apical 4-chamber view, (3) parasternal long-axis view, (4) parasternal short-axis view, (5) pleura right side and (6) pleura left side.

Similarly, the nurse was guided through the examination as described in the FAST protocol and obtained 6-s cineloops for each position. For each volunteer, cineloops were recorded using the curved-array abdominal probe of each of the following positions: (7) subcostal 4-chamber view, (8) peri-hepatic view, (9) peri-splenic view and (10) pelvic view. Finally, cineloops of (11 + 13) lung sliding and (12 + 14) M-mode still images of both lungs were obtained to complete the extended FAST protocol. The setup is summarized in Fig. 3. A research supervisor was present at all times and used a stopwatch to measure the scan time per scanning position. The measurement started when the transducer was placed on the skin and stopped when the onshore expert asked the nurse to store the cineloop or image. When performing the scan, the nurse only received instructions from the onshore expert on how to adjust gain, depth and transducer position. All the cineloops and images where stored on the M-Turbo machine under an alphabetical and numerical code starting with A1, B1, C1, etc. and later transferred to a USB drive.

Data analysis

The data analysis was binate, with one focus on US image quality and another on scanning time. The image quality of the recorded cineloops (stored on a single USB stick) from both the FATE and e-FAST protocols was blindly evaluated by two independent observers (i.e., an independent US expert panel). A previously described method for evaluating image quality of cineloops [30, 31] was used for the FATE and FAST protocols and a YES/NO answer if lung sliding (cineloop) and seashore sign (M-mode still image) could be identified in the e-FAST lung scans. A five-point scale was used [1 = no visible image (i.e., only air artefacts), 2 = poor image quality with no identifiable anatomical structures, 3 = moderate image quality with partly visible anatomical structures, 4 = good image quality with visible anatomical structures and 5 = excellent image quality with highly visible anatomical structures], with a value of 3 representing the cut-off score for images suitable for interpretation [31]. When calculating the fraction of interpretable images, the 5-point scale was dichotomized, with a score of ≥ 3 indicating that clinically useful information could be extracted from the video clips. The extended part of the FAST protocol was to visualize the pleural line. This step was easily achieved in all volunteers, and scoring the image quality of the lungs was considered less important. Therefore, no image score was assigned from positions 11–14 (lung video clips and M-mode still images). Finally, the total time spent for the FATE and e-FAST protocols was calculated by adding the mean scan time for each position 1–6 and 7–10, respectively.

Statistical analysis

The image rating scores were analysed using standard descriptive statistics of central tendencies such as median and mean and associated variation as ± standard deviation (SD), interquartile range and minimum–maximum values. The data were outlined graphically as box plots where the length of the box represented the data between the 25 and 75% percentile, the thickened line inside the box showed the median and "whiskers" showed the min and max values. A breakdown of data by acoustic window (i.e., positions 1–6 for FATE and 7–10 for FAST) was done and presented in tables as the mean ± SD. The fraction of interpretable images by acoustic window and protocol (i.e., FATE and FAST) was calculated as the percentage of images with a score of 3 or higher, indicated in tables, figures and text as $\%^{3\geq}$. Finally, the total scan time was calculated by adding the separate mean scanning times, from probe-on-skin until captured video clip, for positions 1–6, positions 7–10, and positions 11 and 13 for FATE, FAST, and lungs, respectively. All computations were performed using SPSS version 24 (IBM SPSS, Armonk, NY), and data were stored in compliance with current research guidelines.

Results

All offshore workers that volunteered to be scanned were male with a mean age of 48.7 ± 10.3. The mean weight was 86.1 kg ± 13.4 kg. The image quality score of the cineloops was higher with the FATE protocol than the FAST protocol with medians of 4 and 3, respectively. When comparing the percentage of images suitable for interpretation, 96.4% of the cardiac views (i.e., FATE) using the phased-array transducer and 79.1% of the thoraco-abdominal views (i.e., FAST) using the curved-array transducer had an image score equal to or above 3 ($\%^{\geq 3}$). No image scores were calculated for the lungs (i.e., e-FAST) as bilateral lung sliding at the pleural line was easily identified in all participants with $100\%^{\geq 3}$. The median quality scores and fractions of interpretable images for both protocols are outlined as box plots in Fig. 4a, b. Further details about the images' scores and $\%^{\geq 3}$ by acoustic window when performing telementored FATE and FAST are available in Tables 1 and 2.

The mean scan time to complete a full telementored FATE scan comprised six cardio-thoracic views with stored cineloops was 4 min 15 s. Similarly, the mean scan times for FAST comprising four thoraco-abdominal views and bilateral lung scans were 1 min 20 s and 0 min 32 s, respectively. Combined, the mean total scan time to perform a telementored e-FAST was 1 min 52 s. The time measurements for each position were limited to probe-on-skin until image capture. The results for total scan time per protocol, defined as the sum of the mean scan times of each position, are shown in Table 3.

Discussion

It is demonstrated in this study that US examinations combined with audio and camera views can be streamed in real-time via a standard internet connection found onboard offshore installations alongside the Norwegian continental shelf. Furthermore, the results show that an expert user can guide an offshore nurse, novel to US, through PoCUS protocols with a high degree of precision and within an acceptable scanning time. Finally, the vast majority of the stored focused heart, lung and abdominal cineloops are of high-quality images suitable for clinical interpretation. These findings are relevant and may enable telementored US to increase diagnostic accuracy with patients in remote locations.

Although it may not be reasonable to consider PoCUS in all clinical settings, a common theme in austere environments is limited access to healthcare resources and imaging capabilities [3, 10]. As one would expect, many of the US applications found useful in-hospital are equally

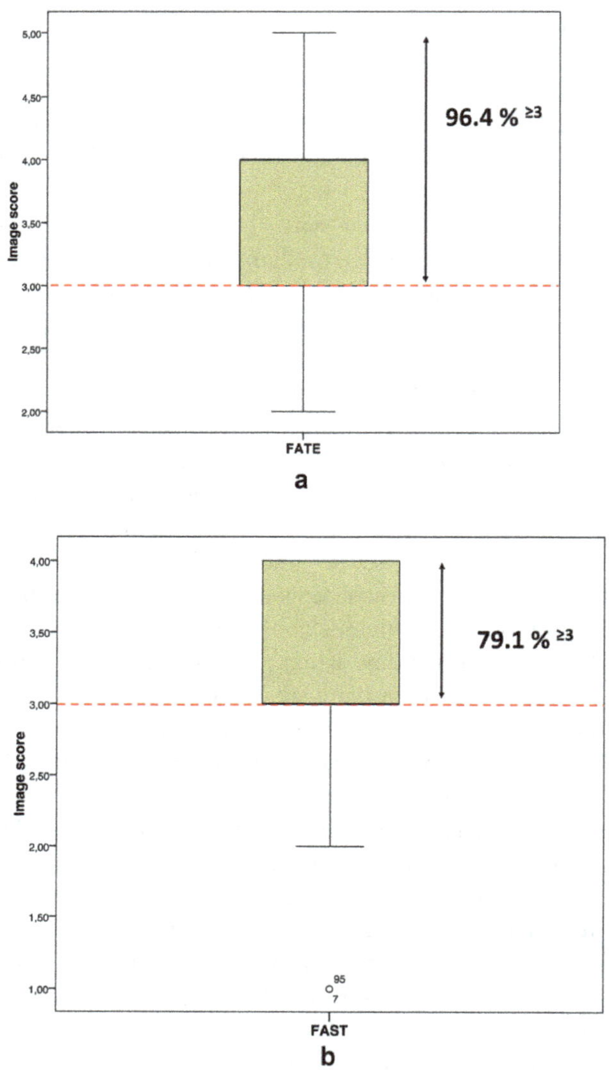

Fig. 4 **a** FATE. Box plot showing the median value, interquartile range, and minimum and maximum values. The box plot is dichotomized by the red dotted line with a score of ≥ 3 indicating that clinically useful information could be extracted from the video clips. Of all images from telementored FATE, 96.4% had a quality score of 3 or higher ($\%^{\geq 3}$). **b** FAST. Box plot showing the median value, interquartile range, and minimum and maximum values. The box plot is dichotomized by the red dotted line, with a score of ≥ 3 indicating that clinically useful information could be extracted from the video clips. Of all images from telementored FAST, 79.1% had a quality score of 3 or higher ($\%^{\geq 3}$). Two defined outliers had an image score of 1

Table 1 Mean image scores by acoustic window of telementored ultrasound in six different cardio-thoracic windows (FATE)

Acoustic window	Position	*n*	Mean[a]	Standard deviation	$\%^{\geq 3,b}$
Subcostal 4-chamber	1	37	3.49	0.65	92
Apical 4-chamber	2	37	3.54	0.56	100
Parasternal long-axis	3	37	3.32	0.58	97
Parasternal short-axis	4	37	3.32	0.58	95
Pleura right side	5	37	4.19	0.46	100
Pleura left side	6	37	3.70	0.62	95

[a] Image quality scoring system: 1 = no visible image, 5 = excellent image quality

[b] $\%^{\geq 3}$ Percentage of images with a score ≥ 3, which was defined as the cut-off score for images with sufficient quality to extract clinical information, *n* number of scans

Table 2 Mean image scores by acoustic window for telementored ultrasound in four different thoraco-abdominal windows (FAST)

Acoustic window	Position	*n*	Mean[a]	Standard deviation	$\%^{\geq 3,b}$
Subcostal 4-chamber	7	37	2.65	0.72	57
Peri-hepatic	8	37	3.35	0.75	84
Peri-splenic	9	37	3.14	0.82	78
Pelvic	10	37	3.73	0.51	97

[a] Image quality scoring system: 1 = no visible image, 5 = excellent image quality

[b] $\%^{\geq 3}$Percentage of images with score of ≥ 3, which was defined as the cut-off score for images with sufficient quality to extract clinical information, *n* number of scans

Table 3 Total scan time per protocol when performing telementored ultrasound

Examination	Number of scanning positions	*N*	Total scan time
FATE	6	222	4 min 15 s
FAST	4	148	1 min 20 s
Lungs	2[a]	74	0 min 32 s

The protocol including lungs is called extended FAST

FATE focus assessed transthoracic echocardiography protocol, *FAST* focused assessment with sonography for trauma

[a] Scanning of each lung to identify lung sliding at the pleural line. The total scan time of the lungs does not include the M-mode scan, *n* number of scans

applicable out-of-hospital. Despite the versatile range of diagnostic and procedural applications, implementation of PoCUS in prehospital care has been slow due to both technical and educational barriers. It is thus important that any equipment carried to a remote location is lightweight, durable and rugged [32]. Many of the current machines are portable and battery-powered and can be brought to the patient regardless of location [31]. They are increasingly cheap, robust and produce high-quality images. Technological advances have led to truly hand-carried PoCUS devices [33]. Another important technical feature of these machines is the capacity for the connections to different platforms, systems and applications [34, 35]. A systematic review by Gopaul et al. [36] lists the lack and cost of formal US training as the main barriers to implementing US in resource-limited settings. Current World Health Organization (WHO) recommendations for US training are quite extensive and involve 300–500 US scans per physician to achieve an acceptable skill level [37]. Our study shows that this educational barrier can be lowered by having experts connect to novice users and guide them through PoCUS protocols. By simply knowing how to operate the on/off button, gain and depth adjustments and save function on the M-Turbo machine, the offshore nurse procured cineloops and images of diagnostic value (score ≥ 3) in 96.4% of the cardiac views and 79.1% of the thoraco-abdominal views. These results clearly indicate that telementored US has the potential to augment clinical decision-making when used as an adjunct to the standard physical examination and perhaps being the only realistic imaging modality available to offshore patients.

In trauma care, it is important to detect the presence of major thoracic and abdominal fluid collection in patients with haemorrhagic shock. The FATE [38] and FAST [39] protocols were developed to efficiently diagnose or rule out a variety of life-threatening conditions. FAST is the basic building block for PoCUS and one of the most studied US tools for haemodynamically unstable patients. Not only it is an effective scan to diagnose free fluid in the thoraco-abdominal cavities and pericardial sac, but it can also be performed quickly and at bedside [39]. The results show that telementored FAST took only 1 min and 20 s, with an additional 32 s to scan the lungs (i.e., extended version of FAST). Although more comprehensive (4 min and 15 s), FATE is one of the most valuable scans for cardiac function, potentially revealing the causes of cardiac arrest and circulatory shock. This protocol has been developed to define the aetiology of circulatory collapse and more specifically to identify reversible causes during ongoing resuscitation (i.e., diagnosing fluid in the pericardial sac or pleural space and evaluating the size, shape and function of the ventricles) [25, 28]. For critically ill and injured patients, time is always critical, and many deaths are preventable if reversible causes are recognized and treated expeditiously [40, 41]. In remote settings, it is important that patients are triaged and transported to the correct level of care. PoCUS examinations performed on-site within a few minutes are thus clinically extremely attractive [3]. The mean scan time for the FATE protocol was longer than FAST but involved obtaining six views rather than four (Table 3). The time recorded in our study was from skin contact to cineloop or image capture, not the time in between the different scanning positions. The reason for this was that the volunteers in this study were on duty when being scanned and consequently had to be available for phone calls and urgent matters if needed. As a result, several of the scanning sessions were disjoined and for this reason the total scan time was not recorded. Total scan time would, therefore, be slightly longer, but both protocols can be performed in a time frame fully comparable to many other diagnostic procedures (e.g., CT, ECG, heart and lung auscultation, arterial and venous blood sampling).

The diagnostic quality of the cineloops obtained from the FATE protocol exceeded those from the FAST protocol, which was a surprise to us, as cardiac scans have been perceived as more cumbersome and difficult to acquire. When looking at the image score by acoustic window for FAST (Table 2), the subcostal 4-chamber view stands out with a much lower $\%^{\geq 3}$ score (57%) than the other three views (84%, 78% and 97%, respectively), bringing the total $\%^{\geq 3}$ score (79%) for this protocol down considerably. The subcostal 4-chamber view is also part of the FATE protocol (Table 1), but the ≥ 3 score was 92%. This discrepancy could be explained by the different transducers used for FAST and FATE. The transducer for the FATE protocol uses phased-array ultrasonics where the US beam can be swept electronically without moving the probe (i.e., beam steering technology). This difference makes it better suited for visualizing a beating heart compared to the more fixed US beam emitted from the curved-array transducer used for the FAST protocol. As an alternative, the phased-array transducer can also be used for FAST. The total FAST $\%^{\geq 3}$ score in our data (Fig. 4b) could, therefore, theoretically increase from 79.1 to 88% if the probes were switched for the subcostal 4-chamber view. However, looking at all data combined, diagnostic information can be extracted from 87.8% of all images ($\%^{\geq 3}$). Furthermore, our study shows that evaluating the lungs is rapid and feasible in all patients. This finding is important as evaluating the pleural line for horizontal sliding (i.e., lung sliding) could distinguish between a normal lung with lung sliding and a pneumothorax without lung sliding [29, 42]. This diagnostic amendment has been added to the standard version of FAST, hence the name e-FAST [43]. In our study, scores were not given for the lung scans (video for lung sliding and M-mode image of the pleural line), but these images and videos were evaluated for whether presence of lung sliding and seashore sign (M-mode) were visible. The expert user found that the pleural line and lung sliding were visible in all images and videos obtained (100%). This high feasibility is likely because the pleural line is located superficially (i.e., close to the anterior chest) in most people, regardless of body state, thus making it easy to visualize with US. However, there are some limitations to lung US, such as the presence of dressings or subcutaneous empyema [44].

Previous literature on telementored US discuss feasibility, technicality and outcomes of having a remote expert guiding novice users in different PoCUS protocols. A selection of relevant studies is shown in Table 4. The research includes a variety of locations where US images

Table 4 Selection of articles showing the use and effect of tele-ultrasound

References	Study design	Type of equipment	No of scans performed	Protocols/anatomy scanned	Main findings
Dyer et al. [49]	Pilot study	Sonix OP Bidirectional videoconference system	20	FAST e-FAST	Installing a tele-ultrasound system for major trauma cases was found to be technically and clinically feasible. The remote expert was able to diagnose pathology with FAST and e-FAST. The technology was also found to enhance ultrasound education and occasionally facilitated important clinical decision-making
Mc Beth et al. [48]	Case series	Sonosite 180 Head camera Laptop w/Skype	N/A	e-FAST	With the use of basic, low-cost cellular networks, it is possible to conduct telementored trauma sonography and produce images of excellent diagnostic quality
Biegler et al. [17]	Feasibility study	Sonosite NanoMaxx Head camera Computer w/Skype	26	Lung	Ultrasound together with simple informatics technologies permits remote telementored ultrasonography as long as internet is available. An ultrasound expert could guide a novice ultrasound user in performing lung ultrasound for detection of pneumothorax post-chest tube removal
Mc Beth et al. [46]	Feasibility study	Sonosite NanoMaxx Head camera Laptop	90	FAST e-FAST	A remote telementored ultrasound system was easy to implement, and with wireless internet, allowed a remote expert to instruct a novice user to obtain diagnostic images for interpretation
Kolbe et al. [22]	Pilot study	Sonosite Titan Laptop w/Skype	132	Foetus/pregnancy Abdomen	Local practitioners in rural areas can, after didactic training, perform POCUS under teleguidance. The implementation of POCUS in a rural village led to a change in management of about half of the patients scanned
Robertson et al. [47]	Feasibility study	Sonosite M-turbo Apple iPhone Apple MacBook Pro	63	Internal jugular vein, lung, heart, bladder	Low-cost commercially available equipment can be used for real-time mentored acquisition and interpretation of high-quality US images that are clinically useful
Olivieri et al. [45]	Pilot study	Sonosite X-porte Tele-ICU program w/camera	40	Heart Lung	After a 60-min training session, a remotely located tele-intensivist could guide a novice US user in performing heart and lung ultrasound. Remote telementored ultrasound could be used to evaluate patients in respiratory failure and/or shock in situations where US-proficient providers are not available at the bedside

had been transferred. The majority of the publications are feasibility studies on healthy volunteers, whereas studies looking at real patients seem to, for practical reasons, take place at hospitals [17, 22, 45]. A study by McBeth et al. [46] also used a phantom to assess the participants' ability to identify simulated pathology. FAST and e-FAST are the most commonly studied protocols, but in a few publications, the US examinations were adapted to meet specific patient needs [22, 47]. The communication equipment used is described as basic and can be bought off-the-shelf, such as laptops with a web camera, mobile phones with FaceTime™ or similar software apps and head-mounted cameras (e.g., Go-Pro™) [17, 22, 46–49]. One exception, similar to our study, is a publication by Olivieri et al. [45] where an already available advanced telecommunication system was used. In all studies, a recurrent theme is that data transmission (i.e., real-time transfer of US and video) is limited by network availability and internet access [3]. Therefore, telementored US may not be suitable for all geographic areas. A systematic review by Marsh-Failey et al. [50] suggests a minimum bandwidth for image transfer of 500 kbps, but the studies described in Table 4 use either a 3G or 4G data network or public wireless network (WiFi), with no significant delay in image transfer reported. In our study, we used a fibre-optic internet line that was part of a deep-sea cable stretched out on the seabed from Statfjord C to an onshore relay station. We did not experience any problems with the transfer of US images from the M-Turbo machine or the roof camera from the hospital bay with both split-screens displayed on the onshore computer (Fig. 2). In contrast, the onshore US expert perceived all PoCUS examinations in real-time with no delay in audio or video signals. The nurse performing the scans could, as described, at all time see the US expert in real-time on the Medical unit screen. The possible impact this might have on the scan performance has not been investigated or analysed. As the videoconference setup allowed for bidirectional video, disabling this function was not considered. It was not crucial for the nurse being able to see the US expert as all instructions given were verbally. The US expert has however stated that he considered it a positive element in guiding process, that both pars could see each other real-time.

Remote oil and gas operations present a multitude of health risks. However, they can be kept as low as reasonably practicable by implementing a number of strategies, such as health risk assessments, medical emergency response planning including medevac, healthcare practitioner competency requirements, remote medical support and telemedicine [5, 6, 12]. To our knowledge, we are the first to explore the use of telementored US in an offshore setting. A few oil companies have, since the data collection period in 2012, installed US in their hospitals, but these installations have almost exclusively been in extremely remote locations (i.e., sites where medical evacuation to a hospital can never be achieved within 4 h, even in the best of circumstances). Increasingly, the energy industry is operating in these environments with the goal of protecting the health of the offshore workers at an equal standard as their non-remote counterparts. As part of their remote healthcare strategy, Equinor ordered an investigation of their offshore medical healthcare systems to describe the use of their SAR helicopters and register the patients' diagnoses or symptoms leading to emergency medevac. This process resulted in a prospective study by Østerås et al. [13] looking at baseline characteristics of all patients ($n=382$) evacuated by SAR from three Equinor offshore installations in the North Sea over a time period of 2 years. The top three diagnoses or symptoms were chest pain ($n=102$), abdominal pain ($n=75$) and trauma ($n=68$), making up 65% of all patients. PoCUS may be used as a diagnostic tool for all these conditions and some others on the list [e.g., cardiac arrhythmia ($n=10$), breathing difficulties ($n=7$), cardiac arrest ($n=4$) and obstetrics ($n=1$)]. Altogether, telementored US could possibly be useful in up to 71% of patients being evacuated from an offshore platform. Furthermore, out of all SAR missions, 71% were a code yellow. This code is used in situations where a patient's condition is not immediately life-threatening (i.e., code red) but often undetermined and may deteriorate. These patients are often evacuated if the offshore nurse and onshore physician feel that further examination and early treatment are necessary. Some patients are even evacuated as a preventive action or simply because of limited access to diagnostic capabilities at the offshore hospitals. There are high costs involved in using the SAR service for medical evacuations, and by adding PoCUS, the nurses might be able to identify and monitor numerous conditions that safely can be treated on-site. Hence, oil and gas companies may prevent health complications, minimize unnecessary medical evacuations (code yellow), facilitate necessary ones (codes yellow and red) and optimize care during transfer (codes yellow and red) if they implement telementored US offshore. Figure 5 shows the setup of an US machine connected to the Medical unit at an offshore hospital today.

From a more global perspective, the World Health Organization (WHO) states that diagnostic imaging is a necessary procedure for accurately treating at least 25% of the worlds' population and that X-ray and US alone can meet over 90% of imaging needs [51]. Therefore, they recommend X-ray and US be available for all patients in primary healthcare settings [52]. However, US technology has several advantages compared to X-ray. It is

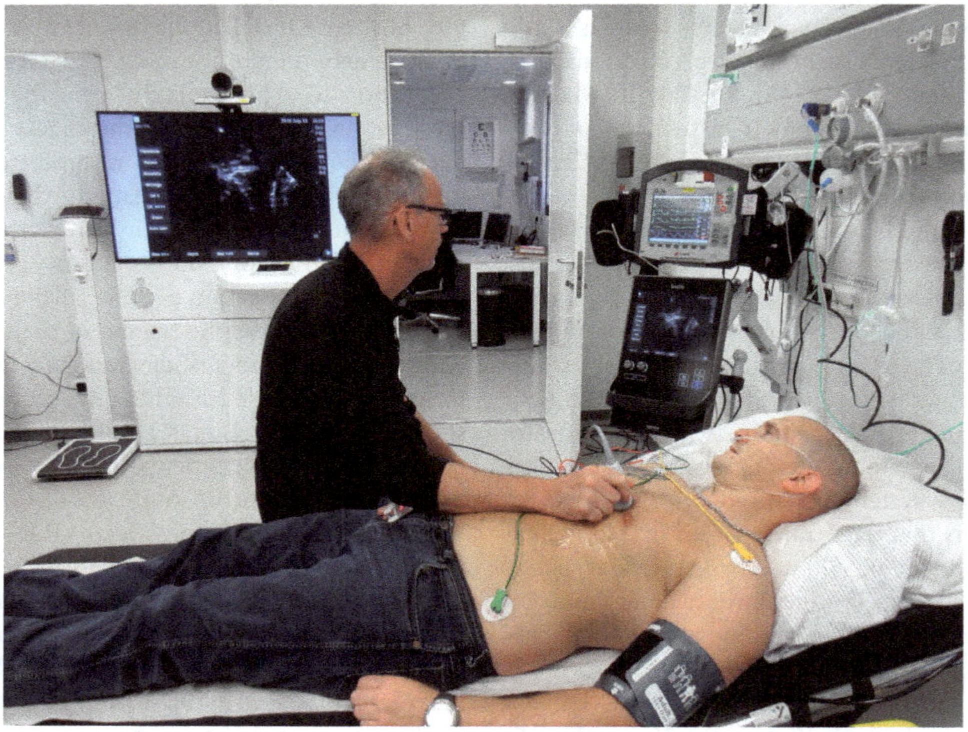

Fig. 5 Telementored ultrasound from the Aasta Hansteen platform in the Norwegian Sea. This oil installation is 300 km from the Norwegian coast, remote from other installations and in an area with extreme weather conditions. Its modern hospital is equipped with a wall-mounted SII Sonosite™ ultrasound machine (bottom) and Corpuls 3™ monitor/defibrillator machine (top), connected to the Medical unit in the background. Telementored ultrasound and live transfer of patient data such as ECG, blood pressure and saturation, make it possible for physicians to monitor and diagnose critically ill and injured patients from onshore hospitals in Norway. Photo: Svein Stalheim

cheaper, portable, battery-powered, dynamic and does not involve ionizing radiation [16]. For all these reasons, telementored US should be part of a global commitment to provide clinical support and overcome geographical barriers with the overall aim of improving health outcomes.

Limitations

First, this study was a small quality assessment study with a limited number of healthy participants ($n = 37$) where all volunteers were male. Second, the telementored US examinations were between the same offshore nurse and onshore expert in all cases which most likely improved the scan time and image quality over the course of the study. However, the data collection was done over a short period of time and for that reason we chose not to analyse the progression potentially reflected in the improved scan time and image quality. Third, the transmission times for audio and video signals (both US and roof camera) were not calculated, but only perceived by the onshore expert to be in real-time without any delays in synchronous streaming. Finally, we used an advanced medical communication unit (Medical unit) connected to the internet via a high-speed fibre-optic cable and did not encounter any issues with the technical equipment during the 2 days of scanning. For these four reasons, the generalizability of our results may be diminished. However, our data analysis is based on a total of 518 telementored US scans, all performed in exactly the same way with the same collaborating nurse and physician. Previous studies have not described the need to use advanced communication systems but rather various cheap and commercially available communication hardware and software (Table 4). Furthermore, a systematic review shows that even a bandwidth speed as low was 500 kbps could be sufficient for synchronous streaming with good image quality [50]. In our study, the US images and videos were retrieved from the US machine to a USB stick and reviewed retrospectively; hence, image degradation due to bandwidth speed was not an issue when evaluating image quality scores. Last, we want to comment on the fact that the data collection was carried out several years ago. There has not been much change with regard to the use of offshore telementored ultrasound and the equipment used in this study is still in use today. We therefore believe that the data are still valid and applicable.

Conclusion

Telementored US using existing communication and network infrastructure available at offshore oil and gas installations in the North Sea is feasible and allows real-time sharing of US cineloops and images. Remotely located experts onshore can guide inexperienced offshore nurses through different PoCUS examinations with ease, such as FATE and e-FAST. Finally, the vast majority of telementored US images and cineloops procured by novices are of high enough quality to visualize relevant anatomical landmarks and to extract diagnostic information. Future research should focus on clinical outcomes of implementing telementored US in remote locations.

Abbreviations

US: Ultrasound; CT: Computerized tomography; MRI: Magnetic resonance imaging; PoCUS: Point-of-care ultrasound; RTMUS: Remote telementored ultrasound; FAST: Focused assessment with sonography for trauma; e-FAST: Extended focused assessment with sonography for trauma; FATE: Focused assessed transthoracic echocardiography; SAR: Search and rescue; Medevac: Medical evacuation; ECG: Electrocardiography; CRP: C-reactive protein; WHO: World Health Organization; NSD: Norwegian Centre for Research Data; REK: Research Ethics Committees; VGA: Video graphics array.

Acknowledgements

The authors acknowledge the energy company Equinor for providing the opportunity to conduct the study at the Statfjord C platform. We would particularly like to thank offshore nurse Svein Stalheim, Statfjord C, Norwegian continental shelf and onshore expert Torvind Naesheim, MD, Tromso, Norway for their contribution to performing all telementored ultrasound scans. Christian A. Frederiksen, MD, PhD and Lars Knudsen, MD, PhD, Aarhus, Denmark, scored all the ultrasound cineloops and images. Finally, we would like to thank all offshore workers from Statfjord C that volunteered as models and made this study possible.

Authors' contributions

VV is the guarantor of the manuscript and takes responsibility for the integrity of the data and the accuracy of the data analysis. VV contributed to the concept and design, the analysis and interpretation of the data, and the drafting, writing, review, revision, and approval of the manuscript. NPO contributed to the concept and design, the analysis and interpretation of the data, the acquisition of the ultrasound data, and the drafting, writing, review, revision, and approval of the manuscript. DK and JC contributed with review and revision of the manuscript. KT and TN contributed to the concept and design and the acquisition of the ultrasound data. All authors read and approved the final manuscript.

Author details

[1] School Health Sciences, Ulster University, Co., Antrim, UK. [2] Faculty of Health Sciences, Department of Quality and Health Technology, University of Stavanger, Stavanger, Norway. [3] Department of Health and Working Environment, Global Business Support, Equinor ASA, Stavanger, Norway. [4] Cardiovascular Research Group, Department of Clinical Medicine, Faculty of Health Sciences, UiT, The Arctic University of Norway, Tromsø, Norway. [5] Department of Anaesthesiology, University Hospital North Norway, Tromsø, Norway. [6] Department of Anaesthesiology and Intensive Care, Stavanger University Hospital, Stavanger, Norway.

References

1. Carpenter AJ (2008) Diagnostic techniques in thoracic trauma. Semin Thorac Cardiovasc Surg 20:2–5
2. Waydhas C, Sauerland S (2007) Pre-hospital pleural decompression and chest tube placement after blunt trauma: a systematic review. Resuscitation 72:11–25
3. Nelson BP, Sanghvi A (2016) Out of hospital point of care ultrasound: current use models and future directions. Eur J Trauma Emerg Surg 42:139–150
4. Blomgren AQC, Austnes-Underhaug R, Harstad AM, Fjose S, Wifstad K, Melbye C, Amble AB, Nyvold DE, Steffensen T, Viggen JR, Iglebæk F, Arnesen T, Hagen SE, Blomgren A, Quale C, Austnes-Underhaug R, Harstad AM, Fjose S, Wifstad K, Melbye C, Amble AB, Nyvold DE, Steffensen T, Viggen JR, Iglebæk F, Arnesen T, Hagen SE (2015) Industribyggerene 2015: en kartlegging av sysselsetting i norske petroleumsrelaterte virksomheter, med er særskilt fokus på leverandørbedriftenes eksportsysselsetting. Rapport IRIS—2015/031. IRIS, Stavanger, Norway
5. Klein S, Mohamed H (2016) Reaching a consensus on the competency and training for healthcare practitioners working in remote oil and gas operations: a collaborative approach. J Inst Remote Health Care 7:6–9
6. Evensen AMC, Brattebø G (2006) Retrospective view and follow up on search and rescue and medical evacuation from oil fields in the Tampen Area, North Sea, Norway. In: Paper presented at the SPE international health, safety & environment conference, Society of Petroleum Engineers, Abu Dhabi, UAE, 1 January 2006
7. Ponsonby W, Mika F, Irons G (2009) Offshore industry: medical emergency response in the offshore oil and gas industry. Occup Med (Lond) 59:298–303
8. Tronsmoen S (1992) He setjenesten offshore. Sykepl Forsk 80:20–21
9. Lyngfoss B, Bjørk IT (2017) Self-evaluation of competence by nurses working offshore. Sykepl Forsk 105:e62873
10. Gillman LM, Ball CG, Panebianco N, Al-Kadi A, Kirkpatrick AW (2009) Clinician performed resuscitative ultrasonography for the initial evaluation and resuscitation of trauma. Scand J Trauma Resusc Emerg Med 17:34
11. Toner S, Wiltens DHA, Berg J, Williams H, Klein S, Marshall S, Nerwich N, Copeland R (2017) Medical evacuations in the oil and gas industry: a retrospective review with implications for future evacuation and preventative strategies. J Travel Med. https://doi.org/10.1093/jtm/taw095
12. Todnem K, Evensen AMC, Oveland N (2012) The implementation of telemedicine as an integrated part of the health service on the statoil operated installations on the Norwegian continental shelf (NCS). Paper presented at the international conference on health, safety and environment in oil and gas exploration and production, Society of Petroleum Engineers, Perth, Australia, 1 January 2012
13. Østerås Ø, Waje-Andreassen A, Brattebø G (2018) Improving medical examination, diagnosis and treatment offshore. Project report 2018. Haukeland University Hospital. Available via ResearchGate. https://www.researchgate.net/publication/335950109. Accessed 29 Apr 2019
14. Cohen HL, Moore WH (2004) History of emergency ultrasound. J Ultrasound Med 23:451–458
15. Ferreira AC, O'Mahony E, Oliani AH, Araujo E Jr, Costa FDS (2015) Teleultrasound: historical perspective and clinical application. Int J Telemed Appl 2015:306259
16. Moore CL, Copel JA (2011) Point-of-care ultrasonography. N Engl J Med 364:749–757
17. Biegler N, McBeth PB, Tiruta C, Hamilton DR, Xiao Z, Crawford I, Tevez-Molina M, Miletic N, Ball CG, Pian L, Kirkpatrick AW (2013) The feasibility of nurse practitioner-performed, telementored lung telesonography with remote physician guidance—'a remote virtual mentor'. Crit Ultrasound J 5:5
18. Carbone M, Ferrari V, Marconi M, Piazza R, del Corso A, Adami D, Lucchesi Q, Pagni V, Berchiolli R (2018) A tele-ultrasonographic platform to collect specialist second opinion in less specialized hospitals. Updates Surg 70:407–413
19. Smith A, Addison R, Rogers P, Stone-McLean J, Boyd S, Hoover K, Pollard M, Dubrowski A, Parsons M (2018) Remote mentoring of point-of-care ultrasound skills to inexperienced operators using multiple telemedicine platforms: is a cell phone good enough? J Ultrasound Med 37:2517–2525
20. Otto C, Hamilton DR, Levine BD, Hare C, Sargsyan AE, Altshuler P, Dulchavsky SA (2009) Into thin air: extreme ultrasound on Mt Everest. Wilderness Environ Med 20:283–289
21. Hamilton DR, Sargsyan AE, Martin DS, Garcia KM, Melton SL, Feiveson A, Dulchavsky SA (2011) On-orbit prospective echocardiography on international space station crew. Echocardiography 28:491–501
22. Kolbe N, Killu K, Coba V, Neri L, Garcia KM, McCulloch M, Spreafico A, Dulchavsky S (2015) Point of care ultrasound (POCUS) telemedicine project in rural Nicaragua and its impact on patient management. J Ultrasound 18:179–185

23. Boniface KS, Raymond A, Fleming K, Scott J, Kerry VB, Haile-Mariam T, Sayeed S, Shokoohi H (2019) The global health service partnership's point-of-care ultrasound initiatives in Malawi, Tanzania and Uganda. Am J Emerg Med 37:777–779
24. Sargsyan AE, Hamilton DR, Jones JA, Melton S, Whitson PA, Kirkpatrick AW, Martin D, Dulchavsky SA (2005) FAST at MACH 20: clinical ultrasound aboard the international space station. J Trauma 58:35–39
25. Jensen MB, Sloth E, Larsen KM, Schmidt MB (2004) Transthoracic echocardiography for cardiopulmonary monitoring in intensive care. Eur J Anaesthesiol 21:700–707
26. Kirkpatrick AW, Sirois M, Laupland KB, Liu D, Rowan K, Ball CG, Hameed SM, Brown R, Simons R, Dulchavsky SA, Hamiilton DR, Nicolaou S (2004) Hand-held thoracic sonography for detecting post-traumatic pneumothoraces: the extended focused assessment with sonography for trauma (EFAST). J Trauma 57:288–295
27. Scalea TM, Rodriguez A, Chiu WC, Brenneman FD, Fallon WF Jr, Kato K, McKenney MG, Nerlich ML, Ochsner MG, Yoshii H (1999) Focused assessment with sonography for trauma (FAST): results from an international consensus conference. J Trauma 46:466–472
28. Via G, Hussain A, Wells M, Reardon R, ElBarbary M, Noble VE, Tsung JW, Neskovic AN, Price S, Oren-Grinberg A, Liteplo A, Cordioli R, Naqvi N, Rola P, Poelaert J, Gulic TG, Sloth E, Labovitz A, Kimura B, Breitkreutz R, Masani N, Bowra J, Talmor D, Guarracino F, Goudie A, Xiaoting W, Chawla R, Galderisi M, Blaivas M, Petrovic T, Storti E, Neri L, Melniker L (2014) International evidence-based recommendations for focused cardiac ultrasound. J Am Soc Echocardiogr 27:683.e1–683.e33
29. Volpicelli G, Elbarbary M, Blaivas M, Lichtenstein DA, Mathis G, Kirkpatrick AW, Melniker L, Gargani L, Noble VE, Via G, Dean A, Tsung JW, Soldati G, Copetti R, Bouhemad B, Reissig A, Agricola E, Rouby JJ, Arbelot C, Liteplo A, Sargsyan A, Silva F, Hoppmann R, Breitkreutz R, Seibel A, Neri L, Storti E, Petrovic T (2012) International evidence-based recommendations for point-of-care lung ultrasound. Intensive Care Med 38:577–591
30. Jakobsen CJ, Torp P, Sloth E (2007) Perioperative feasibility of imaging the heart and pleura in patients with aortic stenosis undergoing aortic valve replacement. Eur J Anaesthesiol 24:589–595
31. Frederiksen CA, Juhl-Olsen P, Larsen UT, Nielsen DG, Eika B, Sloth E (2010) New pocket echocardiography device is interchangeable with high-end portable system when performed by experienced examiners. Acta Anaesthesiol Scand 54:1217–1223
32. Oveland NP, Connolly J (2019) Pre-hospital point-of-care ultrasound. In: Atkinson P, Bowra J, Harris T, Jarman B, Lewis D (eds) Point of care ultrasound for emergency medicine and resuscitation. Oxford University Press, Oxford
33. Constantinescu EC, Nicolau C, Saftoiu A (2018) Recent developments in tele-ultrasonography. Curr Health Sci J 44:101–106
34. McBeth PB, Crawford I, Blaivas M, Hamilton T, Musselwhite K, Panebianco N, Melniker L, Ball CG, Gargani L, Gherdovich C, Kirkpatrick AW (2011) Simple, almost anywhere, with almost anyone: remote low-cost telementored resuscitative lung ultrasound. J Trauma 71:1528–1535
35. Crawford I, McBeth PB, Mitchelson M, Tiruta C, Ferguson J, Kirkpatrick AW (2011) Telementorable "just-in-time" lung ultrasound on an iPhone. J Emerg Trauma Shock 4:526–527
36. Gopaul R, Bearman G, Stevens MP (2018) Ultrasound use in resource-limited settings: a systematic review. J Glob Radiol 4:1–10
37. World Health Organization (1998) Training in diagnostic ultrasound: essentials, principles and standards. Report of a WHO Study Group. World Health Organization, Geneva
38. Harris T, Wond M, French J, Kay S, Atkinson P (2019) The heart and resuscitation. In: Atkinson P, Bowra J, Harris T, Jarman B, Lewis D (eds) Point of care ultrasound for emergency medicine and resuscitation. Oxford University Press, Oxford
39. Bowra J, Loubani O, Atkinson P (2019) The abdomen. In: Atkinson P, Bowra J, Harris T, Jarman B, Lewis D (eds) Point of care ultrasound for emergency medicine and resuscitation. Oxford University Press, Oxford
40. Stocchetti N, Pagliarini G, Gennari M, Baldi G, Banchini E, Campari M, Bacchi M, Zuccoli P (1994) Trauma care in Italy: evidence of in-hospital preventable deaths. J Trauma 36:401–405
41. di Bartolomeo S, Sanson G, Nardi G, Scian F, Michelutto V, Lattuada L (2001) A population-based study on pneumothorax in severely traumatized patients. J Trauma 51:677–682
42. Volpicelli G (2011) Sonographic diagnosis of pneumothorax. Intensive Care Med 37:224–232
43. Kirkpatrick AW, Nicolaou S (2002) The sonographic detection of pneumothoraces. In: Karmy-Jones R, Nathens A, Stern E (eds) Thoracic trauma and critical care. Kluwer Academic Publishers, Boston
44. Lichtenstein D (2014) Lung ultrasound in the critically ill. Curr Opin Crit Care 20:315–322
45. Olivieri PP, Verceles AC, Hurley JM, Zubrow MT, Jeudy J, McCurdy MT (2018) A pilot study of ultrasonography-naive operators' ability to use tele-ultrasonography to assess the heart and lung. J Intensive Care Med. https://doi.org/10.1177/0885066618777187
46. McBeth P, Crawford I, Tiruta C, Xiao Z, Zhu GQ, Shuster M, Sewell L, Panebianco N, Lautner D, Nicolaou S, Ball CG, Blaivas M, Dente CJ, Wyrzykowski AD, Kirkpatrick AW (2013) Help is in your pocket: the potential accuracy of smartphone- and laptop-based remotely guided resuscitative telesonography. Telemed J E Health 19:924–930
47. Robertson TE, Levine AR, Verceles AC, Buchner JA, Lantry JH 3rd, Papali A, Zubrow MT, Colas LN, Augustin ME, McCurdy MT (2017) Remote tele-mentored ultrasound for non-physician learners using FaceTime: a feasibility study in a low-income country. J Crit Care 40:145–148
48. McBeth PB, Hamilton T, Kirkpatrick AW (2010) Cost-effective remote iPhone-teathered telementored trauma telesonography. J Trauma 69:1597–1599
49. Dyer D, Cusden J, Turner C, Boyd J, Hall R, Lautner D, Hamilton DR, Shepherd L, Dunham M, Bigras A, Bigras G, McBeth P, Kirkpatrick AW (2008) The clinical and technical evaluation of a remote telementored telesonography system during the acute resuscitation and transfer of the injured patient. J Trauma 65:1209–1216
50. Marsh-Feiley G, Eadie L, Wilson P (2018) Telesonography in emergency medicine: a systematic review. PLoS ONE 13:e0194840
51. World Health Organization (2009) Telemedicine: opportunities and developments in Member States: report on the second global survey on eHealth. World Health Organization, Geneva
52. World Health Organization (1990) Effective choices for diagnostic imaging in clinical practice. World Health Organization, Geneva

23

Feasibility of renal resistive index measurements performed by an intermediate and novice sonographer in a volunteer population

Mårten Renberg[1,2*], Naima Kilhamn[3], Kent Lund[4], Daniel Hertzberg[1,3], Claire Rimes-Stigare[1] and Max Bell[1,2]

Abstract

Background: The Doppler-derived renal resistive index (RRI) is emerging as a promising bedside tool for assessing renal perfusion and risk of developing acute kidney injury in critically ill patients. It is not known what level of ultrasonography competence is needed to obtain reliable RRI values.

Objective: The aim of this study was to evaluate the feasibility of RRI measurements by an intermediate and novice sonographer in a volunteer population.

Methods: After a focused teaching session, an intermediate (resident), novice (medical student) and expert sonographer performed RRI measurements in 23 volunteers consecutively and blinded to the results of one another. Intraclass correlation coefficients and Bland–Altman plots were used to evaluate interobserver reliability, bias and precision.

Results: Both non-experts were able to obtain RRI values in all volunteers. Median RRI in the population measured by the expert was 0.58 (interquartile range 0.52–0.62). The intraclass correlation coefficient was 0.96 (95% confidence interval 0.90–0.98) for the intermediate and expert, and 0.85 (95% confidence interval 0.69–0.94) for the novice and expert. In relation to the measurements of the expert, both non-experts showed negligible bias (mean difference 0.002 [95% confidence interval -0.005 to 0.009, $p=0.597$] between intermediate and expert, mean difference 0.002 [95% confidence interval -0.011 to 0.015, $p=0.752$] between novice and expert) and clinically acceptable precision (95% limits of agreement -0.031 to 0.035 for the intermediate, 95% limits of agreement -0.056 to 0.060 for the novice).

Conclusions: RRI measurements by both an intermediate and novice sonographer in a volunteer population were reliable, accurate and precise after a brief course. RRI is easy to learn and feasible within the scope of point-of-care ultrasound.

Keywords: Renal resistive index, Point-of-care ultrasound, Ultrasonography, Renal Doppler, Reproducibility of results

Background

Point-of-care ultrasound (POCUS) is ultrasonography (US) performed at the bedside by the clinician, allowing real-time interpretation of the findings [1]. In the last decades, POCUS has become an integral part of clinical decision-making in the fields of emergency medicine, critical- and perioperative care. The Doppler-derived renal resistive index (RRI) has emerged as a promising tool for assessing changes in renal perfusion in a wide range of clinical scenarios in critically ill patients [2–4]. RRI is an index derived from systolic and diastolic blood flow velocities of intrarenal arteries. Normal values are

*Correspondence: marten.renberg@sll.se
[1] Department of Perioperative Medicine and Intensive Care, Karolinska University Hospital, Solna, 171 76 Stockholm, Sweden
Full list of author information is available at the end of the article

around 0.60 [5, 6] with 0.70 considered to be the upper normal threshold in adults [7]. Elevated RRI values have shown promise in early detection of acute kidney injury (AKI) in patients with shock [8–11], as well as in prognosticating intensive care unit (ICU) mortality [12]. Elevated postoperative RRI values seem to be predictive of AKI progression earlier than the conventional diagnostic criteria of oliguria and serum creatinine elevation in a broad range of major surgery [13–19]. The scope of application for RRI is expanding rapidly and the method has recently been proposed to be used in the bedside evaluation of venous congestion and fluid overload in ICU patients [20], as well as a precocious ICU monitoring tool for detecting progression and recovery from severe shock states [21].

To be clinically applicable within a POCUS protocol, RRI measurements need to be obtained by the clinician present at the bedside who may not always be an US expert. In previous studies, the examiners are described as either trained- [11, 13, 14, 17, 18, 20] or expert sonographers [8, 9, 12, 15]. In the only study comparing RRI measurements of non-expert sonographers to that of experts, interobserver reproducibility of RRI values was good after the non-experts had received a half-day course of renal Doppler [22]. These findings from centres with expertise in the RRI method have not been validated in other settings, and it is not known what specific level of US experience is needed to be able to perform RRI measurements at the bedside.

The aim of this study was to evaluate the feasibility of RRI measurements performed by two non-expert examiners, an intermediate and a novice, in a volunteer population after a focused teaching session of renal Doppler. In addition, we evaluated if there was any improvement in the agreement to an expert sonographer when the non-experts had gained practical experience from the first five examinations, hypothesizing a fast progression in the technique of obtaining RRI.

Materials and methods

Study population

The study involved 23 adult volunteers. The study complied with the Declaration of Helsinki and was approved by the Swedish Ethical Review Authority. Written informed consent was obtained before inclusion.

Education of examiners

All measurements and calculations were performed by three examiners of different US experience. The intermediate examiner (MR) was a resident in anaesthesia and intensive care, using US regularly in clinical practice but without any prior experience of renal Doppler. The novice examiner (NK) was a 4th year medical student with prior experience limited to basic theory of US. The expert examiner (KL) was a specialist in clinical physiology, performing US examinations daily with more than 20 years of experience of renal Doppler and RRI measurements. The two non-experts were taught Doppler evaluation of renal perfusion on two separate occasions of 3 h each by the expert. The sessions included a basic theoretical background of renal US and supervised practical training to locate the kidneys, identify the intrarenal vessels using colour-Doppler, and measuring and calculating the RRI.

Data collection

All examinations were performed at the Karolinska University Hospital between June and September 2019. The following variables were recorded from each volunteer: age, weight, height, heart rate, heart rhythm and resting blood pressure. Medical history and ongoing medications were recorded. Each volunteer was examined by all three examiners consecutively, the order of the examiners being random for every session. The examiners were blinded to the examinations and results of one another.

RRI measurement and calculation

In each volunteer, the same designated ultrasound device (GE Vivid S70N, v202CH, US) with a curvilinear probe (1.5–6.0 MHz) was used. The volunteer was positioned on their side and first a complete view of the kidney was obtained. Colour-Doppler was applied to visualize the global organization of intrarenal blood vessels. Pulsed wave Doppler at the smallest possible width between 2 and 5 mm was used to measure flow velocities in an interlobular- or arcuate artery in the upper, middle and lower pole of each kidney. If possible, the examiners obtained a reading with at least three consecutive similar-looking waveforms in each of the three poles for each kidney. RRI was calculated for each of the three poles as [(peak systolic velocity − end diastolic velocity)/peak systolic velocity]. These values were used to compute a total mean RRI (RRI_{total}), a mean RRI for the right kidney (RRI_{dx}) and a mean RRI for the left kidney (RRI_{sin}). If the examiners were unable to obtain a satisfactory measurement in one pole, the mean value was calculated using the measurements obtained. Our protocol for obtaining RRI is in line with previously described protocols [23].

Statistical analysis

Results are described as medians with interquartile range (IQR) and minimum/maximum values (min/max) for continuous variables, or numbers and percentages for categorical variables. Interobserver reliability was assessed calculating the intraclass correlation coefficient (ICC) and their 95% confidence intervals (CI) based on an individual measurement, consistency of agreement,

2-way mixed-effects model [24]. The values were interpreted using the Ko and Li classification system [25] where < 0.5 is poor reliability, 0.50–0.74 is moderate reliability, 0.75–0.89 is good reliability, and ≥ 0.90 is excellent reliability. The mean difference in RRI measurements between non-expert examiners relative to the expert was compared using paired t tests. Bland–Altman plots were constructed plotting the difference of the paired measurements from respective non-expert and the expert (y-axis) against the mean of the two measurements (x-axis) [26]. Bias, reflecting systematic differences, was defined as the mean difference of the paired measurements [27]. Precision, reflecting random differences, was evaluated using the 95% limits of agreement (LoA) (mean difference ±1.96 standard deviations [SD]) between paired measurements. There is no previously agreed definition of acceptable precision for RRI measurements. We considered precision to be clinically acceptable when the percentage error from a proposed normal RRI value of 0.60 was no more than ± 10%, corresponding to an LoA of ± 0.06 for the non-expert examiners in relation to the results of the expert. To evaluate any potential progression in the technique of obtaining RRI in the non-expert examiners, ICC, mean difference, and LoA were again generated after excluding the first five volunteers per examiner. Data analysis was performed using Stata version 15.1 (StataCorp, College Station, US).

Results

Population characteristics

Characteristics of the volunteers are described in Table 1. Two volunteers were being followed in primary care due to slightly increased serum creatinine levels. One volunteer had antihypertensive treatment. Another volunteer was found to have an asymptomatic hypermobile kidney and was referred to specialist care for follow-up.

Table 1 Volunteer characteristics

Number of volunteers	23
Age (years), median (IQR)	38 (31–49)
Female, *n* (%)	14 (61)
Heart rate at examination (beats/min), median (IQR)	59 (56–67)
Systolic blood pressure (mmHg), median (IQR)	117 (109–126)
Diastolic blood pressure (mmHg), median (IQR)	71 (64–83)
History of renal disease, *n* (%)	3 (13)
Elevated s-Cr levels, *n* (%)	2 (9)
Hypertension, *n* (%)	1 (4)
Antihypertensive medication, *n* (%)	1 (4)
Body mass index (kg/m^2), median (IQR)	24 (23–26)

IQR interquartile range, *n* number, *s-Cr* serum creatinine

RRI measurements

All examiners were able to obtain RRI values in all volunteers. Out of 138 possible kidney pole measurements, the intermediate was able to obtain 136 (99%), the novice 134 (97%) and the expert 138 measurements (100%). In all cases where a kidney pole measurement was missing, at least two kidney pole measurements per kidney could be recorded. Measured by the expert, the median RRI_{total} in the study population was 0.58 (IQR 0.52–0.62, min/max 0.46/0.65). All examiners measured RRI values < 0.70 in all volunteers. There was no apparent difference in RRI values obtained from the right or left kidney.

Comparison between non-experts and expert

For RRI means (RRI_{total}, RRI_{dx} and RRI_{sin}) ICC, mean difference between paired measurements, and LoA for respective non-expert in relation to the expert are presented in Table 2a. Interobserver reliability for the intermediate and expert examiners was excellent (ICC ≥ 0.90) for RRI_{total} and in the range of good to excellent (ICC ≥ 0.75) for RRI_{dx} and RRI_{sin}. For the novice and expert examiners, interobserver reliability was in the range of moderate to excellent (ICC ≥ 0.50) for all RRI means. There was no difference in any corresponding RRI means obtained by neither of the non-experts compared to the expert ($p > 0.05$ for all mean differences between paired measurements). Bland–Altman plots for RRI_{total} are presented in Fig. 1. For both non-experts bias was negligible (mean difference 0.002 [95% CI −0.005 to 0.009, $p = 0.597$] between intermediate and expert, mean difference 0.002 [95% CI −0.011 to 0.015, $p = 0.752$] between novice and expert) and precision was clinically acceptable (LoA −0.031 to 0.035 for the intermediate, LoA −0.056 to 0.060 for the novice).

After excluding the first five volunteers, both non-experts were able to obtain 108 measurements (100%) from 108 possible kidney poles. Table 2b presents the repeated analyses for RRI_{total}. ICC for both non-experts in relation to the expert increased, the novice now reaching good to excellent reliability (ICC ≥ 0.75). Bias for both non-experts was still small, and precision was slightly improved.

Discussion

This is the first study to investigate the feasibility of RRI measurements performed by non-expert examiners on different and clearly specified prior US experience levels. In a volunteer population the intermediate examiner, a resident, showed excellent reliability compared to an expert after a brief course of renal Doppler. The novice examiner, a US-naïve medical student, showed moderate to excellent reliability compared to the same

Table 2 Comparison of RRI measurements between respective non-expert and expert examiners

	ICC (95% CI)	Mean difference (95% CI, p value)	LoA
(a) Total study population (*n* = 23)			
RRI_{total}			
INT:EXP	0.96 (0.90–0.98)	0.002 (−0.005 to 0.009, 0.597)	−0.031 to 0.035
NOV:EXP	0.85 (0.69–0.94)	0.002 (−0.011 to 0.015, 0.752)	−0.056 to 0.060
RRI_{dx}			
INT:EXP	0.94 (0.87–0.98)	0.003 (−0.006 to 0.011, 0.508)	−0.035 to 0.040
NOV:EXP	0.86 (0.70–0.94)	0.002 (−0.010 to 0.015, 0.701)	−0.054 to 0.058
RRI_{sin}			
INT:EXP	0.94 (0.87–0.98)	0.001 (−0.007 to 0.010, 0.729)	−0.037 to 0.040
NOV:EXP	0.79 (0.57–0.91)	0.002 (−0.014 to 0.017, 0.836)	−0.070 to 0.073
(b) Study population after excluding first five volunteers (*n* = 18)			
RRI_{total}			
INT:EXP	0.97 (0.92–0.99)	0.004 (−0.004 to 0.012, 0.287)	−0.026 to 0.034
NOV:EXP	0.90 (0.75–0.96)	0.008 (−0.005 to 0.020, 0.223)	−0.042 to 0.058

RRI renal resistive index, *n* number, *ICC* intraclass correlation coefficient, *CI* confidence interval, *LoA* 95% limits of agreement, *INT:EXP* comparison of intermediate and expert examiners, *NOV:EXP* comparison of novice and expert examiners

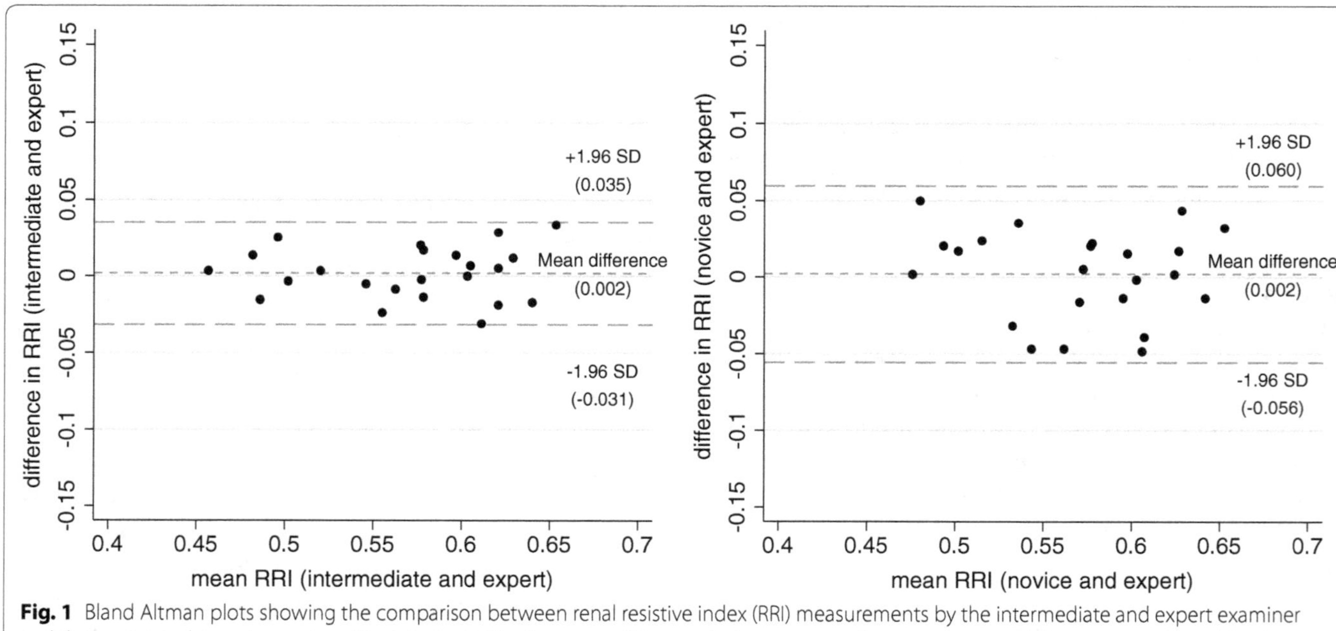

Fig. 1 Bland Altman plots showing the comparison between renal resistive index (RRI) measurements by the intermediate and expert examiner and the novice and expert examiner. Bias is indicated by the mean difference between respective non-expert and the expert, and precision is indicated by the 95% limits of agreement represented by the mean ± 1.96 standard deviations (SD)

expert that increased to the range of good to excellent when the first few examinations were excluded from the analysis indicating a fast progression in the technique of obtaining RRI. The measurements by both non-experts were accurate with clinically acceptable precision. Our results suggest that RRI measurements are feasible for non-expert examiners after only a brief course.

Although several studies have shown good interobserver correlation of RRI measurements between expert sonographers [15, 28–30], only one previous study by Schnell and co-workers [22] did include non-expert examiners. In the Schnell study, residents with prior training in US for critical care patients underwent a comparable course of renal Doppler to that of our study, and then measured RRI in mechanically ventilated patients. ICC in relation to experts was 0.89 (95% CI 0.82–0.93), indicating good to excellent reliability using the Ko and Li classification system [25]. Compared to our study, this is in line with the level of interobserver correlation between the medical student and the expert, whilst the resident instead showed solely excellent reliability compared to the expert from the start. The better correlation of measurements performed by the non-experts in our study could be explained by the fact that our study population consisted of volunteers that were fairly easy to examine, and able to cooperate with breath-hold to minimize motion of the kidneys during measurements. However, measurement conditions in patients on controlled mechanical ventilation could be optimized by initiating an inspiratory- or expiratory pause during the measurement, rendering the kidneys more stationary. It can be argued that RRI values may be hardest to obtain in spontaneously breathing tachypnoeic patients, and the level of US experience and training of renal Doppler needed to obtain reliable RRI values in such a population are still to be investigated.

Only the clinical context can determine the specific demands for precision when comparing RRI values obtained by different examiners. In a study evaluating interobserver variability of RRI measurements in patients with renal allografts, an interobserver interval of −0.035 to 0.044 between two trained sonographers was described as acceptable [31]. Another study on post-operative cardiac surgery patients deemed an LoA as wide as −0.024 to 0.114 comparing a trained sonographer to an expert as adequate [20], though this may be questioned from a clinical standpoint. For example, in ten studies included in a meta-analysis evaluating the role of RRI to predict postoperative AKI, the mean difference of RRI between the group developing AKI and the group that did not was only 0.07 [32]. Whilst the non-expert examiners in the Schnell study [22] showed an evident lack of precision in their RRI measurements compared to experts (LoA −0.107 to 0.105), both non-experts in our study showed far better precision. The very narrow range of the LoA for the intermediate examiner indicates a good precision that would be unlikely to affect decision-making in clinical practice. It is notable that also the novice, without prior US experience, whilst showing a wider LoA than the intermediate still had an acceptable range within ± 0.06 from the results of the expert. Previous studies have shown that US-naïve medical students were able to obtain fair image acquisition of the kidneys after focused courses [33, 34], but this is the first study to investigate and propose that also intrarenal Doppler readings by US-naïve examiners are feasible.

All RRI values obtained by all examiners in our study were within normal range, meaning neither of the non-experts measured an elevated RRI when the expert did not. There was no considerable difference in feasibility if RRI values were obtained from a mean from both kidneys, or only the right or left kidney. However, for measurements obtained from the left kidney the novice showed a worse precision with an LoA that was no longer within the clinically acceptable range. This may suggest a more difficult examination on the left side, which is in line with previous studies where RRI means sometimes were obtained only from the right kidney because it was perceived as technically easier [22, 35].

The results of our study suggest that it is possible to educate non-expert US examiners, and therefore most clinicians working with critically ill patients, the method of RRI during a brief, focused course. However, it must be stressed that interpretation of RRI measurements in these patients is complex and may still need consultation with more experienced clinicians. As POCUS is gaining interest in the management of AKI patients [36] and image acquisition of the kidneys already is part of the curriculum of basic POCUS training [37], it is not unreasonable to add the use of renal Doppler to existing POCUS training programs. Before this can happen, also the input of RRI for monitoring and therapeutic actions in various clinical contexts must be further established.

Our study has several limitations. First, the population size was small, but in line with previous RRI validation studies amongst trained sonographers [31, 38, 39]. Second, since our population consisted only of volunteers, results may not necessarily be transferred to all other hospitalized populations such as ICU patients. However, our results should be transferrable to some previously studied patient populations, for example it has been shown that preoperative RRI obtained under conditions comparable to those of our study could predict postoperative AKI [40]. Third, we only included one non-expert examiner of every experience level. These examiners were perceived as representatives for their respective level of prior US experience but were still individuals from within those groups. Caution should therefore be taken when extrapolating the results to other non-expert examiners. Finally, we did not assess intraobserver variability of RRI measurements in the examiners. Previous studies have shown the intraobserver variability to be low amongst expert- [12, 28] and trained sonographers [17, 31, 41]. The fact that there was good to excellent interobserver correlation in our study whilst examining the subjects consecutively suggests the intraobserver variability was unlikely to be of vast significance.

Conclusions

RRI measurements performed by both an intermediate and novice sonographer in a volunteer population were reliable, accurate and precise after a brief course of renal Doppler. RRI is easy to learn with fast progression, and is feasible within the scope of POCUS.

Abbreviations

POCUS: Point-of-care ultrasound; US: Ultrasonography; RRI: Renal resistive index; AKI: Acute kidney injury; ICU: Intensive Care Unit.

Acknowledgements

We would like to thank all included volunteers for participating in the study.

Authors' contributions

DH, MR and KL conceived the study. MR included the volunteers. MR, NK and KL performed the data collection. NK, DH and MR conducted the analyses and interpretation of the data. MR and NK drafted the manuscript. DH, MB, CRS and KL substantially revised the manuscript. MB supervised the process. All authors read and approved the final manuscript.

Author details

[1] Department of Perioperative Medicine and Intensive Care, Karolinska University Hospital, Solna, 171 76 Stockholm, Sweden. [2] Department of Physiology and Pharmacology, Karolinska Institutet, Stockholm, Sweden. [3] Department of Medicine, Karolinska Institutet, Solna, Stockholm, Sweden. [4] Department of Clinical Physiology, Karolinska University Hospital, Solna, Stockholm, Sweden.

References

1. Moore CL, Copel JA (2011) Point-of-care ultrasonography. N Engl J Med 364:749–757. https://doi.org/10.1056/NEJMra0909487
2. Le Dorze M, Bougle A, Deruddre S, Duranteau J (2012) Renal Doppler ultrasound: a new tool to assess renal perfusion in critical illness. Shock 37:360–365. https://doi.org/10.1097/SHK.0b013e3182467156
3. Schnell D, Darmon M (2015) Bedside Doppler ultrasound for the assessment of renal perfusion in the ICU: advantages and limitations of the available techniques. Crit Ultrasound J 7:24. https://doi.org/10.1186/s13089-015-0024-6
4. Di Nicolo P, Granata A (2019) Renal intraparenchymal resistive index: the ultrasonographic answer to many clinical questions. J Nephrol 32:527–538. https://doi.org/10.1007/s40620-018-00567-x
5. Ponte B, Pruijm M, Ackermann D, Vuistiner P, Eisenberger U, Guessous I, Rousson V, Mohaupt MG, Alwan H, Ehret G, Pechere-Bertschi A, Paccaud F, Staessen JA, Vogt B, Burnier M, Martin PY, Bochud M (2014) Reference values and factors associated with renal resistive index in a family-based population study. Hypertension 63:136–142. https://doi.org/10.1161/hypertensionaha.113.02321
6. Keogan MT, Kliewer MA, Hertzberg BS, DeLong DM, Tupler RH, Carroll BA (1996) Renal resistive indexes: variability in Doppler US measurement in a healthy population. Radiology 199:165–169. https://doi.org/10.1148/radiology.199.1.8633141
7. Tublin ME, Bude RO, Platt JF (2003) Review. The resistive index in renal Doppler sonography: where do we stand? AJR Am J Roentgenol 180:885–892. https://doi.org/10.2214/ajr.180.4.1800885
8. Lerolle N, Guerot E, Faisy C, Bornstain C, Diehl JL, Fagon JY (2006) Renal failure in septic shock: predictive value of Doppler-based renal arterial resistive index. Intensive Care Med 32:1553–1559. https://doi.org/10.1007/s00134-006-0360-x
9. Schnell D, Deruddre S, Harrois A, Pottecher J, Cosson C, Adoui N, Benhamou D, Vicaut E, Azoulay E, Duranteau J (2012) Renal resistive index better predicts the occurrence of acute kidney injury than cystatin C. Shock 38:592–597. https://doi.org/10.1097/SHK.0b013e318271a39c
10. Song J, Wu W, He Y, Lin S, Zhu D, Zhong M (2018) Value of the combination of renal resistance index and central venous pressure in the early prediction of sepsis-induced acute kidney injury. J Crit Care 45:204–208. https://doi.org/10.1016/j.jcrc.2018.03.016
11. Haitsma Mulier JLG, Rozemeijer S, Rottgering JG, Spoelstra-de Man AME, Elbers PWG, Tuinman PR, de Waard MC, Oudemans-van Straaten HM (2018) Renal resistive index as an early predictor and discriminator of acute kidney injury in critically ill patients; a prospective observational cohort study. PLoS ONE 13:e0197967. https://doi.org/10.1371/journal.pone.0197967
12. Boddi M, Bonizzoli M, Chiostri M, Begliomini D, Molinaro A, Tadini Buoninsegni L, Gensini GF, Peris A (2016) Renal Resistive Index and mortality in critical patients with acute kidney injury. Eur J Clin Invest 46:242–251. https://doi.org/10.1111/eci.12590
13. Bossard G, Bourgoin P, Corbeau JJ, Huntzinger J, Beydon L (2011) Early detection of postoperative acute kidney injury by Doppler renal resistive index in cardiac surgery with cardiopulmonary bypass. Br J Anaesth 107:891–898. https://doi.org/10.1093/bja/aer289
14. Guinot PG, Bernard E, Abou Arab O, Badoux L, Diouf M, Zogheib E, Dupont H (2013) Doppler-based renal resistive index can assess progression of acute kidney injury in patients undergoing cardiac surgery. J Cardiothorac Vasc Anesth 27:890–896. https://doi.org/10.1053/j.jvca.2012.11.024
15. Wu HB, Qin H, Ma WG, Zhao HL, Zheng J, Li JR, Sun LZ (2017) Can renal resistive index predict acute kidney injury after acute type A aortic dissection repair? Ann Thorac Surg 104:1583–1589. https://doi.org/10.1016/j.athoracsur.2017.03.057
16. Kararmaz A, Arslantas MK, Aksu U, Ulugol H, Cinel I, Toraman F (2019) Evaluation of acute kidney injury with oxidative stress biomarkers and Renal Resistive Index after cardiac surgery. Acta Chir Belg. https://doi.org/10.1080/00015458.2019.1702371
17. Marty P, Szatjnic S, Ferre F, Conil JM, Mayeur N, Fourcade O, Silva S, Minville V (2015) Doppler renal resistive index for early detection of acute kidney injury after major orthopaedic surgery: a prospective observational study. Eur J Anaesthesiol 32:37–43. https://doi.org/10.1097/eja.0000000000000120
18. Marty P, Ferre F, Labaste F, Jacques L, Luzi A, Conil JM, Silva S, Minville V (2016) The Doppler renal resistive index for early detection of acute kidney injury after hip fracture. Anaesth Crit Care Pain Med 35:377–382. https://doi.org/10.1016/j.accpm.2015.12.013
19. Giustiniano E, Meco M, Morenghi E, Ruggieri N, Cosseta D, Cirri S, Difrancesco O, Zito PC, Gollo Y, Raimondi F (2014) May Renal Resistive Index be an early predictive tool of postoperative complications in major surgery? Preliminary results. Biomed Res Int 2014:917985. https://doi.org/10.1155/2014/917985
20. Beaubien-Souligny W, Benkreira A, Robillard P, Bouabdallaoui N, Chasse M, Desjardins G, Lamarche Y, White M, Bouchard J, Denault A (2018) Alterations in portal vein flow and intrarenal venous flow are associated with acute kidney injury after cardiac surgery: a prospective observational cohort study. J Am Heart Assoc 7:e009961. https://doi.org/10.1161/jaha.118.009961
21. Anile A, Ferrario S, Campanello L, Orban MA, Castiglione G (2019) Renal resistive index: a new reversible tool for the early diagnosis and evaluation of organ perfusion in critically ill patients: a case report. Ultrasound J 11:23. https://doi.org/10.1186/s13089-019-0138-3
22. Schnell D, Reynaud M, Venot M, Le Maho AL, Dinic M, Baulieu M, Ducos G, Terreaux J, Zeni F, Azoulay E, Meziani F, Duranteau J, Darmon M (2014) Resistive Index or color-Doppler semi-quantitative evaluation of renal perfusion by inexperienced physicians: results of a pilot study. Minerva Anestesiol 80:1273–1281
23. Schnell D, Darmon M (2012) Renal Doppler to assess renal perfusion in the critically ill: a reappraisal. Intensive Care Med 38:1751–1760. https://doi.org/10.1007/s00134-012-2692-z
24. Shrout PE, Fleiss JL (1979) Intraclass correlations: uses in assessing rater reliability. Psychol Bull 86:420–428. https://doi.org/10.1037//0033-2909.86.2.420
25. Koo TK, Li MY (2016) A guideline of selecting and reporting intraclass correlation coefficients for reliability research. J Chiropr Med 15:155–163. https://doi.org/10.1016/j.jcm.2016.02.012
26. Bland JM, Altman DG (1995) Comparing methods of measurement: why plotting difference against standard method is misleading. Lancet 346:1085–1087. https://doi.org/10.1016/s0140-6736(95)91748-9
27. Bland JM, Altman DG (1999) Measuring agreement in method comparison studies. Stat Methods Med Res 8:135–160. https://doi.org/10.1177/096228029900800204

28. Dewitte A, Coquin J, Meyssignac B, Joannes-Boyau O, Fleureau C, Roze H, Ripoche J, Janvier G, Combe C, Ouattara A (2012) Doppler resistive index to reflect regulation of renal vascular tone during sepsis and acute kidney injury. Crit Care 16:R165. https://doi.org/10.1186/cc11517
29. Beloncle F, Rousseau N, Hamel JF, Donzeau A, Foucher AL, Custaud MA, Asfar P, Robert R, Lerolle N (2019) Determinants of Doppler-based renal resistive index in patients with septic shock: impact of hemodynamic parameters, acute kidney injury and predisposing factors. Ann Intensive Care 9:51. https://doi.org/10.1186/s13613-019-0525-8
30. Boddi M, Sacchi S, Lammel RM, Mohseni R, Serneri GG (1996) Age-related and vasomotor stimuli-induced changes in renal vascular resistance detected by Doppler ultrasound. Am J Hypertens 9:461–466. https://doi.org/10.1016/0895-7061(96)00027-1
31. Mancini M, Daniele S, Raffio T, Liuzzi R, Sabbatini M, Cianciaruso B, Ferrara LA, Salvatore M (2005) Intra and interobserver variability of renal allograft ultrasound volume and resistive index measurements. Radiol Med 109:385–394
32. Bellos I, Pergialiotis V, Kontzoglou K (2019) Renal resistive index as predictor of acute kidney injury after major surgery: a systematic review and meta-analysis. J Crit Care 50:36–43. https://doi.org/10.1016/j.jcrc.2018.11.001
33. Andersen GN, Viset A, Mjolstad OC, Salvesen O, Dalen H, Haugen BO (2014) Feasibility and accuracy of point-of-care pocket-size ultrasonography performed by medical students. BMC Med Educ 14:156. https://doi.org/10.1186/1472-6920-14-156
34. Steinmetz P, Oleskevich S, Lewis J (2016) Acquisition and long-term retention of bedside ultrasound skills in first-year medical students. J Ultrasound Med 35:1967–1975. https://doi.org/10.7863/ultra.15.09088
35. Darmon M, Schortgen F, Vargas F, Liazydi A, Schlemmer B, Brun-Buisson C, Brochard L (2011) Diagnostic accuracy of Doppler renal resistive index for reversibility of acute kidney injury in critically ill patients. Intensive Care Med 37:68–76. https://doi.org/10.1007/s00134-010-2050-y
36. Beaubien-Souligny W, Denault A, Robillard P, Desjardins G (2019) The role of point-of-care ultrasound monitoring in cardiac surgical patients with acute kidney injury. J Cardiothorac Vasc Anesth 33:2781–2796. https://doi.org/10.1053/j.jvca.2018.11.002
37. Noble VE, Brown DF (2004) Renal ultrasound. Emerg Med Clin North Am 22:641–659. https://doi.org/10.1016/j.emc.2004.04.014
38. Rud O, Moersler J, Peter J, Waliszewski P, Gilfrich C, Hauser H, Burger M, Fritsche HM, Wieland WF, Ahmed AM, Brookman-May S, May M (2012) Prospective evaluation of interobserver variability of the hydronephrosis index and the renal resistive index as sonographic examination methods for the evaluation of acute hydronephrosis. BJU Int 110:E350–E356. https://doi.org/10.1111/j.1464-410X.2012.11087.x
39. Baumgartner I, Behrendt P, Rohner P, Baumgartner RW (1999) A validation study on the intraobserver and interobserver reproducibility of renal artery duplex ultrasound. Ultrasound Med Biol 25:225–231. https://doi.org/10.1016/s0301-5629(98)00142-2
40. Hertzberg D, Ceder SL, Sartipy U, Lund K, Holzmann MJ (2017) Preoperative renal resistive index predicts risk of acute kidney injury in patients undergoing cardiac surgery. J Cardiothorac Vasc Anesth 31:847–852. https://doi.org/10.1053/j.jvca.2016.10.006
41. Samoni S, Nalesso F, Meola M, Villa G, De Cal M, De Rosa S, Petrucci I, Brendolan A, Rosner MH, Ronco C (2016) Intra-Parenchymal Renal Resistive Index Variation (IRRIV) describes renal functional reserve (RFR): pilot study in healthy volunteers. Front Physiol 7:286. https://doi.org/10.3389/fphys.2016.00286

24

Impact of an ultrasound-driven diagnostic protocol at early intensive-care stay

Julio Pontet[1,2,4*], Christian Yic[2], José L. Díaz-Gómez[3], Pablo Rodriguez[1], Igor Sviridenko[1], Diego Méndez[2], Sylvia Noveri[1], Ana Soca[1] and Mario Cancela[2]

Abstract

Background: Point-of-care ultrasound (POCUS) is a tool in increasing use, but there is still a lack of basics for its routine use and evidence of its impact in intensive care.

Objective: To measure the impact of POCUS on resource utilization, diagnostic accuracy, and clinical management in medical-surgical intensive care units (ICUs).

Methods: Prospective, controlled study, in two polyvalent ICUs. The patients were randomly assigned to POCUS or control group.

Interventions: POCUS patients received systematic ultrasound examination of optic nerve, lung/pleura, heart, abdomen, and venous system, performed at the bedside by trained intensivists. Control patients were treated by critical care specialists who do not perform ultrasound in their clinical practice.

Results: We included 80 patients, 40 per group. There were no significant differences in age, sex, APACHE II score, or admission diagnosis. POCUS group used fewer resources per patient in the first 5 days of hospitalization: chest radiography (2.6 ± 2.0 vs 4.1 ± 3.5, $P = 0.01$), additional ultrasound evaluations performed by a radiology specialist (0.6 ± 0.7 vs 1.1 ± 0.7, $P = 0.002$), and computed tomography studies (0.5 ± 0.6 vs 0.9 ± 0.7, $P = 0.007$). Time to perform any requested ultrasound evaluation after ICU admission was 2.1 ± 1.6 h versus 7.7 ± 6.7 h ($P = 0.001$). Systematic ultrasound evaluation led to better characterization of ICU admission diagnosis in 14 (35%) patients and change in clinical management in 24 (60%). POCUS group had lower fluid balance at 48 and 96 h after admission ($P = 0.01$) and spent less time mechanically ventilated (5.1 ± 5.7 days vs 8.8 ± 9.4, $P = 0.03$).

Conclusions: Systematic application of POCUS may decrease utilization of conventional diagnostic imaging resources and time of mechanical ventilation, and facilitate meticulous intravenous fluid administration in critically ill patients during the first week of stay in the ICU.

Trial registration ClinicalTrials.gov Identifier: NCT03608202.

Keywords: Clinical impact, Critical care, Diagnostic techniques and procedures, Point-of-care ultrasound, Point-of-care systems, Ultrasound protocol

*Correspondence: jpontet2003@gmail.com
[4] Larravide 2458, Montevideo, Uruguay
Full list of author information is available at the end of the article

Introduction

Ultrasonography is currently considered almost essential in the management of patients in shock, acute respiratory failure, or multiorgan dysfunction [1–4]. There is still a broad field of research aimed at generating a transformational change based on scientific evidence in critical care ultrasound [5, 6]. Given the inherent limitations for an accurate physical examination of the critically ill, imaging modalities such as chest, abdominal radiography, and computed tomography (CT) are considered more reliable, useful, and impactful in the critical care setting. However, their portability, versatility, and costs are less than ideal [1], with unnecessary delays in obtaining a diagnosis in the critically ill, and increased risk for hypoxemia or refractory arterial hypotension during transportation [3]. In contrast, ultrasound, a widely available, simpler technique that can be performed with portable equipment at the bedside, has gained progressive acceptance [4].

Recent investigations have demonstrated that multiorganic ultrasound decreases resource utilization and guides clinical management of critical ill patients while enhancing diagnostic accuracy [7–11]. Nevertheless, these previous publications lack a randomized and controlled trial methodology. We hypothesize that routine use of methodic, multisystemic ultrasound protocol in critically ill patients at admission to the intensive-care unit (ICU) reduces utilization of diagnostic resources and consultation and time to definitive diagnosis and tracheal extubation. Thus, the aims of our investigation were to analyze diagnostic and therapeutic implications of a point-of-care ultrasound (POCUS)-driven protocol during the first 5 days of ICU admission.

Materials and methods

Study design

Our prospective, randomized, controlled study was conducted at two major referral hospitals, Asociación Española Primera de Socorros Mutuos and Hospital Pasteur, Administración de Servicios de Salud del Estado. Patients admitted to a 12-bed medical-surgical ICU and 8-bed stepdown unit in those institutions were included in the study. The study protocol was approved by the Institutional Ethics Committee, and informed consent was obtained prior to each patient's enrollment.

Patients

We screened patients between February 1, 2017 and May 31, 2017, admitted to the ICUs. Inclusion criteria to the study were: (1) 18 years of age or older; (2) mechanical ventilation (MV) required at ICU admission. Patients with more than 24 h of hospitalization and those considered with low likelihood of survival by the treating intensivist at ICU admission were excluded.

Clinical data

We collected pertinent clinical data, including Acute Physiology and Chronic Health Evaluation, second version (APACHE II) score at admission, reason for admission to the ICU, and other relevant physiologic data.

The Distensibility index of inferior vena cava (%) was utilized as the primary measure for fluid responsiveness based on a previous investigation [12] (Table 1). In addition, we routinely used invasive MAP monitoring, capillary filling, hourly diuresis, central venous saturation, arteriovenous CO_2 difference, and plasma lactate measurement alongside measure of cardiac output and LVEF as supportive parameters of the clinical-decision making of administering intravenous fluids to patients suffering from shock.

Intervention

Two groups were compared; the study group received routine evaluation with an ultrasound-driven protocol (POCUS group), while a control group received conventional management according to the pre-established protocols in the ICU (in sepsis, pneumonia, postoperative care, heart failure and myocardial ischemia, trauma, COPD, etc.).

Patients were randomly assigned by permuted blocks to either the POCUS group or the control group.

The POCUS protocol is shown in Table 1; the following variables were evaluated: confirmation of initial diagnosis; change in initial diagnosis; new unsuspected finding; lack of change in initial diagnosis, inability to rule out a condition, and no changes in treatment; association with wrong diagnosis; and association with subsequent pharmacologic, medical, procedural, or surgical measures. In addition, these resource- and outcome-related variables were analyzed for comparison between the two groups: number of additional radiologic, ultrasound, and CT studies; number and type of procedures or interventions ordered; time to for ultrasound evaluation; duration of MV; length of stay in the ICU; and mortality rate.

POCUS studies were conducted with Logiq-e (General Electric Healthcare Japan Corporation) system with digital image storage capacity. Clinical data were saved in the SPSS Statistics 23 program (International Business Machines Corp.).

Statistical analysis

With a sample size of 40 patients per group for an annual population of 400 patients admitted to each ICU, we estimated a margin of error of 14% (95% CI). The qualitative

Table 1 POCUS protocol

Type of ultrasound	Instruments questions	Theoretic considerations
Optical behavior	Diameter optic nerve: right eye (mm); left eye (mm)	A diameter > 5.7 is a noninvasive indication of intracranial hypertension
Neck anatomy	Visualization of great vessels (jugular vein, carotid artery): normal or abnormal	Detection of patency (thrombosis) and anatomical variants or abnormalities
Pulmonary	Lung ultrasound score, 0–36 points	Score increases as pulmonary water increases; indicates pulmonary edema
Pleural	Presence of pleural occupation and estimation of pleural effusion (mL)	Confirmation of diagnosis, volume evaluation and follow-up
Echocardiography overall function	Estimation of left-ventricular systolic function by LVEF (%) and right-ventricular systolic function by TAPSE (mm)	LVEF > 50% and TAPSE > 15 mm is considered normal
Prediction of volume responsiveness	Distensibility index of inferior vena cava (%)	An index > 12% indicates response to intravenous fluid challenges
Estimation of CO	CO (L/min) estimated by left ventricular outflow tract by velocity time integral and diameter	Normal values, 4–6 L/min
Abdominal screening	FAST protocol for presence or absence of intraperitoneal free fluid	Presence of free fluid is abnormal
Biliary	Presence of lithiasis or dilated biliary tract	Biliary tract pathology may be an incidental finding or the cause of critical illness
Renal	Presence of urinary lithiasis or dilated urinary tract	Urinary tract pathology may be an incidental finding or the cause of critical illness
Ultrasound-guided invasive procedures	Venous or arterial access, pleural or abdominal drainage	Ultrasound-guided invasive procedures are more secure, with fewer adverse effects

CO cardiac output, *FAST* focused assessment with sonography in trauma, *IH* intracranial hypertension, *LVEF* left-ventricular ejection fraction, *POCUS* point-of-care ultrasound, *TAPSE* tricuspid annular plane systolic excursion

variables were records as percentages and the quantitative as mean ± standard deviation. For the comparison of mean between groups, either the Student's *t* test for independent groups or Mann–Whitney test was applied according to the case; and binaries in contingency tables by χ^2 or Fisher's exact test. A *P* value < 0.05 was considered significant in all tests.

Results

Patient demographics

We included 80 patients, 40 in each group. In the POCUS group, 24 were men (61%) and 16 were women (39%); similarly, in the control group, there were 25 men (62%) and 15 women (38%). There were no statistical differences between the groups regarding age, sex, APACHE II score at 24 h after admission, or reason for admission to ICU (Table 2).

Clinical information or decision-making following POCUS

The POCUS protocol was performed in 15–30 min in all cases.

In the POCUS group, 48 clinical decisions were made in 36 of 40 patients (90%). Furthermore, 35% of these observations were related to the diagnostic category, and either due to new or changed diagnosis. Modifications in pharmacologic therapy occurred in 24 patients (60%), and invasive maneuvers or procedures were necessary in 9 (23%) (Table 3).

Utilization of additional diagnostic testing

Overall, there was lower utilization of resources per patient during the first 5 days of ICU stay in the POCUS group compared with the control group (Table 4): lower number of chest radiography requested (2.6 ± 2.0 vs 4.1 ± 3.5, respectively, $P = 0.01$); lower utilization of additional ultrasound ICU imaging per radiology specialist (0.6 ± 0.7 vs 1.1 ± 0.7, respectively, $P = 0.002$); and fewer CT scans performed (0.5 ± 0.6 vs 0.9 ± 0.7, respectively, $P = 0.007$).

Analysis of delay times

We measured time from admission to first ultrasound (delay time). The delay in performing diagnostic ultrasound was significantly reduced in the POCUS group versus control (2.1 ± 1.6 h vs 7.7 ± 6.7, $P = 0.001$). In the control group, all diagnostic ultrasound evaluations were performed by radiology specialists available via telephone.

Table 2 Demographic data and diagnosis at admission in each group

Groups ($N=80$)	POCUS ($n=40$)	Control ($n=40$)	*P* value
Age, median ± SD, y	60 ± 15	57 ± 15	0.99
Sex, no. (%), male	24 (60.0)	23 (57.5%)	0.99
APACHE II, median ± SD	27 ± 9	26 ± 7	0.99
Diagnosis at admission, no. (%)			0.99
Respiratory sepsis	6 (15.0)	4 (10.0)	
Severe community-acquired pneumonia	5 (12.5)	3 (7.5)	
Decompensated heart failure	5 (12.5)	4 (10.0)	
Peritoneal sepsis	4 (10.0)	4 (10.0)	
Pulmonary tuberculosis	2 (5.0)	1 (2.5)	
Guillain–Barré syndrome	2 (5.0)	1 (2.5)	
Sepsis unknown origin	1 (2.5)	0 (0.0)	
Third-degree AV block	1 (2.5)	2 (5.0)	
Stroke	3 (7.5)	3 (7.5)	
COPD exacerbation	2 (5.0)	5 (12.5)	
Acute myocardial infarction	2 (5.0)	2 (5.0)	
Severe trauma	2 (5.0)	3 (7.5)	
Suicide attempt	2 (5.0)	3 (7.5)	
Acute bacterial meningitis	1 (2.5)	0 (0.0)	
Pulmonary embolism	1 (2.5)	1 (2.5)	
Thyrotoxicosis	1 (2.5)	0 (0.0)	
Enteric sepsis	0 (0.0)	2 (5.0)	
Acute encephalitis	0 (0.0)	1 (2.5)	
Status epilepticus	0 (0.0)	1 (2.5)	

APACHE II Acute Physiology and Chronic Health Evaluation II, *AV* atrioventricular, *COPD* chronic obstructive pulmonary disease, *POCUS* point-of-care ultrasound

Table 3 Description of changes in clinical information or decisions led by ultrasound

Modification in diagnosis and therapeutic decisions led by US	No. changes	No. patients
Related to clinical decision-making, total	48	36
New or unidentified diagnosis: Pneumonia, 2; significant pleural effusion, 5; pneumothorax, 1; significant pericardial effusion, 1; cholecystitis, 1	10	8
Clinical diagnosis: Pneumonia to respiratory distress due to biliary sepsis, 1; pneumonia to heart failure, 2; asthma to pneumonia, 1	4	4
Pharmacological therapy: Fluid challenges, 6; start diuretics, 5; dobutamine, 5; noradrenaline, 2; antibiotics, 5; alteplase, 1	24	16
Invasive procedures: Thoracic drainage, 5; emergency bronchoscopy, 2; laparotomy, 1; suprapubic bladder catheterization, 1	9	7
Alveolar recruitment maneuver, 1	1	1
No changes	0	4

US ultrasound

Clinical outcomes

Fluid management

The POCUS-driven decision of fluid management in each patient was left at treating intensivist discretion. Similarly, clinical decisions on fluid, inotropic, or vasopressor therapy, and adjustments to MV were made based on POCUS assessment. Fluid balance (FB) was much lower in the POCUS group than in the control at 48 and 96 h after ICU admission (-1600 ± 2750 mL vs -400 ± 2130 mL, $P=0.03$, and -3200 ± 3510 mL vs -890 ± 3900 mL, $P=0.006$, respectively). There was a significant positive linear correlation between left-ventricular ejection fraction (LVEF) and FB at 48 (Pearson correlation $r=0.57$, $P=0.002$) (Fig. 1) and 96 h ($r=0.58$, $P=0.03$).

Table 4 Comparison of resource utilization, length of stay and mortality in ultrasound-driven evaluation versus conventional management in ICU

Variable	POCUS group (mean ± SD)	Control group (mean ± SD)	*P* value
Chest radiography[a]	2.6 ± 2.0	4.1 ± 3.5	0.01
US requested outside of ICU[a]	0.6 ± 0.7	1.1 ± 0.7	0.002
Computed tomography[a]	0.5 ± 0.6	0.9 ± 0.7	0.007
Mechanical ventilation, days	5.1 ± .7	8.8 ± 9.4	0.03
Length of stay in ICU, d	9 ± 8	13 ± 10	0.05
Mortality, no. (%)	7 (17)	6 (15)	>0.99

Echo echocardiography, *ICU* intensive-care unit, *US* ultrasound

[a] During the first 5 days of intensive-care unit stay

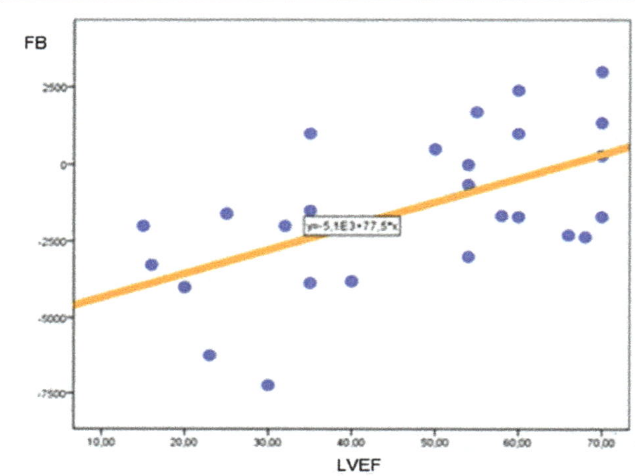

Fig. 1 Linear correlation between fluid balance at 48 h and left-ventricular ejection fraction. Pearson correlation $r = 0.57$, $P = 0.002$. *FB* fluid balance, *LVEF* left-ventricular ejection fraction

Duration of MV

The POCUS group showed a lower duration of MV than the control (5.1 ± 5.7 days vs 8.8 ± 9.4 days, $P = 0.03$) (Table 4). There was no significant correlation between the time spent on MV and FB, or between the time spent on MV and LVEF.

Length of stay in ICU and mortality

Mortality rates did not differ between POCUS and control groups. Of note, there was a tendency for decreased ICU length of stay with POCUS (Table 4).

Discussion

We demonstrated the direct impact of a routine POCUS-driven protocol in patients during the early phase after admission to medical–surgical ICUs. A systematic application of POCUS resulted in decreased utilization of conventional diagnostic imaging resources and time of MV, and facilitated a judicious intravenous fluid administration in critically ill patients during the first week of ICU hospitalization. Application of routine POCUS appears to be safe if utilized by appropriately trained intensivist as no complications were directly associated with POCUS use in the study group.

Previous investigations [2, 5] applying particular ICU-sound protocol led to more accurate admission diagnosis in 25.6% to 24.9%. They had an observational design, but are comparable to the 22% accuracy rate of new or corrected diagnoses in our study. Moreover, the majority of our patient population suffered from sepsis. Manno et al. [2] proposed that septic patients may be the most favored subgroup of patients receiving a POCUS protocol because of the myriad of information and therapies that can be tailored to each individual patient.

The main effect of routine utilization of our POCUS protocol was the clinical decision-making, more specifically in pharmacologic management adjustments in shock patients (60%) and ordering of ultrasound-guided procedures (23%). In our study, we found that 23% of our population required ultrasound-guided invasive procedures, which is similar to the 21.6% reported by the Manno group [2]. Vignon et al. [13] described a change in therapeutic management of patients in 51% of the cases, and Bernier-Jean et al. [5] in 44%.

Management of intravascular volume status can be a difficult decision at the bedside. Meticulous fluid management in treating shock patients with heart disease is desirable. In our case, the most common clinical decision was related to fluid management. Similar findings have been described in an observational study [13], but we emphasize the randomized-controlled design of our study. Nonetheless, our direct comparison of timely ultrasound-driven versus conventional management allows us to represent the current practice in the majority of medical centers due to lack of routine utilization of ultrasound by intensivists. Furthermore, positive fluid responsiveness test does not indicated necessity of further fluid administration, our clinical-decision making was determined by the echocardiography measurements (LVEF, IVC distensibility index) in addition to systemic perfusion surrogates (central venous saturation, arteriovenous CO2 difference, and plasma lactate measurements). Finally, in cases of heart failure, we guided restriction of fluids by signs of pulmonary and systemic congestion. However, we acknowledge tolerance to fluids must be assessed with diastolic function parameters and may be in addition to lung ultrasonography [14–16].

Our POCUS protocol led to a significantly lower utilization of chest radiography, ultrasound performed by non-intensivist specialists, and CT scans (up to 56% reduction in CT requests). We found a reduction of radiology evaluation utilization from 4.1 in the control group to 2.6 in the POCUS group (63% reduction). This finding differs from other groups reporting 22% to 26% reduction in radiography utilization [17, 18]. Possible explanations include intensivist discretion versus specific protocol, considerable critical care ultrasound expertise by attending intensivist at time of the study, and more availability of fully capable ultrasound devices. Of note, the American College of Radiology expert panel recommended daily radiology for each intubated patient [17]. The direct clinical implications of our findings were associated with lower radiation exposure, less intra-hospital transportation of unstable patients, and inherent economic savings with more sophisticated evaluations, including in improved imaging suites workflow and reduced necessity for personnel to transport patients [19–21].

We found a significant correlation between cardiac function (left systolic ventricle function measured by LVEF index) and a negative FB in the first 5 days of ICU management. This might indicate that judicious fluid management and decisions in administration of diuretic agents are facilitated with real-time utilization of POCUS since ICU admission. We did not find a significant correlation between time spent on MV and FB or between duration of MV and LVEF. This can possibly be explained by the heterogeneity of our population. However, there was correlation between lower LVEF and negative FB, since patients with low LVEF are likely to receive less fluids and more diuretics.

We acknowledge several limitations in the current investigation. First, our small patient population avoids finding significant differences in meaningful clinical outcomes, such as mortality. Second, we analyzed only the first 5 days of ICU stay. However, as patients stay longer in the ICU, additional confounding factors not necessarily related with admission diagnosis can affect the outcomes (late-onset, ventilator-associated pneumonia). Mortality was similar between both groups, but it should be noted that future studies with larger patient populations having a shorter time of MV as found in the POCUS group could potentially determine a decrease in mortality related to MV complications. Third, we did not find a significant correlation between normal or high ejection fraction and pulmonary B profile in our study that can imply possible tolerance to fluid administration. However, patients with CHF and preserved EF can be only characterized with advanced echocardiography parameters of diastolic function. We recognize that the lack of diastolic function assessment is another limitation of this study. However, we aimed to evaluate a practical approach for assessment of ventricular function and fluid responsiveness, so we propose further investigation of the correlation between normal or high ejection fraction and pulmonary B profile in addition to diastolic function assessment in septic shock patients.

Finally, the absence of a reposition protocol guided by pre-established ultrasound should be endorsed in multicentric studies.

Conclusions

A systematically applied POCUS protocol upon admission to the ICU can guide diagnostic and therapeutic decisions in critically ill patients. This potentially leads to greater resourcefulness and shorter duration of MV. Definitive associations, such as ultrasound-driven fluid resuscitation and improved outcomes, remain to be proven in larger multicenter studies. Diastolic function assessment can improve overall evaluation of fluid tolerance to the fluid management of septic shock patients.

Acknowledgements

Stella Calvo, MD for his technical help in the elaboration of the manuscript.

Preliminary results and abstract presented at 13th WINFOCUS World Congress, Argentina, September 2017, and received the Golden Probe Award as Best Poster Presentation.

Authors' contributions

JP and CY have made substantial contributions to the conception and design of the work, the acquisition, analysis, and interpretation of data, and have drafted the work. JLD have made contributions to the analysis and interpretation of data and substantively revised it. PR, IS, and DM have made contributions to the acquisition and analysis of data. SN, AS, and MC have made contributions to the analysis and interpretation of data and substantively revised it. All authors read and approved the final manuscript.

Author details

Intensive Care Unit, Hospital Pasteur, Administración de Servicios de Salud del Estado, Montevideo, Uruguay. [2] Intensive Care Unit, Asociación Española Primera de Socorros Mutuos, Montevideo, Uruguay. [3] Department of Critical Care Medicine, Mayo Clinic, Jacksonville, USA. [4] Larravide 2458, Montevideo, Uruguay.

References

1. Frankel HL, Kirkpatrick AW, Elbarbary M et al (2015) Guidelines for the appropriate use of bedside general and cardiac ultrasonography in the evaluation of critically ill patients—part I: general ultrasonography. Crit Care Med 43:2479–2502
2. Manno E, Navarra M, Faccio L et al (2012) Deep impact of ultrasound in the intensive care unit: the "ICU-sound" protocol. Anesthesiology 117:801–809
3. Moore CL, Copel JA (2011) Point-of-care ultrasonography. N Engl J Med 364:749–757
4. Narasimhan M, Koenig SJ, Mayo PH (2016) A whole-body approach to point of care ultrasound. Chest 150:772–776
5. Bernier-Jean A, Albert M, Shiloh AL, Eisen LA, Williamson D, Beaulieu Y (2017) The diagnostic and therapeutic impact of point-of-care ultrasonography in the intensive care unit. J Intensive Care Med. 32:197–203
6. Bossone E, DiGiovine B, Watts S et al (2002) Range and prevalence of cardiac abnormalities in patients hospitalized in a medical ICU. Chest 122:1370–1376
7. Kristensen MS, Teoh WH, Graumann O, Laursen CB (2014) Ultrasonography for clinical decision-making and intervention in airway management: from the mouth to the lungs and pleurae. Insights Imaging. 5:253–279
8. Laursen CB, Sloth E, Lassen AT et al (2014) Point-of-care ultrasonography in patients admitted with respiratory symptoms: a single-blind, randomised controlled trial. Lancet Respir Med. 2:638–646
9. Oks M, Cleven KL, Cardenas-Garcia J et al (2014) The effect of point-of-care ultrasonography on imaging studies in the medical ICU: a comparative study. Chest 146:1574–1577

10. Pontet J, Yic C, Diaz-Gomez J, et al. Ultrasonografía En Medicina de Urgencias, Terapia Intensiva Y Anestesia. 1st ed: Montevideo; 2016
11. Volpicelli G, Lamorte A, Tullio M et al (2013) Point-of-care multiorgan ultrasonography for the evaluation of undifferentiated hypotension in the emergency department. Intensive Care Med 39:1290–1298
12. Feissel M, Michard F, Faller JP, Teboul JL (2004) The respiratory variation in inferior cava diameter as a guide to fluid therapy. Intensive Care Med 30(9):1834–1837
13. Vignon P, Frank MB, Lesage J et al (2004) Hand-held echocardiography with Doppler capability for the assessment of critically-ill patients: is it reliable? Intensive Care Med 30:718–723
14. Geri G, Vignon P, Aubry A, Fedou AL, Charron C, Silva S, Repessé X, Vieillard-Baron A (2019) Cardiovascular clusters in septic shock combining clinical and echocardiographic parameters: a post hoc analysis. Intensive Care Med 45(5):657–667
15. Nair S, Sauthoff H (2019) Assessing extravascular lung water with ultrasound: a tool to individualize fluid management? J Intensive Care Med. https://doi.org/10.1177/0885066619855000 **(Epub ahead of print)**
16. Orme RM, Oram MP, McKinstry CE (2009) Impact of echocardiography on patient management in the intensive care unit: an audit of district general hospital practice. Br J Anaesth 102:340–344
17. Expert Panel on Thoracic Imaging, McComb BL, Chung JH et al (2016) ACR appropriateness criteria routine chest radiography. J Thorac Imaging. 31:W13–15
18. Krinsley JS (2003) Test-ordering strategy in the intensive care unit. J Intensive Care Med. 18:330–339
19. Expert Round Table on Echocardiography in ICU (2014) International consensus statement on training standards for advanced critical care echocardiography. Intensive Care Med 40:654–666
20. Kue R, Brown P, Ness C, Scheulen J (2011) Adverse clinical events during intrahospital transport by a specialized team: a preliminary report. Am J Crit Care. 20:153–161 **(quiz 162)**
21. Smith I, Fleming S, Cernaianu A (1990) Mishaps during transport from the intensive care unit. Crit Care Med 18:278–281

25

Sonographic exploration for fascial exploration (SEFE) in necrotizing fasciitis

Jessica Fozard, Krystle Shafer* and Thompson Kehrl

Abstract

Background: Necrotizing skin and soft tissue infections are life-threatening cond tions. Reliance on gas in tissue planes leads to worsened outcomes in patients with non-gas forming types of necrotizing fasciitis (NF).

Case presentation: We present a case of Group A Strep (GAS) necrotizing fasciitis, which was identified at bedside with point-of-care ultrasound (US) including an area of subfascial fluid. Computerized tomography only revealed diffuse cellulitic changes. Patient was taken to the operating room where fascial exploration was not performed at the concerning area seen on ultrasound and thus falsely negative. The patient subsequently developed multi-system organ failure and required amputation of the limb due to rapid spread of GAS NF.

Conclusion: We suggest an US protocol to help identify optimal areas for fascial exploration—sonographic exploration for fascial exploration (SEFE).

Keywords: Point-of-care ultrasound, Necrotizing fasciitis, Musculoskeletal ultrasound

Background

Utilization of CT scan for diagnosis of NF is supported only by small studies that which focus on images using IV contrast enhancement. The most common CT finding is focal subcutaneous fat infiltration and fascial thickening [1]. These findings lack specificity and can be seen with non-necrotizing infections and even non-inflammatory conditions [2]. MRI is considered to be the current gold standard imaging testing, with a sensitivity of 93% in detecting NF [3]. This imaging modality, however, can be time consuming to obtain in a rapidly fatal disease. With regard to US, there are emerging research and approaches for the diagnosis of necrotizing soft tissue infections as there have been multiple case reports that demonstrated accurate diagnosis of NF with US where as CT and MR only demonstrated changes consistent with cellulitis [4]. The STAFF exam provides a simple and memorable acronym for identifiable signs of necrotizing soft tissue infection (NSTI) on US—subcutaneous thickening, air, and fascial fluid [5]. With regard to fascial fluid amount, the best cut-off to diagnose NF is reported as 2 mm of fluid accumulation, which has a sensitivity of 75% and a specificity of 70.2% [6]. However, data with US is limited as well, and a negative US exam, much like a negative CT scan or LRINEC (laboratory risk indicator for necrotizing fasciitis) score, does not exclude the diagnosis [5]. US is reported to have a sensitivity of 88.2%, specificity of 93.3%, a positive predicative value of 83.3%, a negative predictive value of 95.4% and an accuracy of 91.9% in the diagnosis of NF [7]. Surgical exploration remains the gold standard for both diagnosis and treatment and was appropriately performed in this patient case [8]. The time to successful surgical debridement is considered the single most important variable influencing mortality in this patient population [9]. What is unique about our case goes beyond using US for diagnosis, but also using this modality to help identify the muscle compartment to be explored during surgery. If the US results were utilized

*Correspondence: kshafer@wellspan.org
WellSpan York Hospital Emergency Medicine Residency Program, WellSpan York Hospital, York, PA, USA

in this case to aid the site of surgical exploration, the ultimate outcome of this patient may have been different.

With regard to the surgical decisions on areas of debridement for NF, examination of surgical reference textbooks reveals vague allusions to "immediate and extensive surgical debridement", but without any specific technique mentioned [10, 11]. A surgical review article on NF states to make an incision over any "overtly necrotic area", and when this is not evident, to make an incision over the area "deemed to be the center of the disease process", without any further elaboration [12]. This lack of standardization is particularly concerning in early NSTIs when the skin may be spared and not exhibit any impressive or obvious appearance of underlying pathology. Our patient in this case is an example of this, as her skin changes were misleading in the operating room (her entire left lower extremity was mottled) and led to two negative biopsies. The specific location of the infection was correctly identified on bedside ultrasound and but not on CT. Unfortunately, the compartment identified on ultrasound was not explored during the initial operation.

The utility of US to help guide surgical debridement with regard to the extent or timeliness has yet to be defined in the literature. In this particular case described below, US would have been helpful in guiding the surgeons toward a specific anatomic location for their surgical incision and drainage. Other than the STAFF exam, there does not appear to be any unified or systematic process for evaluating a limb or area for underlying NF when the area involved is either extensive or uncertain. In a review of the US literature, we found a routine approach to soft tissue ultrasound that could be applied by trained physicians to systematically evaluate an extremity. The same principles could be applied to other areas of the body as well. Primarily, scanning an unaffected area/contralateral extremity, as well as over areas that are concerning for pathology [13] should be considered. Scanning in multiple planes is also recommended for localization and providing as much information as possible [13]. We propose combining both approaches to create a protocolized US to help identify optimal areas for fascial exploration—sonographic exploration for fascial exploration (SEFE) (Table 1).

Case presentation

An 80-year-old female presented to the Emergency Department (ED) via ambulance with altered mental status. Her family reported the patient developed rapid onset of and worsening lethargy that started shortly after she awoke in the morning. Emergency medical services (EMS) noted the patient to be tachycardic and hypotensive en route. Upon arrival to the ED, she was somnolent but arousable to voice and unable to provide any details. Her past medical history included diabetes and hypertension. Vital signs upon presentation included a temperature of 38.4 °C, heart rate 128 beats per minute, blood pressure 100/64 mm Hg, respiratory rate 32, and pulse oximetry of 97% on room air. On exam she was noted to have a mottled left lower extremity (Fig. 1) with intact distal dorsal pedal and posterior tibial pulses. No crepitus or bullae were noted. Palpation of her entire left lower

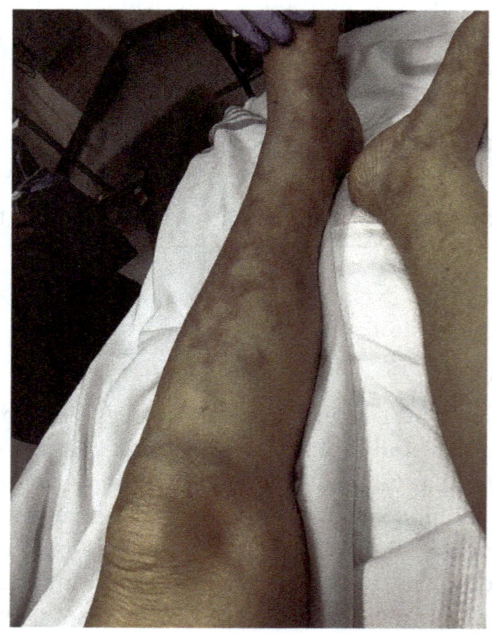

Fig. 1 Left lower extremity upon presentation to the emergency department. Note mottling of skin but no bullae

Table 1 Explanation of the steps to perform a SEFE examination

SEFE examination
Step 1: Scan all fascial compartments (such as anterior, lateral, superficial posterior and deep posterior in the lower extremity) even if skin changes are not present
Step 2: Do you have BOTH diffuse subcutaneous thickening AND fascial fluid > 2 mm present? = If so, this is diagnostic for NF
Step 3: Additionally look for supporting, but not mandated findings such as subcutaneous air or abnormal architecture of the muscle tissue
Step 4: Mark area of US findings on patient skin and consult surgery for exploration

extremity appeared to be painful, especially in her groin and proximal calf area.

Laboratory analysis included white blood cell count of 12.2 and a significantly elevated venous lactic acid at 9.8. Acute renal failure was noted with a serum creatinine of 3.05 (baseline 1.00). Sodium was 140 and glucose 167. A venous blood gas showed pH 7.21, pCO_2 32, and HCO3 13. Blood cultures were sent. Left lower leg X-rays showed mild soft tissue edema, but no gas in tissue planes. A point-of-care ultrasound (US) was performed (SonoSite, Bothell, WA) and showed thickened subcutaneous tissue with fluid accumulating superficial to the deep fascial layer > 4 mm in the superficial posterior compartment of the left lower leg. Distal to the popliteal fossa on the posterior aspect of the left leg deep to the fascial layer there was an anechoic fluid pocket with swirling of fluid noted with transducer compression (Additional file 1: Video 1). Abnormal sonographic architecture of the gastrocnemius muscle was noted as well (Fig. 2). Additional file 2: Video 2 displays a normal lower extremity ultrasound for comparison purposes.

Patient was diagnosed with necrotizing fasciitis and ordered broad-spectrum antibiotics: vancomycin, clindamycin, and piperacillin–tazobactam. She was resuscitated with intravenous fluids. Surgical consultation was obtained. Recommendations included computerized tomography (CT) of the left lower extremity of which was obtained (Fig. 3). This was performed without intravenous contrast and showed soft tissue swelling, subcutaneous fatty standing and mildly enlarged lymph nodes in the left inguinal region with possible small hematoma. The radiologist's differential diagnosis included cellulitis or anasarca. Diffuse subcutaneous fatty stranding was noted in the left calf, ankle and foot region, with edema being most likely.

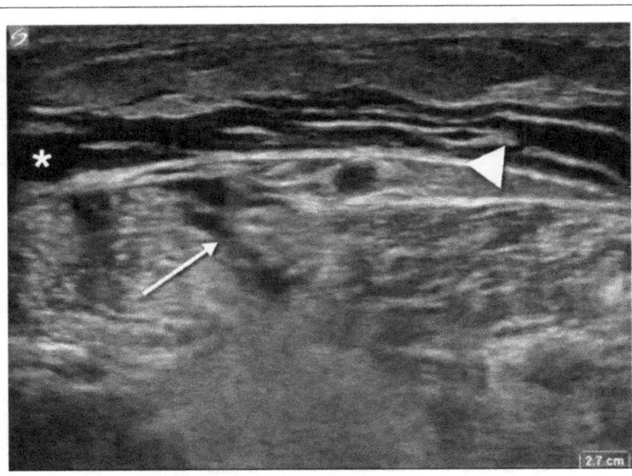

Fig. 2 Transverse view of posterior left lower extremity distal to popliteal crease. Fascia is indicated by arrowhead. Anechoic fluid collection is noted anterior to fascia (*). Deep to fascial layer, a complex fluid collection is noted (arrow) with diffuse hyperechogenicity of gastrocnemius

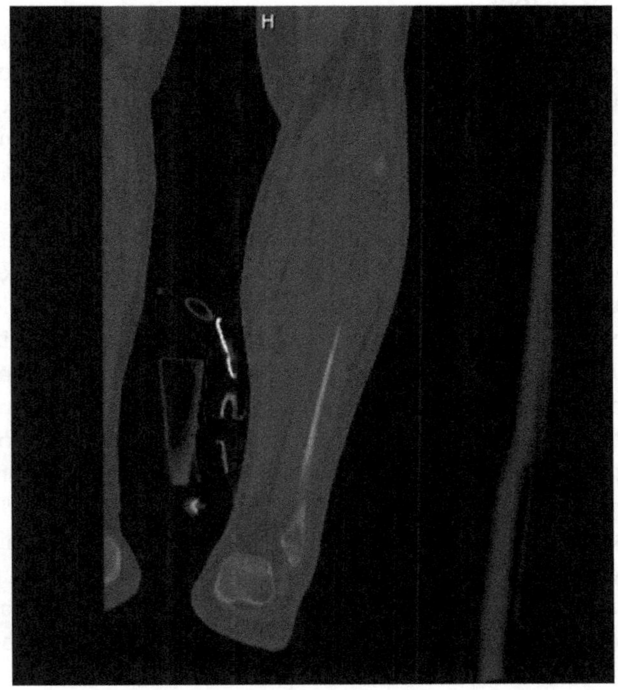

Fig. 3 CT sagittal view of the left lower extremity which reveals mild diffuse fatty stranding

She was taken to the operating room by the surgical service where two incisions were made. The first surgical incision was made on the left lateral leg just anterior to the greater trochanter and was taken down to the level of the fascia. Fascial planes appeared intact and there was no evidence of necrotizing process. A second incision was made just :nferior to the head of the fibula in the lateral compartment and again taken down to the level of the fascia, which was not entered. Intra-operative compartment pressures were measured and noted to be normal. The left lower leg incision was closed with staples and a vacuum dressing was placed on the left thigh incision.

Post-operatively, her clinical condition worsened. Both blood and intra-operative cultures grew Group A *Streptococcus*. She returned to the operating room on hospital day #2. Her lateral calf incision was extended proximally and distally; the fascia was opened up in all four lower extremity compartments and necrotic tissue was noted diffusely. Because o: extent of necrosis in the left lower extremity, a below the knee guillotine amputation was performed. She returned to the operating room on hospital day #3 for further extensive debridement. On hospital day #4 her condition continued to worsen and she expired.

Conclusions

When the diagnosis of necrotizing fasciitis is made and involves a location with multiple potential muscle compartments as potential etiologies (such as the lower extremity) and CT/X-ray imaging does not reveal obvious location, we recommend the following approach: using the distal lower extremity as the example, we recommend scanning all four fascial compartments (anterior, lateral, superficial posterior and deep posterior) regardless of skin findings on clinical exam. A linear transducer should be utilized and each compartment should be scanned in multiple planes. Specific attention should be paid attention to subcutaneous tissue and fascial planes. As identified by the STAFF exam, the examiner should look for subcutaneous thickening, air, and fascial fluid. Additional findings may include abnormal architecture of the muscle tissue as was identified in our patient case. Applying this technique has the potential to serve as both an additional diagnostic tool and as guidance for successful operative exploration and debridement. However, it should be noted that more data are needed on this topic such as a prospective clinical trial and ultrasound should never be used as a rule-out test. While we should use every tool at our disposal to diagnose this rapidly fatal condition and point-of-care ultrasound findings can be integrated with the clinical picture, it still remains that surgical exploration is the gold standard for diagnosis of NF.

Supplementary information

Additional file 1: Video 1. Transverse view of the patient's posterior left lower extremity in same anatomic site as Fig. 2. Note swirling of complex fluid deep to fascia

Additional file 2: Video 2. Transverse view of a normal posterior left lower extremity in same anatomic site as Fig. 2.

Abbreviations

NF: Necrotizing fasciitis; GAS: Group A Strep; US: Ultrasound; SEFE: Sonographic exploration for fascial exploration; ED: Emergency Department; EMS: Emergency medical services; CT: Computerized tomography; NSTI: Necrotizing soft tissue infection; LRINEC: Laboratory risk indicator for necrotizing fasciitis.

Acknowledgements

There are no acknowledgements.

Authors' contributions

All three authors were involved in the writing and editing of this manuscript. All authors read and approved the final manuscript.

References

1. Hayeri M, Ziai P, Shehata M, Teytelboym O, Huang B (2016) Soft-tissue infection and their imaging mimics: from cellulitis to necrotizing fascitis. Radiographics 36:6
2. Malghem J, Lecouvet F, Omoumi P, Maldague B, Vande Berg B (2013) Necrotizing fascitis: contribution and limitations of diagnostic imaging. Joint Bone Spine 80(2):146–154
3. Ali S, Srinivasan S, Peh W (2014) MRI in necrotizing fasciitis of the extremities. Br J Radiol 87(1033):20130560
4. Misiakos E, Bagias G, Patapis P, Sotiropoulos D, Kanavidis P, Machairas A (2014) Current concepts in the management of necrotizing fasciitis. Front Surg 1:36
5. Castleberg E, Jenson N, Dinh V (2014) Diagnosis of necrotizing fasciitis with bedside ultrasound: the STAFF exam. West J Emerg Med 15(1):111–113
6. Lin C, Hsiao C, Chang C, Huang T, Hsiao K, Chen Y, Fann W (2019) The relationship between fluid accumulation in ultrasonography and the diagnosis and prognosis of patients with necrotizing fasciitis. Ultrasound Med Biol 45(7):1545–1550
7. Yen Z, Wang H, Ma H, Chen S, Chen W (2002) Ultrasonographic screening of clinically-suspected necrotizing fasciitis. Acad Emerg Med 9(12):1448–1451
8. Bonne S, Kadri S (2017) Evaluation and management of necrotizing soft tissue infections. Infec Dis Clin North Am 31(3):497–511
9. Bellapianta J, Ljungquist K, Tobin E, Uhl R (2009) Necrotizing fasciitis. J Am Acad Orthop Surg 17(3):174–182
10. Marcucci L, Moritz MJ, Chen H (2006) Avoiding common surgical errors. Lippincott Williams & Wilkins, Philadelphia
11. Michael WM et al; illustrations by Holly R. Fischer. (2006). Greenfield's surgery: scientific principles and practice. Philadelphia: Lippincott Williams & Wilkins
12. Hakkarainen T, Kopari N, Pham T, Evans H (2014) Necrotizing soft tissue infections: review and current concepts in treatment, systems of care, and outcomes. Curr Probl Surg 51(8):344–362
13. Kaplan P, Matamoros A Jr, Anderson J (1990) Sonography of the musculoskeletal system. Am J Roentgenol 155(2):237–245

26

Sonographic features of carotid artery dissection due to extension of aortic dissection

Christian Boßelmann[1] and Sven Poli[2*]

Abstract

Background: Carotid artery dissection due to extension of aortic dissection (CAEAD) is a severe complication of acute aortic dissection. The risk of ischemic stroke is increased. Early sonographic detection and repeat evaluation are necessary to guide clinical management.

Case presentation: A 58-year-old male patient presents with sudden, tearing retrosternal pain. Point-of-care carotid ultrasound is used to establish the diagnosis of CAEAD. We describe a number of sonographic features and compare ultrasound to other imaging modalities.

Conclusions: Bedside carotid ultrasound enables rapid, sensitive and safe hemodynamic assessment, especially in critically ill patients.

Keywords: Neurology, Ultrasound, Point-of-care systems, Carotid artery dissection

Background

Aortic dissection (AD) is a clinical emergency. A tear in the tunica intima, the innermost layer of the vessel, is propagated by blood flowing into the false lumen. This dissection membrane can further extend into the aortic branches, including the carotid arteries. This is referred to as carotid artery extension of aortic dissection (CAEAD). Cerebral malperfusion can result from the dissection membrane restricting or occluding blood flow, akin to a carotid stenosis or large-vessel occlusion. Alternatively, artery-to-artery embolization or progressive stenosis from mural thrombosis may occur. Hence, rapid diagnosis and repeat hemodynamic evaluation are necessary to guide clinical management [1].

Case presentation

A 58-year-old male patient presented with sudden tearing retrosternal pain and dyspnea. No traumatic injury was reported. Chest computed tomography angiography (CTA) displayed an acute aortic dissection (Stanford type A, DeBakey type I), extending from the aortic sinus to both common iliac arteries and all supra-aortic branches (Fig. 1). The patient underwent emergency supracoronary ascending aorta replacement and aortic valve repair.

Postoperatively, dynamic evaluation through pulsed-wave mode Doppler (8 MHz, vascular probe) and brightness-mode (B-mode) ultrasound demonstrated several sonographic features typical of a dissection. Notably, a dissection membrane was seen extending from the proximal right common carotid artery (CCA) to the distal ICA (Fig. 2, Additional file 1: Video S1). Flow direction in the true lumen was orthograde. No collateral flow was noted on transcranial Doppler, i.e., both the ophthalmic artery and the anterior cerebral artery were found to have normal, orthograde flow. Thus, distal high-grade stenosis or occlusion was excluded.

The left carotid arteries were also examined. On B-mode ultrasound, no dissection membrane or any of

*Correspondence: sven.poli@uni-tuebingen.de
[2] Department of Neurology and Stroke, and Hertie-Institute for Clinical Brain Research, Eberhard-Karls University of Tübingen, Hoppe-Seyler-Straße 3, 72076 Tübingen, Germany
Full list of author information is available at the end of the article

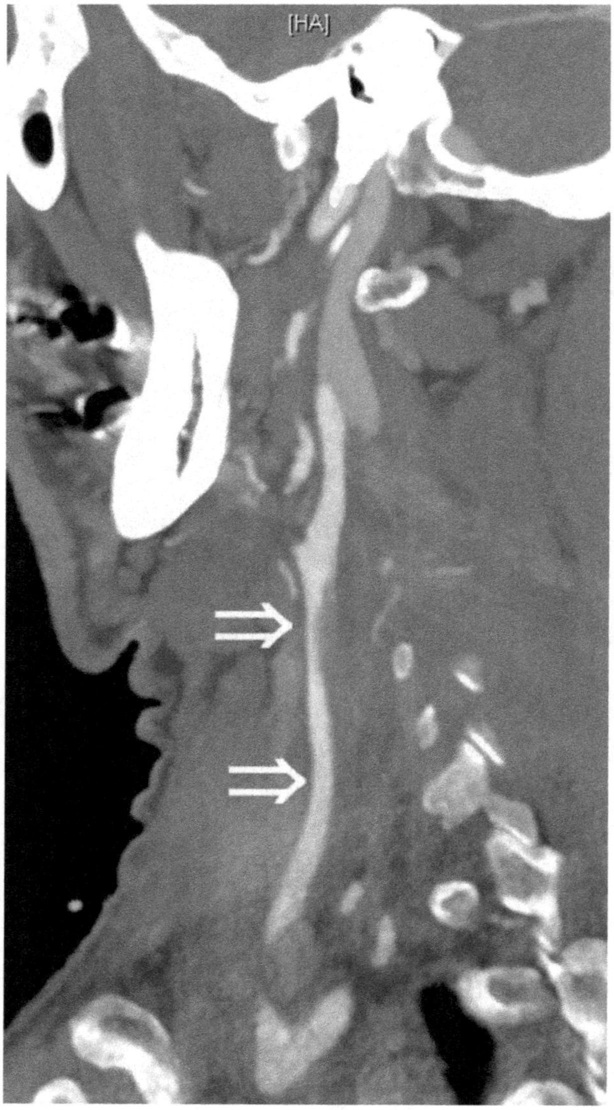

Fig. 1 Computed tomography angiography. On sagittal oblique maximum intensity projection (MIP), an extended and smoothly tapering stenosis of the right common carotid artery is seen (arrows)

the features described above were observed. However, Doppler ultrasound demonstrated a high peak systolic flow velocity of 470 cm/s in the proximal left CCA (reference range 29–178 cm/s [2]), indirectly suggesting bilateral CCA dissection (not pictured).

Discussion

Here, we report a case where bedside carotid ultrasound enabled early detection and hemodynamic assessment of CAEAD in a critically ill patient. A number of sonographic features are shown, such as luminal stenosis, a perfused false lumen, and a dissection membrane. Features not present include a thickened and hypoechogenic vessel wall, intracranial stenosis or occlusion, and pseudoaneurysm [3].

Four imaging modalities are primarily used in the diagnosis of carotid dissections. Digital subtraction angiography (DSA), i.e., contrast-enhanced invasive vascular imaging, remains the gold standard. Dynamic magnetic resonance angiography (MRA) may also be performed, especially in patients with iodinated contrast allergy or renal impairment. Fat-saturation sequences are useful to detect intramural hematoma, even if the lumen itself is not narrowed. Compared to DSA, MRA offers a variable performance at a sensitivity of 50–100% and a specificity of 29–100% [4] and is considered by the American Heart Association and the American Stroke Association to be the best initial screening test [5]. However, the speed of image acquisition is slow and MRA is not always feasible in intensive care unit (ICU) patients. Conversely, CTA is widely available, offers rapid image acquisition and compares favorably with DSA at a sensitivity of 64–100% and specificity of 67–100% [6].

Carotid ultrasound offers a number of advantages over static vessel imaging. Doppler mode yields information on flow characteristics including the peak systolic as well as diastolic flow velocities. This method is used to diagnose and grade stenosis and is especially valuable in the indirect assessment of the petrous ICA segment, where CTA is limited due to vessel wall calcifications or skull base artifacts. Using additional brightness-mode (B-mode) imaging with color-coded Doppler significantly increases the sensitivity in detecting carotid dissections, as compared to MRA, with no false-positive diagnoses [7]. Carotid ultrasound is also portable, which enables bedside examination and avoids unnecessary transports in ICU patients, which are associated with a number of serious adverse events [8]. Lastly, carotid ultrasound is the least invasive method, avoiding radiation exposure or the administration of a contrast agent. Hence, bedside carotid ultrasound is a safe and effective imaging modality in carotid dissections, suitable for use in critically ill patients.

Limitations may apply. Minor vessel damage, such as an intimal tear or small mural hematoma, may not be readily apparent on ultrasound. This applies especially to locations where B-mode imaging cannot be carried out, such as the skull base. Here, alternate imaging modalities, such as fat-saturation MRI or (contrast-enhanced) MRA, may be useful as complementary diagnostic tools.

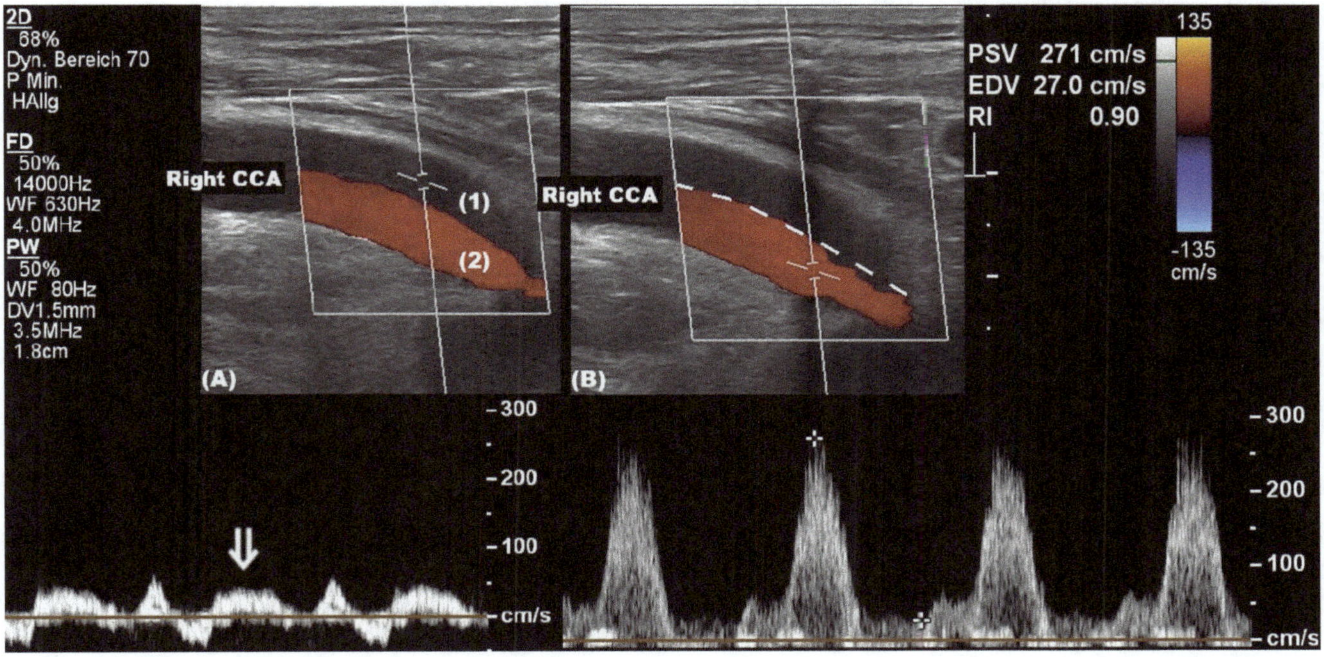

Fig. 2 Duplex sonography of the right common carotid artery. Note the dissection membrane (dashed line) separating two distinct lumina, each with different flow profiles. The false lumen (1) exhibits systolic and diastolic orthograde flow (arrow). The true lumen (2) also displays orthograde flow, but is narrowed to a luminal stenosis of 50% (peak systolic velocity 271 cm/s, reference range 29–178 cm/s [2])

Conclusion

This case study demonstrates the effective use of bedside carotid ultrasound to diagnose carotid artery dissection due to extension of aortic dissection (CAEAD). This enabled rapid decision-making in regards to further medical management.

Supplementary information

Additional file 1: Video S1. B-mode ultrasound of the right common carotid artery, examined continuously, starting in the proximal segment and moving the transducer distally. (A) Transverse view. (B) Sagittal view. Note the dissection membrane, a linear and mobile hyperechogenic structure, extending from the proximal CCA to the distal ICA, separating the false (1) and true (2) lumina.

Abbreviations

AD: aortic dissection; CAEAD: carotid artery extension of aortic dissections; CCA: common carotid artery; CTA: computed tomography angiography; DSA: digital subtraction angiography; ECA: external carotid artery; ICA: internal carotid artery; ICU: intensive care unit; MRA: magnetic resonance angiography.

Acknowledgements

The authors thank Julia Wittlinger (Eberhard-Karls University of Tübingen, Department for Neurology) for her technical assistance.

Authors' contributions

CB and SP performed ultrasound imaging and contributed to data collection and analysis. CB drafted the manuscript. SP reviewed and edited the manuscript. Both authors read and approved the final manuscript.

Author details

[1] Department of Neurology and Epileptology, and Hertie-Institute for Clinical Brain Research, Eberhard-Karls University of Tübingen, Hoppe-Seyler-Straße 3, 72076 Tübingen, Germany. [2] Department of Neurology and Stroke, and Hertie-Institute for Clinical Brain Research, Eberhard-Karls University of Tübingen, Hoppe-Seyler-Straße 3, 72076 Tübingen, Germany.

References

1. Laser A, Drucker CB, Harris DG et al (2017) Management and outcomes of carotid artery extension of aortic dissections. J Vasc Surg 66(2):445–453
2. Blackshear WM, Phillips DJ, Chikos PM, Harley JD, Thiele BL, Strandness DE (1980) Carotid artery velocity patterns in normal and stenotic vessels. Stroke 11(1):67–71
3. Baumgartner RW (2006) Handbook on neurovascular ultrasound. Front Neurol Neurosci. 21:70–84
4. Provenzale JM, Sarikaya B (2009) Comparison of test performance characteristics of MRI, MR angiography, and CT angiography in the diagnosis of carotid and vertebral artery dissection: a review of the medical literature. AJR 193(4):1167–1174
5. Brott TG, Halperin JL, Abbara S, Bacharach JM, Barr JD, Bush RL et al (2011) ASA/ACCF/AHA/AANN/AANS/ACR/ASNR/CNS/SAIP/SCAI/SIR/SNIS/SVM/SVS guideline on the management of patients with extracranial carotid and vertebral artery disease. A report of the American College of Cardiology Foundation/American Heart Association Task Force on Practice Guidelines, and the American Stroke Association, American Association of Neuroscience Nurses, American Association of Neurological Surgeons, American College of Radiology, American Society of Neuroradiology, Congress of Neurological Surgeons, Society of Atherosclerosis Imaging and Prevention, Society for Cardiovascular Angiography and Interventions, Society of Interventional Radiology, Society of NeuroInterventional Surgery, Society for Vascular Medicine, and Society for Vascular Surgery. Circulation 124(4):e54–e130

6. Hakimi R, Sivakumar S (2019) Imaging of carotid dissection. Curr Pain Headache Rep 23(1):2. https://doi.org/10.1007/s11916-019-0741-9
7. Clevert DA, Jung EM, Johnson T, Kubale R, Rupp N, Schoenberg SO, Reiser M (2007) Cervical artery dissection: improved diagnosis by B-Flow ultrasound. Clin Hemorheol Microcirc. 36(2):141–153
8. Jia L, Wang H, Gao Y, Liu H, Yu K (2016) High incidence of adverse events during intra-hospital transport of critically ill patients and new related risk factors: a prospective, multicenter study in China. Crit Care 20:12

27

ABCDE of prehospital ultrasonography

Rein Ketelaars[1,2*], Gabby Reijnders[3], Geert-Jan van Geffen[1,2], Gert Jan Scheffer[1] and Nico Hoogerwerf[1,2]

Abstract

Prehospital point-of-care ultrasound used by nonradiologists in emergency medicine is gaining ground. It is feasible on-scene and during aeromedical transport and allows health-care professionals to detect or rule out potential harmful conditions. Consequently, it impacts decision-making in prioritizing care, selecting the best treatment, and the most suitable transport mode and destination. This increasing relevance of prehospital ultrasonography is due to advancements in ultrasound devices and related technology, and to a growing number of applications. This narrative review aims to present an overview of prehospital ultrasonography literature. The focus is on civilian emergency (trauma and non-trauma) setting. Current and potential future applications are discussed, structured according to the airway, breathing, circulation, disability, and environment/exposure (ABCDE) approach. Aside from diagnostic implementation and specific protocols, procedural guidance, therapeutic ultrasound, and challenges are reviewed.

Keywords: Prehospital, Ultrasonography, Diagnostic imaging, Emergency medical services, Air ambulances, Emergency medicine, Review

Introduction

Point-of-care ultrasound (PoCUS) refers to a sign or symptom-based ultrasonography (US) examination either at the bedside or wherever patients are being treated [1]. The use of PoCUS by nonradiologists is being adopted in prehospital emergency care. It may help health-care professionals of emergency medical services (EMS) to diagnose or rule out potential life-threatening or otherwise harmful conditions [2–4]. Prehospital point-of-care ultrasonography (PHUS) may have an impact on decision-making in prioritizing initial treatment and choosing the most appropriate hospital and mode of transportation [5, 6]. Besides deploying PHUS for diagnostic purposes, it is used for procedural and therapeutic interventions.

Although the use of PHUS is increasing, its added value is still under debate. In 2010, Jørgensen was unable to conclude that PHUS improves treatment of trauma patients [5]. Five years later, O'Dochartaigh found only moderate evidence to support the use of PHUS in physician-staffed prehospital systems [6]. A recent Cochrane review concluded that, at best, abdominal US has no negative impact on mortality and morbidity, although it might reduce ordered computed tomography (CT)-scans [7]. Rudolph et al. found that PHUS may improve patient management with respect to diagnosis, treatment, and hospital referral [8]. However, they were unable to assess the effect of PHUS on patient outcomes based on the current body of evidence.

The image quality, size, and weight of portable ultrasound devices are improving. Costs for equipment are decreasing, while the number of indications for PHUS is increasing. The result is an exponentially growing body of publications, including some narrative reviews, with varying perspectives [9–11].

This narrative review is based on relevant papers selected from an extensive search in the Ovid MEDLINE® database. We added additional papers found in the references and from the authors' personal libraries.

The aim is to present an overview of the literature on PHUS in a civilian emergency (trauma and non-trauma) setting. The first part deals with current PHUS applications structured according to the familiar airway,

*Correspondence: Rein.Ketelaars@radboudumc.nl
[1] Radboud Institute for Health Sciences, Department of Anesthesiology, Pain, and Palliative Medicine, Radboud university medical center, Geert Grooteplein-Zuid 10, 6525 GA Nijmegen, The Netherlands
Full list of author information is available at the end of the article

breathing, circulation, disability, and exposure/environment (ABCDE) approach [12]. The second part will discuss interventions, procedures, challenges, and potential future applications.

PHUS in general

The use of PHUS provides diagnostic and therapeutic benefit, and it does not delay patient management [3, 8, 13–15]. It has been found to be feasible to enhance clinical assessment in a variety of out-of-hospital settings [15]. Price was among the first to show that ultrasonography (US) is also feasible during helicopter transport and that focused assessment with sonography for trauma (FAST) can be rapidly performed in-flight and has no influence on aircraft avionics [16].

Physicians and paramedics without being educated as a radiologist can be trained effectively to perform PoCUS. Lyon et al. demonstrated that prehospital critical care providers could learn to detect the sonographic sliding lung sign with a high level of sensitivity (97%) and specificity (94%) and retain their skill over time [17]. Forty physicians participated in a 4-h hands-on training and demonstrated significant improvements in the ability to perform US examinations [18]. Although the initial learning curve for FAST is steep, it starts to flatten after 30–100 scans [19]. Probably even more training and experience is required for advanced applications such as transcranial Doppler for ischemic stroke or specific triage protocols.

With the right education and mentorship, paramedics can obtain ultrasound images of sufficient quality to positively identify significant pathologies in critically ill patients [20]. A recent Canadian study found that PHUS performed by both physicians and non-physicians supported interventions in both trauma and medical patients [21].

The reported diagnostic accuracy of PHUS varies widely. Some reported a sensitivity of 85–90% and a specificity of 96–100% for chest, abdominal, and cardiac US. Positive predictive value (PPV) and negative predictive value (NPV) were 100 and 95.5% [3, 13]. Diagnostic accuracy during transportation also varies. For PHUS during transfer by ground ambulance and PHUS on-scene, Brun reported a sensitivity of 94.7 and 95.2%, respectively [22]. In-flight ultrasound examinations of the lung, abdomen, and pericardium yielded a sensitivity of only 50–64.7% when compared to pathology that required an intervention, rather than to all positive findings [23]. Others found a sensitivity of 78.6% for in-flight extended FAST (eFAST) compared to CT scan [24]. Because of the high specificity, the activation of a trauma surgery team is justified for positive PHUS findings [23].

Despite the range in diagnostic accuracy, PHUS is still highly reliable compared to clinical assessment [3, 5]. In 169 non-trauma patients, PHUS improved the diagnostic accuracy based on traditional clinical examination to 67% compared to the final in-hospital diagnosis. Diagnostic accuracy was improved in 90% of patients in whom the initial diagnosis was uncertain (n = 115) [25]. Blaivas found that PHUS improved the certainty of the diagnosis in 68% of 25 mainly non-trauma patients [26].

PHUS potentially impacts life-saving procedures, priorities in the care for one or many patients, and the most appropriate destination. Indications exist that PHUS benefits outcome, but evidence is still lacking [5]. Nevertheless, O'Dochartaigh and Jørgensen noted that PHUS impacted and streamlined in-hospital treatment [5, 6]. The impact was not quantified, but O'Dochartaigh suggested that PHUS-supported interventions were more frequent in the more severely injured patients.

Diagnostic applications

A—Airway

First-attempt success rates of prehospital rapid sequence intubations vary between 46 and 85% [27]. An attempt fails when the endotracheal tube (ETT) cannot be placed between the vocal cords in the trachea or is inadvertently placed in the esophagus. It is of paramount importance to acknowledge esophageal intubation as soon as possible.

The use of tracheal and cricothyroid ultrasound can be very useful to confirm correct ETT placement. This was first described in neonates by Slovis in 1986 [28]. Fourteen years later, Dreschler was the first to also visualize the esophagus and to detect esophageal intubation in five out of five cadaver models [29]. A recent review showed a pooled sensitivity and specificity of, respectively, 98 and 94% of transtracheal US in emergency intubations [30]. Therefore, the confirmation of correct ETT position by PoCUS in the prehospital setting is likely to be beneficial [12, 31, 32]. Although capnography is considered the gold standard to confirm a correct tube position, it does not discriminate between endotracheal and endobronchial intubation [33]. Furthermore, in a prehospital setting, chest radiography is impossible, and auscultation is not always feasible. Therefore, PHUS might be a valuable tool to assess the airway [34].

Zadel et al. confirmed endotracheal tube position by the detection of bilateral lung sliding and bilateral diaphragmatic excursion in 124 out-of-hospital patients [32]. Esophageal intubation occurred in 13 patients (10.5%), of which only 30% was detected visually or by auscultation before waveform capnography was recorded. Both sensitivity and specificity of PHUS for a correct tube position was 100%. The performance of PHUS took a median of 30 s (sd = 8–120 s). A prospective study in pediatrics preferred the assessment of bilateral diaphragmatic excursions to confirm proper ETT placement [35]. Therefore, the assessment of lung sliding and diaphragmatic excursions is of value in the absence of chest radiography or capnography.

B—Chest, pulmonary

The cause of acute dyspnea is not immediately apparent, especially in the prehospital setting. Caregivers must differentiate between a cardiac or a pulmonary cause. In an emergency department (ED) study, Kajimoto proposed a quick method to integrate (1) lung ultrasound, (2) cardiac ultrasound, and (3) measurements of the inferior vena cava (LCI) [36]. Lung ultrasound is performed in eight chest areas (four anterior and four lateral). Cardiac ultrasound estimates the global left ventricular function and mitral or tricuspid valve regurgitation. Subsequently, collapsibility of the inferior vena cava is determined. The LCI integrated examination will take only up to 3 min. The sensitivity and specificity were 94.3 and 91.9% for acute heart failure syndromes, compared to the traditional methods of differentiating between pulmonary and cardiac causes including electrocardiogram, chest X-ray, and B-type natriuretic peptide (BNP).

A similar *triple scan* consisting of basic echocardiography, lung ultrasound, and assessment of inferior vena cava collapsibility was proposed by Mantuani et al. [37]. They included 57 patients with acute dyspnea caused by acute decompensated heart failure (ADHF), chronic obstructive pulmonary disease (COPD), and pneumonia. After the triple scan, the accuracy of the diagnosis, based on history and physical examination, increased from 53 to 77%. Sensitivity and specificity of the triple scan for ADHF were 100 and 84%.

Lichtenstein's bedside lung ultrasound in emergency (BLUE) protocol allows rapid diagnosis of acute respiratory failure and can be completed in under 3 min [38, 39]. Four standardized points on either side of the chest are assessed for ten signs indicative of normal lung surface, pleural effusions, lung consolidations, alveolar–interstitial syndrome, and pneumothorax. For simplicity, echocardiography is not included. Distinct profiles are recognized for the main causes of respiratory distress: pneumonia, congestive heart failure, COPD, asthma, pulmonary embolism, and pneumothorax as summarized in Table 1. It has a diagnostic accuracy of > 90% [40].

The LCI, *triple scan*, and BLUE protocol all might be relevant and valuable in the prehospital setting because of simplicity and nominal time investment. With the help of these protocols, the EMS caregiver can accurately differentiate between causes and direct treatment and avoid unnecessary or harmful interventions.

Besides the diagnosis of dyspnea, lung US may be used to support prehospital continuous positive airway pressure (CPAP) treatment [41]. In 20 ADHF patients, a physician-staffed EMS sonographically assessed 15 chest wall regions before and after CPAP treatment compared to standard treatment. The number of B-lines (explained in Table 1 and shown in Figs. 1, 2) was significantly lower in the CPAP group, and their respiratory and hemodynamic variables improved after CPAP. The number of B-lines correlates with the amount of extravascular lung water (EVLW) and NT-proBNP levels and thus with the severity of ADHF. They develop at a pulmonary artery occlusion pressure (PAOP) > 18 mmHg [42].

In high-altitude medicine, Wimalasena described the value of lung US in the early detection of high-altitude pulmonary edema (HAPE) before symptoms appear, and in differentiating HAPE from other causes of dyspnea such as pneumonia or pneumothorax [43]. The number of B-lines, indicating an increased amount of EVLW, is inversely correlated with the oxygen saturation and both values improve on (early) treatment [44].

B—Chest, traumatic

Pneumothorax

Using PoCUS for detecting pneumothorax is feasible, fast, without any radiation, has a steep learning curve and high diagnostic accuracy, and it allows for dynamic and repeated examinations [45, 46].

A pneumothorax is characterized by the abolition of lung sliding, the absence of B-lines, and the appearance of the A-line sign [39]. Lung sliding is the representation of the visceral and parietal pleura sliding against each other during respiration. B-lines are the result of the accumulation of fluid in the pulmonary interstitium. Therefore, the presence of B-lines on PoCUS rules out a pneumothorax. Horizontal A-lines are reflections of the pleural line caused by gas below the parietal pleura either within or outside of the lung. These signs are explained further in Table 1; adapted from Lichtenstein's paper on the BLUE and FALLS protocol [39]. A normal lung US image is shown in Figs. 1, 2, and 3. Images of pneumothorax are shown in Figs. 4, 5, and Additional file 1: Video 1.

An important implication of detecting or excluding pneumothorax is the subsequent decision to perform (or withhold) a tube thoracostomy. An evaluation of prehospital chest US in 281 patients revealed that the acute medical management changed in 21%. The intention to introduce a tube thoracostomy was abandoned in 4% (n = 10) and the transport destination changed in another 4% [4]. Similarly, Mazur found that chest US examinations (n = 60) performed in preparation for air transport helped them prevent four (8%) chest tube thoracostomies [47].

Table 1 BLUE protocol profiles. Lichtenstein [39]

P#	Profile name	Location	Appearance	Implication/diagnosis
1	A-profile	Anterior chest wall	Lung sliding—visualization of the movement of the visceral pleura against the parietal pleura with respiration A-lines—an indication of the presence of air below the parietal pleura[a]	Normal lung surface
2	B-profile		Lung sliding Lung rockets—a pattern of three vertical B-lines caused by edema in the interlobular septa[b]	Pulmonary edema
3	B'-profile		No lung sliding—in the B' profile lung sliding is abolished by the deposition of fibrin caused by pneumonia Lung rockets	Pneumonia
4	A/B-profile		Unilateral lung rockets—indicative for a (unilateral) pneumonia and does not correspond with generalized pulmonary edema	Pneumonia
5	C-profile	Anterior chest wall	Anterior lung consolidation—anteriorly located, therefore unlike to be caused by hemodynamic pulmonary edema or embolism	Pneumonia
6	A-profile without DVT[c]		Lung sliding A-lines[a] No DVT	Normal
	A-no-V-PLAPS profile	Posterolateral chest wall	Lung sliding A-lines[a] No DVT PLAPS[e]—posterolateral alveolar and/or pleural syndrome—pulmonary consolidation and pleural effusion	Pneumonia
7	A-profile with DVT[c]		Lung sliding A-lines[a] DVT	Pulmonary embolism
8	A'-profile	Anterior chest wall	No lung sliding—lung sliding abolished by separation of the visceral pleura from the parietal pleura A-lines—an indication of the presence of air below the parietal pleura[a]	Pneumothorax when the mandatory 'lung point'[d] is visualized
9	A-profile without DVT and no PLAPS (nude profile)		Lung sliding A-lines[a] No DVT No PLAPS	Asthma or COPD

The bedside lung ultrasound in emergency (BLUE) protocol defines nine profiles. They are defined by their sonographic appearance and are associated with the different diagnoses as described in the right-most column

[a] A-lines = Horizontal repetition of the pleural line appearing below the pleural line at multiples of the skin–pleural line distance. Their appearance is an indication of air below the parietal pleura, either in or outside of the lung. They are particularly apparent in the absence of B-lines potentially obscuring the A-lines

[b] B-lines = A long, well-defined, hyperechoic comet tail artifact arising from the pleural line that obliterates the A-lines

[c] DVT = Deep venous thrombosis. Has to be separately found or excluded at the lower extremities

[d] Lung point = The location where the visceral pleura is only partially in contact with the parietal pleura. With respirations, the A' profile (without lung rockets) is intermittently replaced with the A-profile (lung rockets are possible). The lung point is a pathognomonic sign for the diagnosis of pneumothorax! See Additional file 1: Video 1

[e] PLAPS = Posterolateral alveolar and/or pleural syndrome (posterolateral consolidations or pleural effusions)

Detection of pneumothorax during flight

In some EMS systems, patients are evaluated and treated while in-flight in a helicopter or fixed-wing aircraft. In prehospital and flight medicine, lung US was found to be feasible and safe [16, 24, 48]. For instance, M-mode (Figs. 3, 5) ultrasonography was used to successfully evaluate a pleural interface model on board a helicopter while stationary, with rotor rotation before take-off, and at level flight [49]. Madill reported the case of a blast injury patient in whom an in-flight chest US examination identified an untreated pneumothorax. This directed the decision to perform a successful in-flight thoracentesis and tube thoracostomy [50]. In 2013, Roline was reported to be the first to evaluate in-flight chest US in a helicopter emergency medical service (HEMS) operation [51]. They performed 41 chest US examinations in 71 patients. Expert sonographers reviewed the images and reached substantial agreement with the providers. Image quality was good or poor in 54 and 46%, respectively. Challenges consisted of the

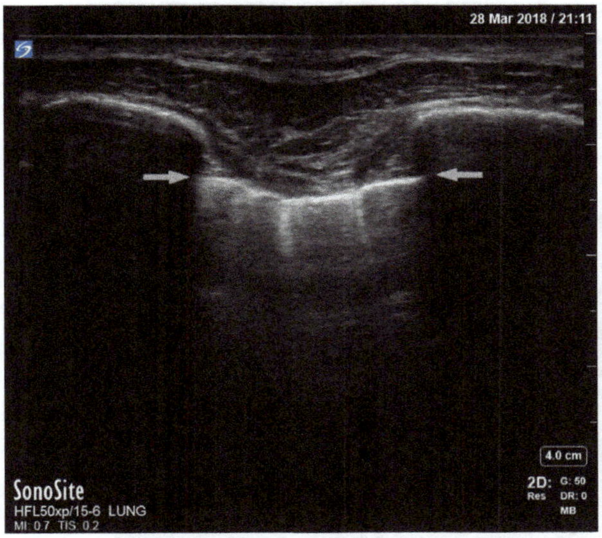

Fig. 1 Normal lung. A normal lung ultrasound image acquired with a 15–6 MHz linear transducer. The ribs are visible with their anechoic shadows on both sides of the image. The pleural line is shown in between the ribs, indicated with two horizontal arrows. Emanating down from the pleural line are comet tails. B-lines (not visible here) also start at the pleural line, but extend all the way down to edge of the image

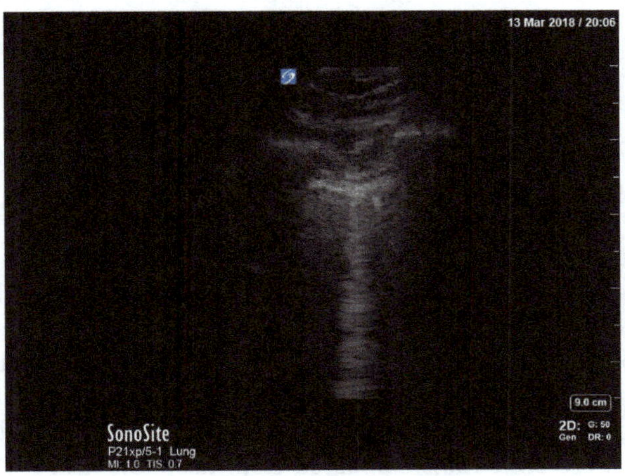

Fig. 2 Normal lung + B-line. A normal lung ultrasound image acquired with a 5–1 MHz phased-array cardiac transducer. In the middle of the image, one B-line is seen. This is also seen in healthy subjects and a single B-line is without meaning

lack of time, limited aircraft space, and, less frequently, the presence of pacer pads. They concluded that in-flight chest US is feasible, has a steep learning curve, and that additional training is needed to improve image quality. Quick et al. found that the diagnostic accuracy of in-flight US for pneumothorax is nearly similar to US in the ED: 91 and 96%, respectively [52].

These reports suggest that PHUS augment the diagnostic capabilities of prehospital aeromedical providers, also when in-flight, and might lead to better outcomes.

Hemothorax

No studies with substantial data on the diagnostic performance of PHUS and hemothorax are available. Ketelaars described that PHUS detected one hemothorax in seven cases specifically assessed for hemothorax with 100% accuracy [4]. In a 2007 *best evidence topic report* the authors concluded that ultrasound is a sensitive, specific, and accurate method to detect the presence of hemothorax in trauma patients [53]. A more recent meta-analysis of hospital studies revealed a pooled sensitivity and specificity of 67 and 99% of PoCUS for hemothorax. For radiography, these were 54 and 99% [54]. Therefore, PoCUS for hemothorax may be valuable in both in-hospital and prehospital settings. Future studies might demonstrate the added value of early, prehospital, detection of hemothorax although an early chest tube thoracostomy is rarely required [55]. Still, PHUS yields valuable information to include in the prearrival notification to the receiving trauma center.

Diaphragmatic rupture

Diaphragmatic rupture occurs in up to 5% of blunt abdominal trauma patients and may be present despite a negative FAST scan [56]. Ultrasonographic signs may be poor movement (on M-mode) or elevation of the diaphragm, a liver sliding sign (at the right chest wall), subphrenic effusion, or the presence of an intrathoracic spleen or liver [57–59]. In addition, Gangahar introduced *Rip's absent organ sign* as an indirect marker: nonvisualization of the spleen or heart caused by displacement of abdominal contents anteriorly to these organs [60, 61].

B—Gastric tube

The only indication for a gastric tube (GT) in the prehospital setting is to relieve gastric distention that is often caused or aggravated by bag-valve-mask ventilation. Traditionally, correct positioning is verified by injecting air in the tube while listening for air bubbles, or by aspiration of gastric contents. These methods are unreliable, especially in the noisy prehospital environment, and the recommended pH measurements and chest X-rays are not feasible [62]. Chenaitia et al. estimated the diagnostic accuracy of PHUS confirming GT placement in 130 prehospital intubated patients, compared to in-hospital chest X-ray. They positioned the probe subxiphoidal in the transverse plane, oriented toward the left hypochondrium to visualize the GT tip in the gastric antrum. Examination time was limited to 1 min. Sensitivity and

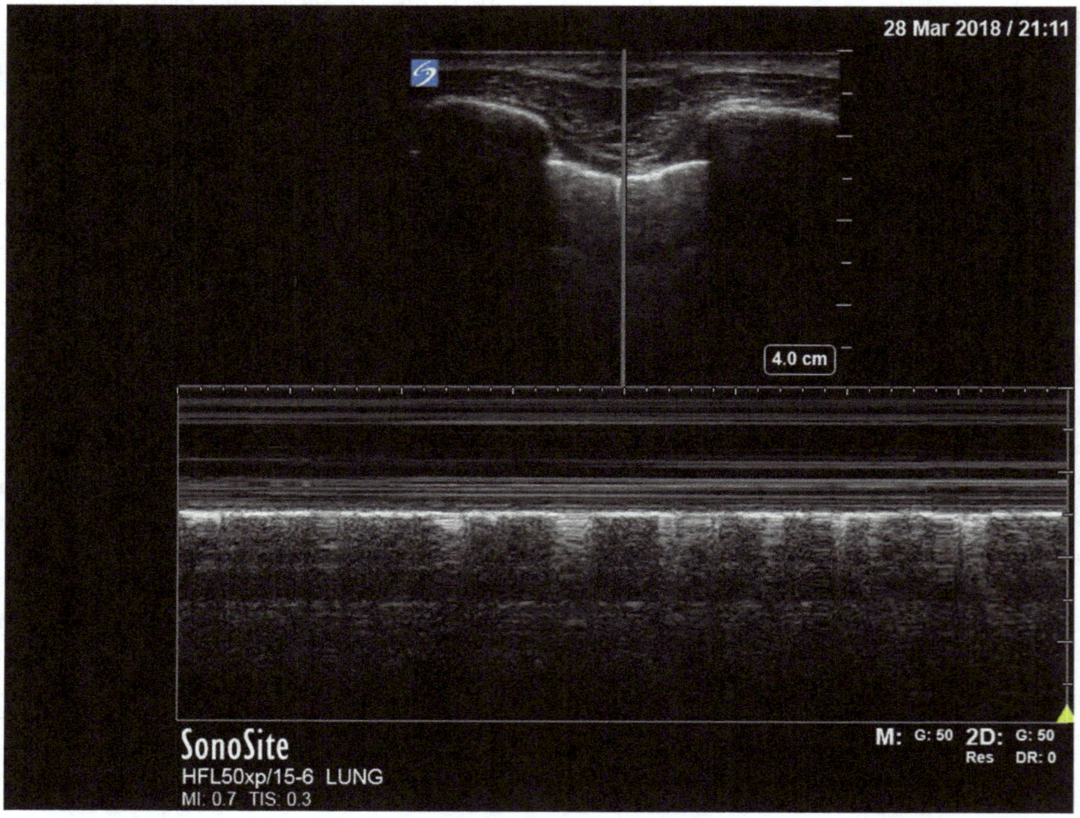

Fig. 3 Normal lung—M-mode ultrasound image. The ultrasound reflections on the vertical line in the upper part of the image are sequentially displayed from left to right in the lower part as time progresses. It allows to capture the motion of the upper 2D image in the stationary image below. A normal M-mode image of the chest wall and pleura is displayed here. The stationary chest wall produces straight horizontal lines above the pleural line. The lung sliding and movement of the artifacts below produces a grainy image. This is called the seashore sign

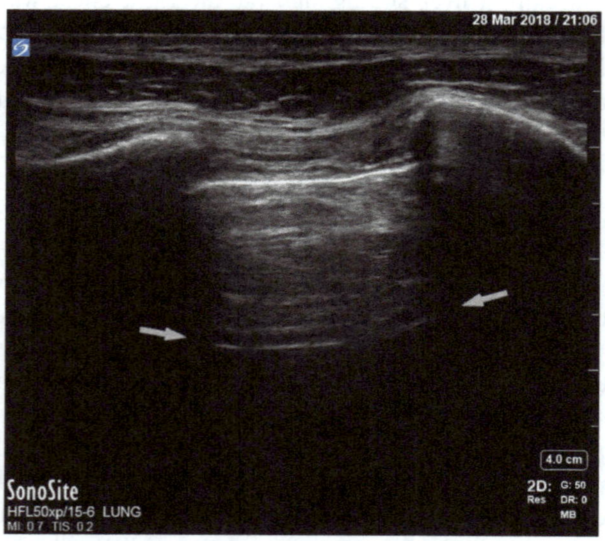

Fig. 4 Pneumothorax + A-line. A-lines are reflections of the pleural line caused by gas below the parietal pleura. An A-line is indicated by the arrows. The A is for "air" either within or outside of the lung. In case of a pneumothorax, there are no B-lines (Fig. 2) that may obscure the A-lines making them stand out more clearly

specificity were 98.3 and 100%. PPV and NPV were 100 and 85.7% [63].

In a follow-up study they added an esophageal view at the anterior neck during and after GT insertion. In case the GT was visualized in the esophagus but not in the stomach, 50 ml of air was inserted. An intragastric position of the tip was visualized or assumed when gastric air entry was observed as *dynamic fogging*: an expanding volume of hyperechoic 'fog'. Sensitivity and specificity were both 100% compared to in-hospital chest X-ray [64]. When US is only performed after GT insertion, it is as fast as the traditional air insufflation and aspiration method.

C—Circulation–cardiac arrest

Current European resuscitation guidelines state that there is no doubt that focused cardiac ultrasound (FoCUS)—using specific protocols for US evaluation—has the potential to detect reversible causes of cardiac arrest [12]. FoCUS can help distinguish the PEA type, identify the cause of the arrest, choose a suitable

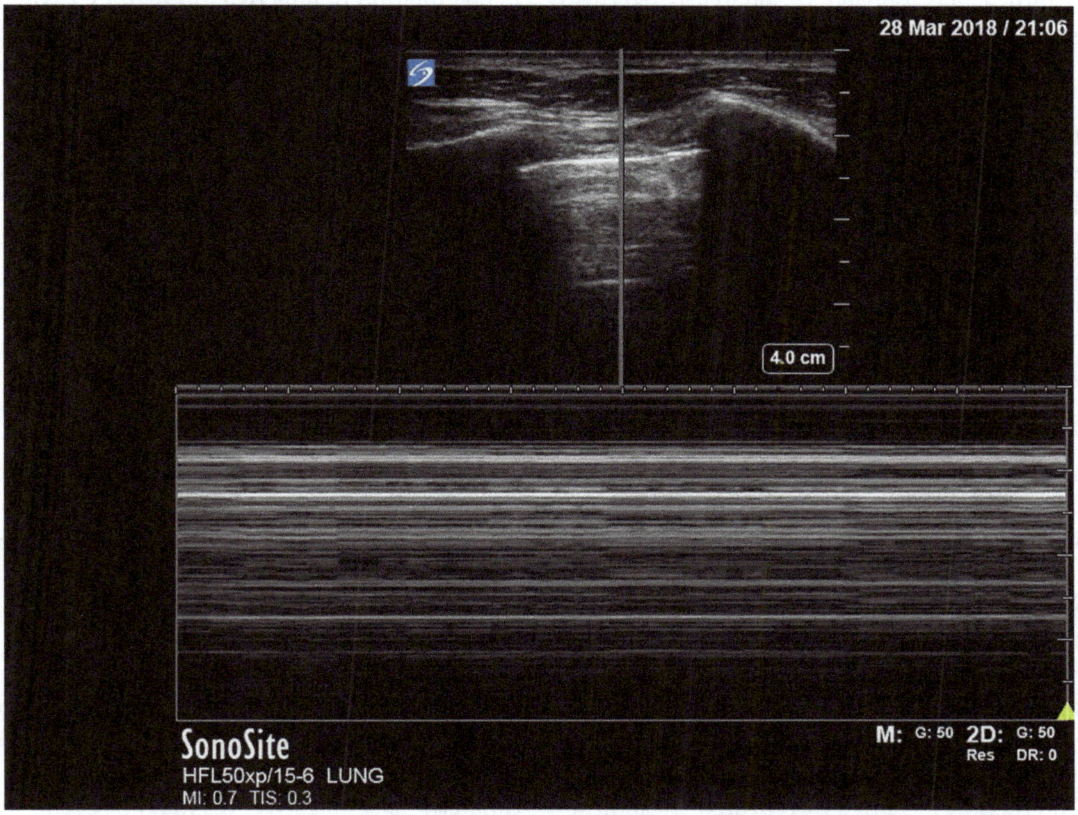

Fig. 5 Pneumothorax—M-mode ultrasound image. There is no visible movement above or below the pleural line. Because all tissue and artifacts are stationary, the M-mode image appears as horizontal straight lines throughout the image. This is called a barcode sign or stratosphere sign

treatment, and make the right decision on cardiopulmonary resuscitation (CPR) termination [65]. In 75% of the patients with pulseless electrical activity (PEA), FoCUS showed coordinated cardiac motion (pseudo-PEA) in a prehospital peri-resuscitation care study [66]. Pseudo-PEA is strongly associated with increased survival compared to a true PEA. Treatable causes were reduced ventricular function (59%), pericardial tamponade (9.8%), a significantly dilated right ventricle (7.8%), and hypovolemia (3.9%) [66]. A return of spontaneous circulation (ROSC) was indeed achieved after pericardiocentesis. Three of five tamponade patients survived to hospital admission.

Similarly, cardiac motion in PEA patients in the ED is positively associated with ROSC. Salen found that in 8 of 11 (73%) patients with sonographic cardiac activity, ROSC was achieved but in none of 23 without cardiac activity [67]. A retrospective analysis of 318 pulseless trauma patients revealed that the survival of pulseless traumatic arrest patients without sonographic cardiac activity is rare [68]. In non-trauma ED patients, cardiac standstill on FoCUS during CPR correlated with death with a PPV of 97.1% and an NPV of 57.1% [69]. However, the timing and the duration of the FoCUS examination could be very important.

Termination of resuscitation (TOR) may be considered in out-of-hospital cardiac arrest patients when these four criteria are met: no ROSC before transport, no shock delivered, no bystander CPR, and an unwitnessed arrest [70]. Goto developed a similar TOR rule: no prehospital ROSC, non-shockable initial rhythm, and unwitnessed by bystanders. Their rule is a > 99% predictor of death within 1 month after out-of-hospital cardiac arrest (OHCA) [71]. Cardiac standstill on initial FoCUS may predict non-ROSC and could be used in the decision for the termination of treatment [67, 72]. However, a 2016 study in non-traumatic OHCA patients undergoing serial FoCUS confirmed ROSC could occur within 10 min after initial cardiac standstill [73]. However, after a cardiac standstill of 10 min or longer, no ROSC occurred. These findings suggest that PHUS might play an important role here: consider TOR after 10 min of sonographic cardiac standstill?

In addition to uncovering treatable causes of cardiac arrest, FoCUS is invaluable in confirming mechanical ventricular capture (as opposed to electrical capture) during transcutaneous cardiac pacing [74].

C—Shock

Although the cause of shock may not be apparent, FoCUS might guide therapy such as intravenous fluid administration, inotropic therapy, and the choice of destination hospital. FoCUS directly altered treatment in 51% of the cardiac arrest and peri-resuscitation patients in Breitkreutz's prehospital study [66]. This implies that every hemodynamically unstable patient could potentially benefit from PHUS.

Non-traumatic shock

To evaluate critically ill patients with acute circulatory failure, Lichtenstein devised the fluid administration limited by lung sonography (FALLS)-protocol aimed at reducing the mortality from septic shock [39]. It aims to sequentially rule out (1) obstructive, (2) cardiogenic, and (3) hypovolemic shock for expediting the diagnosis of distributive (usually septic) shock, displayed in Fig. 6. When other causes of shock are eliminated and distributive shock (sepsis) remains, fluid therapy and vasopressors are indicated. Fluid therapy is guided by repeated chest ultrasound based on the appearance of the so-called B-profile as defined in the BLUE protocol (Table 1).

The rapid ultrasound in shock (RUSH) examination involves a three-part assessment simplified as (1) the pump, (2) the tank, and (3) the pipes [75]. *The pump* refers to an evaluation of the pericardial sac, left ventricular contractility, and the relative size of the right ventricle to the left ventricle. *The tank* refers to the determination of effective intravascular volume status by measuring the inferior vena cava (IVC) and assessment of the lung, pleural and abdominal cavity. *The pipes* refer to scanning for an aneurysm or dissection of the thoracic and abdominal aorta, and deep venous thrombosis.

Both the FALLS and RUSH protocol combine familiar US scans proven to be feasible in the prehospital setting. Although we are unaware of any reports, these protocols are potentially valuable in prehospital care.

Traumatic shock

In traumatic shock, the (extended) FAST protocol may be used to detect a hemoperitoneum. A US image of a normal hepatorenal recess and one with a hemoperitoneum are displayed in Figs. 7, 8. In abdominal trauma, its sensitivity and specificity are comparable between in-hospital and prehospital: 100 and 97.5% in-hospital and 90 and 99% prehospital, respectively [2]. The feasibility and efficiency of the extended FAST were also comparable, with no significant difference in US duration [22].

In shocked blunt abdominal trauma patients, expeditious PoCUS should take a minimum amount of time. Clarke found that mortality increases by 1% for every 3-min delay of a necessary intervention [76, 77]. Unfortunately, false-negative results do occur and they do most frequently in scans performed early in the disease process [22, 78]. Therefore, when FAST is negative it is recommended to repeat the examination every 15 min [2, 77]. Repeated abdominal US scans may lead to a 50% reduction of false negatives [79]. However, a hemorrhage in the retroperitoneum or any solid organ injuries cannot be detected reliably with FAST. So, a negative FAST

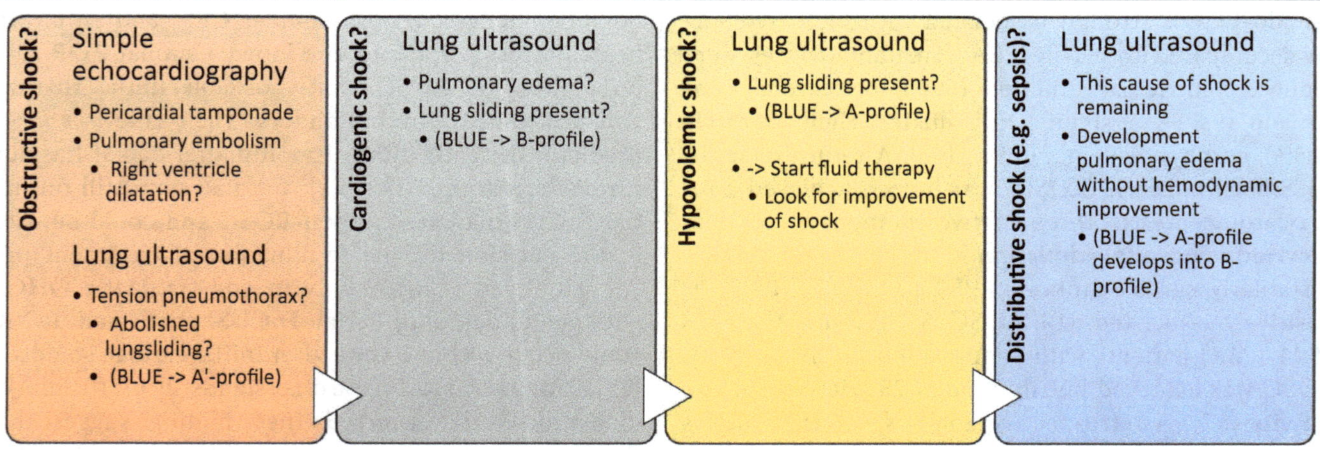

Fig. 6 FALLS protocol. This diagram is an adaptation of the work by Dr. Lichtenstein [39]. Firstly, this diagram shows the type of shock the focus is on. Secondly, the type of ultrasound examination is shown. Thirdly, possible diagnoses to consider are shown including their appearance in terms of the BLUE protocol. Every cause of shock is sequentially excluded for expediting the diagnosis of distributive (septic) shock. *FALLS* fluid administration limited by lung sonography, *BLUE* bedside lung ultrasound in emergency, BLUE and the A, B, and A' profile are explained in Table 1, items 1, 2, and 8, respectively

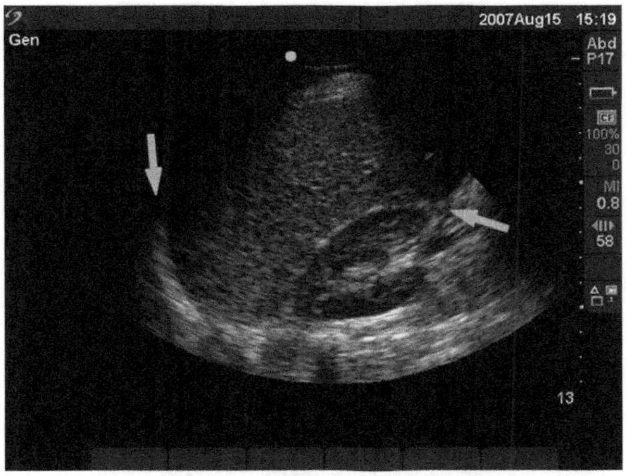

Fig. 7 Normal hepatorenal recess. A normal ultrasound image of the hepatorenal recess (Morison's pouch). A phased-array cardiac transducer was used with the abdominal settings. The left arrow indicates the diaphragm. The right arrow indicates the hepatorenal recess. The liver is shown above this line and the right kidney below

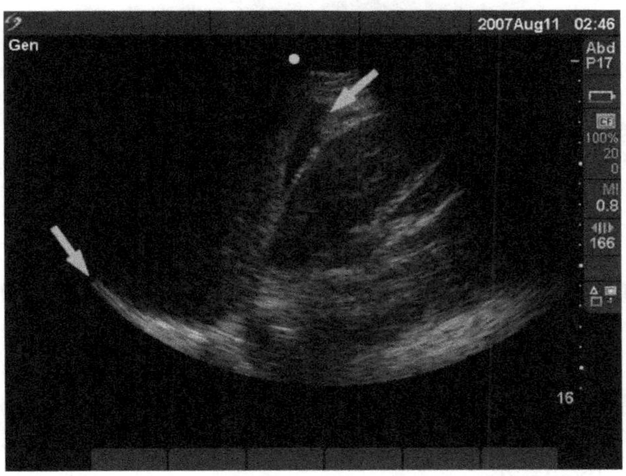

Fig. 8 Hemoperitoneum at the splenorenal recess. An ultrasound image of the splenorenal recess (Koller's pouch). A phased-array cardiac transducer was used with the abdominal settings. The left arrow indicates the diaphragm. The right arrow indicates the splenorenal recess with a hypoechoic collection between the spleen (left) and the left kidney (right). This is the image of free intraperitoneal fluid and is very suggestive for intraperitoneal hemorrhage when encountered in a trauma victim

does not compensate for a high suspicion of abdominal hemorrhage.

A (non) traumatic pneumoperitoneum is almost invariably caused by gastrointestinal perforation. When detected prehospitally, this might steer early treatment and transportation. Sensitivity and specificity of abdominal US for pneumoperitoneum is 85–90% and 100%. In experienced hands it can be as good as CT; an amount as small as 1 ml of free air can be detected [80–82]. Thus, it appears plausible to use PHUS also for this indication.

In their meta-analysis, Stengel et al. concluded that US for blunt abdominal trauma does not decrease the laparotomy rate or mortality. Nevertheless, the number of ordered CT scans decreased by 50%. However, this might reflect a false sense of security due to the low sensitivity of abdominal ultrasound for both free fluid and organ lacerations [77]. Montoya also reported that US led to fewer CT scans. In addition, however, they found a decreased time to appropriate interventions, shortened hospital stay, and decreased use of healthcare resources [78].

C—Abdominal aortic aneurysm

US is feasible and suitable to assess for an aneurysm of the abdominal aorta in symptomatic patients. An ED study showed a sensitivity and specificity of 100 and 98% [83]. Prehospitally this is also feasible, reported Heegaard et al. Trained ambulance paramedics performed PHUS scans of the abdominal aorta in 20 symptomatic patients. A blinded expert also judged the images and agreed 100% with the paramedics' judgment [84].

D—Central nervous system

Stroke—transcranial US

Reducing the interval between ischemic stroke and intravenous thrombolysis is associated with reduced mortality, reduced symptomatic intracranial hemorrhage, and higher rates of independent ambulation at discharge and discharge to home [85, 86]. Unfortunately, prehospital delays lead to missed opportunities to initiate treatment within the preferred 90 min after the onset of symptoms [87]. For instance, in an American study, only 38% of patients arrived within 2 h of the onset of their symptoms [88].

Early prehospital detection of ischemic stroke may be beneficial to a favorable outcome. Prehospital caregivers could allocate patients to the most appropriate hospital, provide a prearrival notification, and initiate stroke-specific therapies such as sonothrombolysis and neuroprotective strategies [87, 89, 90]. Intravenous thrombolysis, however, is only administered safely after a CT or magnetic resonance imaging (MRI) scan excludes an intracranial hemorrhage.

Herzberg et al. evaluated the diagnostic accuracy of prehospital neurological examination supported by transcranial color-coded sonography (TCCS) [89]. The TCCS consisted of color-mode visualization and flow measurements in the proximal M-1 segment of both middle cerebral arteries (MCA) to find an occlusion. When desired, they scanned the anterior and posterior cerebral arteries or administered an intravenous ultrasound contrast agent (UCA). Sensitivity and specificity were 95 and 48%; PPV and NPV were 82 and 77% for the prehospital diagnosis of 'any stroke' compared to in-hospital CT angiography (CTA) and magnetic resonance angiography (MRA). With appropriate training, telemedicine, and UCAs, these results might still improve [89].

In their prehospital study, Schlachetzki found that 36% of the physicians used microbubbles as a UCA to save time or to increase the diagnostic confidence when temporal window anatomy did not allow an optimal visualization of the MCAs. The sensitivity and specificity of ultrasound for MCA occlusions were 90 and 98%. PPV and NPV were 90 and 98% [90].

Besides arterial occlusions, vasospasm due to aneurysmal subarachnoid hemorrhage may be detected by transcranial US. However, its diagnostic accuracy varies widely depending on the vessel, the diagnostic criteria, and timing [91]. Anecdotal evidence exists on other intracranial pathologies which may be detected by PHUS such as intracranial hematomas and ventricular system enlargement [92, 93].

The biggest limitation of the application of transcranial US is the ability to obtain US images through the temporal window (Fig. 9). This is the thinnest part of the temporal bone that allows penetration of the US beam at a suitable angle and distance in relation to basal portions of the major cerebral arteries and the circle of Willis. This procedure may be very demanding and requires training and experience. Therefore, transcranial US might not be suitable for every ultrasound-equipped (H)EMS service.

The therapeutic applications of transcranial US in ischemic stroke are discussed in the *interventions* section of this paper.

ONSD

Both optic disc edema detected by fundoscopy and an increased optic nerve sheath diameter (ONSD) are indications of increased intracranial pressure (ICP) [94]. The ONSD can easily be measured using US, although the use of a UCA might enhance the recognition of relevant anatomy [95]. ONSD measurements, using a cutoff value of 5.0 mm, have a sensitivity and specificity of 100 and 95% in predicting an elevated ICP compared to CT [96]. Moretti et al. compared US to invasive ICP measurements. Using a cutoff value of 5.2 mm, they found a sensitivity and specificity of 93.1 and 73.9% for an ICP $\geq$ 20 mmHg [97]. More recently, Maissan et al. measured the ONSD in ICP-monitored traumatic brain injury (TBI) patients before, during, and after routine suctioning of the endotracheal tube leading to a transient ICP rise. With a cutoff value of 5.0 mm they found the sensitivity and specificity to be 94 and 98% for a rise in ICP [98].

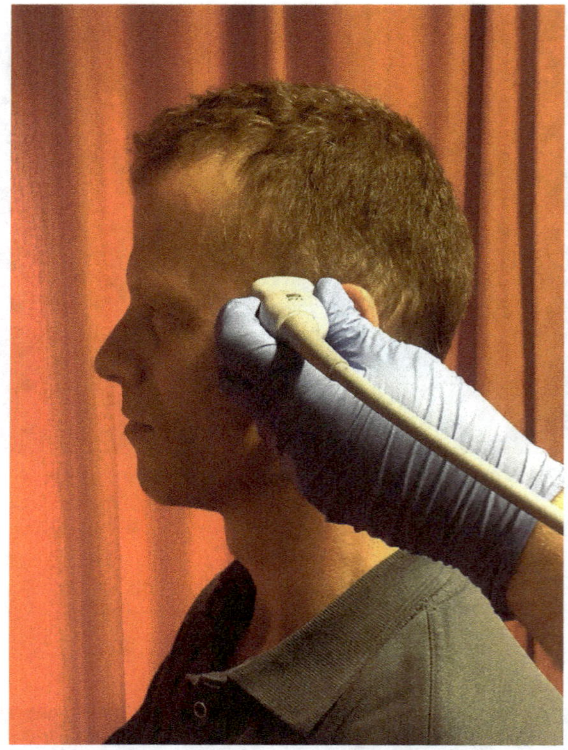

Fig. 9 Ultrasound transducer positioned at the temporal window. The ultrasound transducer is positioned at the site where the temporal bone is thinnest and the ultrasound beam is least obstructed penetrating the skull (Reproduced with permission from Rob Stoffels and Yvonne Houben)

Like US in ischemic stroke, the benefit of prehospital ONSD measurements might be to start neuroprotective strategies, to determine the need for neurosurgical care, or to provide a prearrival notification. However, the evidence on prehospital feasibility and benefit is still negligible.

E—Injuries

Fractures

Dulchavsky concluded that non-physicians in the ED (cast technicians) can reliably diagnose orthopedic injury with an accuracy of 94% after a brief PoCUS training. This was more reliable for fractures of the humerus, forearm, femur, and lower leg than for hand and foot fractures, and tendon injuries [99].

Bozorgi et al. evaluated US in 108 ED patients with 158 fractures in the extremities. The overall sensitivity was 68.3%. Sensitivity for femoral fractures and humeral fractures was 100 and 76.2%, respectively. The detection of intra-articular fractures was the most difficult with a sensitivity of only 48% [100].

In the civilian prehospital setting, PHUS for fractures is probably feasible. It is useful for (long) bone fractures in the upper and lower arm, and leg. Advantages in the prehospital setting could be early reduction and splinting, triage, and selecting the best destination provided with a specific prearrival notification.

Foreign objects

In the wilderness environment, Paziana described two cases where PHUS was successfully used to aid in the removal of foreign objects from soft tissue [101]. PHUS may determine the exact location and depth of a foreign object despite that some are radiolucent. The location and size of the incision can be determined, and the removal may take place under direct US visualization.

Ocular ultrasonography

Besides ONSD measurements, ocular US appears useful and feasible in the prehospital setting. It is useful to diagnose penetrating globe injury, foreign body retention, retinal detachment, vitreous detachment, central retinal artery occlusion, lens dislocation, retrobulbar hematoma, and retinal and vitreous hemorrhage [102, 103]. The eye can be accurately assessed without the need to open the eyelid in case of swelling. An austere environment case report described PHUS helping to diagnose a retinal detachment after a facial gunshot wound. Immediate evacuation was arranged to facilitate appropriate follow-up care [104].

Interventions

Here, many diagnostic applications of PHUS have been discussed. Besides its diagnostic applications, PHUS has been shown to be potentially valuable in guiding interventions or as a therapeutic intervention in its own right.

Interventions—airway

Emergency percutaneous cricothyroidotomy may be unsuccessful or produce a tear in the posterior tracheal wall. Siddiqui et al. compared anatomical orientation by either digital palpation or US for performing a percutaneous cricothyroidotomy with the Portex® device. In cadavers in which palpation of the cricothyroid ligament is difficult, US increased the probability of a correct device insertion by 5.6 times and reduced the incidence of laryngeal and tracheal injury from 100 to 33%. A possible disadvantage of US may be the prolonged time to airway insertion [105].

In the emergency prehospital setting, the open cricothyroidotomy is the preferred approach in invasive airway management. Whether a US-guided percutaneous technique should be used in an emergency at all is a matter of debate. Nevertheless, Curtis et al. found a US-guided bougie-assisted open cricothyroidotomy to be a rapid and reliable technique. Cricothyroidotomy was successful in 20 of 21 cadavers, with a median time to completion of 26.2 s [106].

Interventions—breathing

Medical patients with severe symptomatic pleural effusion might require early pleural aspiration in the prehospital setting. Pleural US is useful in the diagnosis and localization of fluid. US-guided thoracentesis is a safer and more effective method to relieve symptoms than a blind approach [107, 108].

Interventions—circulation

To guide interventions, PHUS is most frequently used for (central) venous access. It was the second most used PHUS application overall (after assessment of blunt abdominal trauma) in an Australian retrieval team [47]. Intraosseous access is the most appropriate approach in time-critical emergencies. However, for less urgent but difficult to obtain peripheral intravenous access, US guidance is faster and more effective than traditional catheter insertion [109].

Symptomatic pericardial effusion might need prompt treatment in the prehospital setting. US-guided pericardiocentesis under continuous visualization using a multi-angled needle guide was found to be effective, safe, and easy to perform [110].

First described in 1954, resuscitative endovascular balloon occlusion of the aorta (REBOA) is a technique to stabilize patients suffering hemodynamic shock by temporarily interrupting blood flow to non-compressible hemorrhage in the chest, abdomen, or pelvis [111, 112]. In animal studies, REBOA resulted in a 74% mortality risk reduction [113]. After 40 min of occlusion, however, the risks start outweighing the benefits [113, 114]. In 2014, the London HEMS was the first to report a prehospital performed REBOA in a patient with a pelvic fracture resulting in successful hemorrhage control [115].

Chaudery found that the use of US improved the correct placement of REBOA catheters, shortened the time until correct placement, and improved the participants' confidence in catheter placement of Zone III (infrarenal aorta) REBOA catheters in 20 porcine cadavers [116].

These developments are promising for future prehospital US-guided REBOA hemorrhage control. However, future research is needed on prehospital feasibility, variations in body habitus, and zone I (intrathoracic aorta) placement.

Interventions—disability

In the aforementioned *disability* section, we highlighted the value of TCCS in diagnosing ischemic stroke. A therapeutic application of ultrasound in ischemic stroke patients is continuous transcranial Doppler (TCD) to enhance the thrombolytic activity of tissue plasminogen activator (t-PA) [117]. In a phase II multicenter randomized trial (CLOTBUST), transducers were applied over the temporal bone in a head frame. The investigators applied TCD (or placebo TCD) on maximum power output continuously for 2 h and simultaneously started intravenous t-PA treatment in all patients. Two hours after starting thrombolysis, recanalization or almost full recovery was observed in 49% in the continuous TCD group versus 30% in the control group. However, clinical recovery after 24 h and outcome after 3 months was similar [117]. In 2014, another analysis of the CLOTBUST trial, including more subjects, revealed 38.6% complete recanalization in the sonothrombolysis group and 17.1% in the intravenous t-PA group [118]. A phase III trial is underway [119]. Tsivgoulis concluded in a meta-analysis that high-frequency ultrasound (both TCD and TCCS) combined with t-PA was associated with a higher likelihood of complete recanalization (pooled OR = 2.99) than t-PA alone [120]. They found no increased risk of symptomatic intracerebral hemorrhage.

Probably, transcranial US combined with microbubbles but without t-PA is effective as well [121, 122]. Microbubbles consist of an injectable aqueous suspension of small (1.5–4.7 μm) bubbles of a high molecular-weight gas that is used as a US contrast agent to improve the visualization of blood vessels [123]. In a meta-analysis, Saqqur indeed concluded that sonothrombolysis with or without microbubbles or t-PA was effective and safe [124]. These findings allow the exploration of early prehospital initiation of sonothrombolysis in suspected ischemic stroke without needing a CT or MRI scan. Hölscher already suggested that PHUS could serve to 'precondition' the culprit clot to increase its therapeutic sensitivity to t-PA or neuro intervention while providing neuroprotection for tissue at risk [121].

Interventions—regional anesthesia

US-guided regional anesthesia is a common technique for providing perioperative pain relief for elective surgical procedures of the extremities. These techniques can also be employed in the prehospital setting to provide effective analgesia for extremity injuries and avoid the side effects associated with the administration of systemic analgesics. For instance, ultrasound-guided femoral nerve blocks effectively provide pain relief in hip fractures [125]. Also, PHUS might facilitate already successful prehospital fascia iliaca compartment blocks [126]. Similarly, Lippert et al. suggested the added value of US-guided nerve blocks to improve pain control in disaster settings [127].

The transversus abdominis plane (TAP) block is an effective technique for pain relief in pelvic fractures and because of its ease and safety it may be applicable in the prehospital setting [128]. Blocking the nerves that supply the anterior abdominal wall relaxes the abdominal wall muscles that will subsequently reduce the traction on the ischium and pubis. The 'flank bulge sign' is a direct consequence of this relaxation [129].

Disaster triage

In a multiple casualty incident (MCI), resources are limited. Triage systems are used to determine treatment priority of the injured patients based on history and physical examination. PoCUS was reported to be valuable in the

Table 2 The CAVEAT protocol. Stawicki et al. [135]

Urgency	Step	Examination	Focus on	Looking for
CAVEAT protocol				
Primary assessment (mandatory)	1	Evaluation of the pleura	Chest	Pneumothorax
	2	Complete FAST examination	Abdomen Costophrenic recesses	Hemoperitoneum Hemothorax
	3	Inferior Vena Cava assessment	Collapsibility index	Volume depletion
Secondary assessment (optional)	4	Upper- and lower extremities	Long bones; regions of pain, tenderness, or deformity	Major fractures eligible for more accurate reduction and stabilization Fractures to prioritize utilization of radiographic resources, or achieve even more accurate triage

CAVEAT sonographic evaluation of the chest, abdomen, vena cava, extremities for acute triage, *FAST* focused assessment with sonography for trauma

This table shows the suggested order of examinations in the CAVEAT protocol. Specific components may depend on the operators' skill level and on the individual patient's injuries

triage process during several earthquake disasters [130–134]. Stawicki proposed a protocol that integrates some common PoCUS applications to evaluate the chest, abdomen, vena cava, and extremities as an adjunct to acute triage (CAVEAT) and to be executed during the secondary survey [135]. The protocol will take approximately 5 min longer than a traditional FAST scan. It is explained in more detail in Table 2. Although the merits of its component parts have been described extensively, the benefit of the protocol is yet to be established.

Future applications

Sonothrombolysis

As we have discussed in the *interventions* section, early prehospital sonothrombolysis in ischemic stroke patients might be safe and effective. The CLOTBUST investigators have developed a hands-free headframe containing 18 ultrasound transducers positioned at the temporal occipital bone windows to deliver operator-independent ultrasound energy directly to the culprit clot. It was successfully applied to and well tolerated by 15 volunteers and is currently evaluated in stroke patients [136]. It may facilitate and enhance early thrombolysis because of its portability and that no formal ultrasound training is needed.

Telemedicine

With improving data communication technologies, telemedicine is a promising technique for remotely evaluating ultrasound clips acquired by less experienced operators. They might even be coached in real time supported by remotely operating the ultrasound device settings in complex scenarios [137]. Kolbe introduced a PoCUS curriculum in a one-room medical clinic in rural Nicaragua. Despite limited resources, after the first introduction the ultrasound instructors used telemedicine to remotely view the ultrasound images in real time [138]. In 2016, Kirkpatrick demonstrated the feasibility of remotely telementoring ultrasound-naïve firefighters using trauma ultrasound for free fluid detection on a phantom [137]. Remote telementored ultrasound was feasible to coach untrained and inexperienced nurse practitioners to assess patients for pneumothorax immediately after removal of their tube thoracostomy [139]. Rubin demonstrated the feasibility of remote review and interpretation of TCD and carotid ultrasound data in healthy volunteers dubbed “teleneurosonology” [140].

Integrating telemedicine concepts in PoCUS-enhanced disaster triage might be promising and feasible in the light of progressing technological advancements.

Wearable US

Mierzwa developed a flat and flexible 5 MHz US probe designed to wear on a fingertip to aid in US-guided vascular access, for instance. The device can be configured as a linear or curvilinear transducer array and it can be mounted directly onto the body as an adhesive patch or wearable device. They speculate on many applications such as point-of-care imaging, combat casualty care, ultrasound therapy, and patient monitoring [141]. A specific prehospital application might also be a US patch for continuous cardiac visualization during cardiopulmonary resuscitation.

Assessment of intraosseous needle position

Tsung demonstrated the feasibility of US to determine the location of an intraosseous needle in six resuscitation cases. He argues that every intraosseous access should be verified with color Doppler because a correct position cannot be accurately confirmed by the aspiration of blood, blood on the stylet tip, the needle being firmly in place, or the absence of soft tissue extravasation [142].

Predicting outcomes in resuscitative thoracotomy (RT)

In some countries, a prehospital or ED resuscitative thoracotomy (RT) is performed on patients with a penetrating (sometimes also blunt) thoracic injury decompensating into cardiac arrest. The goal is to treat a cardiac tamponade or major injuries of the heart, control intrathoracic bleeding, clamp the thoracic aorta, or perform direct cardiac massage or defibrillation. The RT is an invasive and last-resort treatment. Inaba found that FoCUS was a predictor of futile care in these patients [143]. In 187 RT patients, only 6 survived and 3 were eligible organ donors. All survivors and organ donors had visible cardiac motion before RT was performed. If no cardiac motion or pericardial effusion on US was observed, the survival was zero. Thus, utilizing US would have avoided a considerable number of RTs that were ultimately futile [143]. Because of these findings, PHUS would be a valuable addition to prehospital RT protocols.

US-guided cannulation for extracorporeal life support (ECLS)

Lamhaut concluded in 2013 that prehospital implementation of ECLS by non-surgeons was safe and feasible [144]. Four years later their group described a case of ECLS cannulation in the Louvre museum in Paris in which they used a hybrid surgical/Seldinger technique [145, 146]. Another future PHUS application might be US-guided percutaneous ECLS cannulation that may be easier, faster, and less invasive. It could be complemented by (contrast enhanced) echocardiography to verify correct placement of the venous catheter tip [147, 148].

Challenges of prehospital ultrasonography

PHUS is subject to specific challenges in the prehospital environment: ambient lighting, confined space, extremes of temperature, precipitation, dressings, splints, and rapid transport times [3, 6].

Diagnostic ultrasound is generally considered harmless. However, it may heat up tissue depending on these factors: exposure duration, the acoustic output, and tissue characteristics. For instance, some unique properties of the eye such as high absorption of ultrasound and the absence of cooling blood supply may cause the lens to heat up faster than other tissues [149, 150]. Therefore, this has to be considered in ocular ultrasound or ONSD measurements.

PHUS is used by nonradiologists mainly to answer simple yes/no questions and to guide treatment decisions. Sensitivity for solid organ injuries is low and small quantities of blood early in the post-injury phase may be missed. Traumatic aortic pathology cannot be detected by chest or abdominal US; therefore, PHUS is not a valid replacement for CT angiography in patients subjected to high-energy thoracic trauma [78]. False negatives will occur; therefore, negative findings should not indicate a final exclusion of diagnoses [3]. Thus, for some indications, the sensible choice might be to use PHUS only as a 'rule-in' tool not to be falsely reassured by (false) negative test results.

Another concern of PHUS is the potential delay in treatment. In general, a slight delay might occur when PHUS is performed on-scene. However, delays are nonexistent when performed in parallel with other procedures, while in-flight, or during ground ambulance transport. Busch found the median PHUS duration to be 2.5 min (range 1–3) [13]. For a range of PHUS examinations, Hoyer measured a mean of 1 min 54 s, decreasing to 56 s during the 3-year study period [3]. In their review, Jørgensen et al. reported a delay of 0–6 min. Examination time depends on the protocol and the results: positive findings will reduce the examination time [5].

Although a slight delay may occur, this might easily be outweighed by the advantage of improved diagnostic and therapeutic accuracy, and the potential time gains by transporting the patient directly to the most appropriate hospital.

Conclusions

We have provided a comprehensive summary of the literature on prehospital applications of diagnostic and therapeutic ultrasound structured according to the ABCDE approach. Also, we have highlighted in-hospital PoCUS procedures that appear useful and plausible for prehospital use, current challenges in PHUS, and potential future applications. It may be commendable to revise this review in the near future when, undoubtedly, additional useful PHUS applications will have emerged.

Improvements in portability, quality, and price of handheld ultrasound systems add to the accessibility and its feasibility for prehospital use. PHUS improves the diagnostic capabilities of prehospital health-care providers and might improve treatment decisions, prearrival notifications, and transport mode and destination. As new PoCUS techniques and applications are being researched, new protocols are being tested for diagnostics, procedural guidance, and therapeutic use.

However, prehospital caregivers should unabatedly be aware of the limitations of PHUS. The time investment will not always pay off and diagnostic accuracy is not perfect. Diagnostic accuracy is quite dependent on training and experience of the providers.

The diagnostic and therapeutic possibilities of PoCUS are increasing. With promising techniques, such as sonothrombolysis in ischemic stroke, we are bringing the hospital-level medical care to prehospital patients to an ever-increasing extent [119].

Additional file

Additional file 1: Video 1. Lung point.

Abbreviations

ABCDE: airway, breathing, circulation, disability, exposure/environment; ADHF: acute decompensated heart disease; BLUE: bedside lung ultrasound in emergency; BNP: B-type natriuretic peptide; CAVEAT: chest, abdomen, vena cava, and extremities as an adjunct to acute triage; COPD: chronic obstructive pulmonary disease; CPAP: continuous positive airway pressure; CPR: cardiopulmonary resuscitation; CT: computed tomography; CTA: CT angiography; ECLS: extracorporeal life support; ED: emergency department; eFAST: extended FAST; EMS: emergency medical service; ETT: endotracheal tube; EVLW: extravascular lung water; FALLS: fluid administration limited by lung sonography; FAST: focused assessment with sonography for trauma; FoCUS: focused cardiac ultrasound; GT: gastric tube; HAPE: high-altitude pulmonary edema; HEMS: helicopter emergency medical service; ICP: intracranial pressure; IVC: inferior vena cava; LCI: lung ultrasound; cardiac ultrasound; inferior vena cava measurements; MCA: middle cerebral artery; MCI: multiple casualty incident/mass casualty incident; M-mode: motion mode; MRA: magnetic resonance angiography; MRI: magnetic resonance imaging; NPV: negative predictive value; OHCA: out-of-hospital cardiac arrest; ONSD: optic nerve sheath diameter; PAOP: pulmonary artery occlusion pressure; PEA: pulseless electrical activity; PHUS: prehospital ultrasound; PoCUS: point-of-care ultrasound; PPV: positive predictive value; REBOA: resuscitative endovascular balloon occlusion of the aorta; ROSC: return of spontaneous circulation; RT: resuscitative thoracotomy; RUSH: rapid ultrasound in shock; TAP: transversus abdominis plane (block); TBI: traumatic brain injury; TCCS: transcranial color-coded sonography; TCD: transcranial Doppler; TOR: termination of resuscitation; UCA: ultrasound contrast agent; US: ultrasound.

Authors' contributions

All authors contributed substantially to the manuscript and all agree with this definitive version. RK and GR were responsible for conceiving the paper and have collected all the source papers, analyzed all abstracts and full articles, and written the manuscript. RK, GR, and NH formulated the literature search strategies. All authors have contributed to the design, the writing, and revising of the manuscript drafts. All authors read and approved the final manuscript.

Authors' information

RK, GJvG, and NH are anesthesiologists and experienced HEMS physicians at the Lifeliner 3 station at the Volkel Air Force Base, The Netherlands. GR is employed as a resident in intensive care medicine with a special interest in anesthesiology and prehospital emergency medicine. GJS is an anesthesiologist and chair of the anesthesiology department.

Author details

[1] Radboud Institute for Health Sciences, Department of Anesthesiology, Pain, and Palliative Medicine, Radboud university medical center, Geert Grooteplein-Zuid 10, 6525 GA Nijmegen, The Netherlands. [2] Radboud Institute for Health Sciences, Helicopter Emergency Medical Service Lifeliner 3, Radboud university medical center, Geert Grooteplein-Zuid 10, 6525 GA Nijmegen, The Netherlands. [3] Department of Intensive Care, Catharina Hospital, Michelangelolaan 2, 5623 EJ Eindhoven, The Netherlands.

Acknowledgements

We would like to thank Rob Stoffels and Yvonne Houben for their demonstration of transcranial sonography.

References

1. Moore CL, Copel JA (2011) Point-of-care ultrasonography. N Engl J Med 364(8):749–757
2. Walcher F, Weinlich M, Conrad G, Schweigkofler U, Breitkreutz R, Kirschning T, Marzi I (2006) Prehospital ultrasound imaging improves management of abdominal trauma. Br J Surg 93(2):238–242
3. Hoyer HX, Vogl S, Schiemann U, Haug A, Stolpe E, Michalski T (2010) Prehospital ultrasound in emergency medicine: incidence, feasibility, indications and diagnoses. Eur J Emerg Med 17(5):254–259
4. Ketelaars R, Hoogerwerf N, Scheffer GJ (2013) Prehospital chest ultrasound by a Dutch helicopter emergency medical service. J Emerg Med 44(4):811–817
5. Jorgensen H, Jensen CH, Dirks J (2010) Does prehospital ultrasound improve treatment of the trauma patient? A systematic review. Eur J Emerg Med 17(5):249–253
6. O'Dochartaigh D, Douma M (2015) Prehospital ultrasound of the abdomen and thorax changes trauma patient management: a systematic review. Injury 46(11):2093–2102
7. Stengel D, Rademacher G, Ekkernkamp A, Guthoff C, Mutze S (2015) Emergency ultrasound-based algorithms for diagnosing blunt abdominal trauma. Cochrane Database Syst Rev 9:CD004446
8. Rudolph SS, Sorensen MK, Svane C, Hesselfeldt R, Steinmetz J (2014) Effect of prehospital ultrasound on clinical outcomes of non-trauma patients—a systematic review. Resuscitation 85(1):21–30
9. El Sayed MJ, Zaghrini E (2013) Prehospital emergency ultrasound: a review of current clinical applications, challenges, and future implications. Emerg Med Int 2013:531674
10. Sun J-T, Huang C-Y, Huang Y-S, Sim S-S, Chong K-M, Wang H-P, Lien W-C (2014) Prehospital ultrasound. J Med Ultrasound 22(2):71–77
11. Nelson BP, Sanghvi A (2016) Out of hospital point of care ultrasound: current use models and future directions. Eur J Trauma Emerg Surg 42(2):139–150
12. Soar J, Nolan JP, Bottiger BW, Perkins GD, Lott C, Carli P, Pellis T, Sandroni C, Skrifvars MB, Smith GB, Sunde K, Deakin CD (2015) Adult advanced life support section C. European Resuscitation Council Guidelines for Resuscitation Section 3. Adult advanced life support. Resuscitation 2015(95):100–147
13. Busch M (2006) Portable ultrasound in pre-hospital emergencies: a feasibility study. Acta Anaesthesiol Scand 50(6):754–758
14. Kirkpatrick AW, Breeck K, Wong J, Hamilton DR, McBeth PB, Sawadsky B, Betzner MJ (2005) The potential of handheld trauma sonography in the air medical transport of the trauma victim. Air Med J 24(1):34–39
15. Nelson BP, Melnick ER, Li J (2011) Portable ultrasound for remote environments, part I: feasibility of field deployment. J Emerg Med 40(2):190–197
16. Price DD, Wilson SR, Murphy TG (2000) Trauma ultrasound feasibility during helicopter transport. Air Med J 19(4):144–146
17. Lyon M, Walton P, Bhalla V, Shiver SA (2012) Ultrasound detection of the sliding lung sign by prehospital critical care providers. Am J Emerg Med 30(3):485–488
18. Krogh CL, Steinmetz J, Rudolph SS, Hesselfeldt R, Lippert FK, Berlac PA, Rasmussen LS (2016) Effect of ultrasound training of physicians working in the prehospital setting. Scand J Trauma Resusc Emerg Med 24:99
19. Gracias VH, Frankel HL, Gupta R, Malcynski J, Gandhi R, Collazzo L, Nisenbaum H, Schwab CW (2001) Defining the learning curve for the Focused Abdominal Sonogram for Trauma (FAST) examination: implications for credentialing. Am Surg 67(4):364–368
20. Brooke M, Walton J, Scutt D (2010) Paramedic application of ultrasound in the management of patients in the prehospital setting: a review of the literature. Emerg Med J 27(9):702–707
21. O'Dochartaigh D, Douma M, MacKenzie M (2017) Five-year retrospective review of physician and non-physician performed ultrasound in a Canadian Critical Care Helicopter Emergency Medical Service. Prehosp Emerg Care 21(1):24–31
22. Brun PM, Bessereau J, Chenaitia H, Pradel AL, Deniel C, Garbaye G, Melaine R, Bylicki O, Lablanche C (2014) Stay and play eFAST or scoop and run eFAST? That is the question! Am J Emerg Med 32(2):166–170
23. Press GM, Miller SK, Hassan IA, Alade KH, Camp E, Junco DD, Holcomb JB (2014) Prospective evaluation of prehospital trauma ultrasound during aeromedical transport. J Emerg Med 47(6):638–645
24. Yates JG, Baylous D (2017) Aeromedical ultrasound: the evaluation of point-of-care ultrasound during helicopter transport. Air Med J 36(3):110–115
25. Lapostolle F, Petrovic T, Lenoir G, Catineau J, Galinski M, Metzger J, Chanzy E, Adnet F (2006) Usefulness of hand-held ultrasound devices in out-of-hospital diagnosis performed by emergency physicians. Am J Emerg Med 24(2):237–242
26. Blaivas M, Kuhn W, Reynolds B, Brannam L (2005) Change in differential diagnosis and patient management with the use of portable ultrasound in a remote setting. Wilderness Environ Med 16(1):38–41
27. Peters J, van Wageningen B, Hendriks I, Eijk R, Edwards M, Hoogerwerf N, Biert J (2015) First-pass intubation success rate during rapid sequence induction of prehospital anaesthesia by physicians versus paramedics. Eur J Emerg Med 22(6):391–394
28. Slovis TL, Poland RL (1986) Endotracheal tubes in neonates: sonographic positioning. Radiology 160(1):262–263
29. Drescher MJ, Conrad FU, Schamban NE (2000) Identification and description of esophageal intubation using ultrasound. Acad Emerg Med 7(6):722–725
30. Das SK, Choupoo NS, Haldar R, Lahkar A (2015) Transtracheal ultrasound for verification of endotracheal tube placement: a systematic review and meta-analysis. Can J Anaesth 62(4):413–423
31. Grmec S (2002) Comparison of three different methods to confirm tracheal tube placement in emergency intubation. Intensive Care Med 28(6):701–704
32. Zadel S, Strnad M, Prosen G, Mekis D (2015) Point of care ultrasound for orotracheal tube placement assessment in out-of hospital setting. Resuscitation 87:1–6
33. Li J (2001) Capnography alone is imperfect for endotracheal tube placement confirmation during emergency intubation. J Emerg Med 20(3):223–229
34. Hunt RC, Bryan DM, Brinkley VS, Whitley TW, Benson NH (1991) Inability to assess breath sounds during air medical transport by helicopter. JAMA 265(15):1982–1984
35. Kerrey BT, Geis GL, Quinn AM, Hornung RW, Ruddy RM (2009) A prospective comparison of diaphragmatic ultrasound and chest radiography to determine endotracheal tube position in a pediatric emergency department. Pediatrics 123(6):e1039–e1044
36. Kajimoto K, Madeen K, Nakayama T, Tsudo H, Kuroda T, Abe T (2012) Rapid evaluation by lung-cardiac-inferior vena cava (LCI) integrated ultrasound for differentiating heart failure from pulmonary disease as the cause of acute dyspnea in the emergency setting. Cardiovasc Ultrasound 10(1):49
37. Mantuani D, Frazee BW, Fahimi J, Nagdev A (2016) Point-of-care multi-organ ultrasound improves diagnostic accuracy in adults presenting to the emergency department with acute dyspnea. West J Emerg Med 17(1):46–53
38. Lichtenstein D (2009) Lung ultrasound in acute respiratory failure an introduction to the BLUE-protocol. Minerva Anestesiol 75(5):313–317

39. Lichtenstein DA (2015) BLUE-protocol and FALLS-protocol: two applications of lung ultrasound in the critically ill. Chest 147(6):1659–1670
40. Lichtenstein DA, Meziere GA (2008) Relevance of lung ultrasound in the diagnosis of acute respiratory failure: the BLUE protocol. Chest 134(1):117–125
41. Strnad M, Prosen G, Borovnik Lesjak V (2016) Bedside lung ultrasound for monitoring the effectiveness of prehospital treatment with continuous positive airway pressure in acute decompensated heart failure. Eur J Emerg Med 23(1):50–55
42. Lichtenstein DA, Meziere GA, Lagoueyte JF, Biderman P, Goldstein I, Gepner A (2009) A-lines and B-lines: lung ultrasound as a bedside tool for predicting pulmonary artery occlusion pressure in the critically ill. Chest 136(4):1014–1020
43. Wimalasena Y, Windsor J, Edsell M (2013) Using ultrasound lung comets in the diagnosis of high altitude pulmonary edema: fact or fiction? Wilderness Environ Med 24(2):159–164
44. Fagenholz PJ, Gutman JA, Murray AF, Noble VE, Thomas SH, Harris NS (2007) Chest ultrasonography for the diagnosis and monitoring of high-altitude pulmonary edema. Chest 131(4):1013–1018
45. Lichtenstein DA, Meziere G, Lascols N, Biderman P, Courret JP, Gepner A, Goldstein I, Tenoudji-Cohen M (2005) Ultrasound diagnosis of occult pneumothorax. Crit Care Med 33(6):1231–1238
46. Schaal JV, Pasquier P, Renner J, Dubost C, Merat S (2014) Ultrasounds for prehospital recognition of tension pneumothorax. Injury 45(6):1019
47. Mazur SM, Pearce A, Alfred S, Sharley P (2007) Use of point-of-care ultrasound by a critical care retrieval team. Emerg Med Australas 19(6):547–552
48. Lichtenstein D, Courret JP (1998) Feasibility of ultrasound in the helicopter. Intensive Care Med 24(10):1119
49. Lyon M, Shiver SA, Walton P (2012) M-mode ultrasound for the detection of pneumothorax during helicopter transport. Am J Emerg Med 30(8):1577–1580
50. Madill JJ (2010) In-flight thoracic ultrasound detection of pneumothorax in combat. J Emerg Med 39(2):194–197
51. Roline CE, Heegaard WG, Moore JC, Joing SA, Hildebrandt DA, Biros MH, Caroon LV, Plummer DW, Reardon RF (2013) Feasibility of bedside thoracic ultrasound in the helicopter emergency medical services setting. Air Med J 32(3):153–157
52. Quick JA, Uhlich RM, Ahmad S, Barnes SL, Coughenour JP (2016) In-flight ultrasound identification of pneumothorax. Emerg Radiol 23(1):3–7
53. McEwan K, Thompson P (2007) Ultrasound to detect haemothorax after chest injury. Emerg Med J 24(8):581–582
54. Rahimi-Movaghar V, Yousefifard M, Ghelichkhani P, Baikpour M, Tafakhori A, Asady H, Faridaalaee G, Hosseini M, Safari S (2016) Application of ultrasonography and radiography in detection of hemothorax; a systematic review and meta-analysis. Emergency 4(3):116–126
55. Wells BJ, Roberts DJ, Grondin S, Navsaria PH, Kirkpatrick AW, Dunham MB, Ball CG (2015) To drain or not to drain? Predictors of tube thoracostomy insertion and outcomes associated with drainage of traumatic hemothoraces. Injury 46(9):1743–1748
56. Blaivas M, Brannam L, Hawkins M, Lyon M, Sriram K (2004) Bedside emergency ultrasonographic diagnosis of diaphragmatic rupture in blunt abdominal trauma. Am J Emerg Med 22(7):601–604
57. Kim HH, Shin YR, Kim KJ, Hwang SS, Ha HK, Byun JY, Choi KH, Shinn KS (1997) Blunt traumatic rupture of the diaphragm: sonographic diagnosis. J Ultrasound Med 16(9):593–598
58. Rattan KN, Magu S, Agrawal K, Ratan S (2005) Traumatic diaphragmatic herniation. Indian J Pediatr 72(11):985–986
59. Kirkpatrick AW, Ball CG, Nicolaou S, Ledgerwood A, Lucas CE (2006) Ultrasound detection of right-sided diaphragmatic injury; the "liver sliding" sign. Am J Emerg Med 24(2):251–252
60. Gangahar R, Doshi D (2010) FAST scan in the diagnosis of acute diaphragmatic rupture. Am J Emerg Med 28(3):387-e1
61. Brun PM, Bessereau J, Levy D, Billeres X, Fournier N, Kerbaul F (2014) Prehospital ultrasound thoracic examination to improve decision making, triage, and care in blunt trauma. Am J Emerg Med 32(7):817-e1
62. Walker LJ (2005) Methods to correct placement of a nasogastric tube: beware of the pitfalls. Age Ageing 34(6):655
63. Chenaitia H, Brun PM, Querellou E, Leyral J, Bessereau J, Aime C, Bouaziz R, Georges A, Louis F, France WG (2012) Ultrasound to confirm gastric tube placement in prehospital management. Resuscitation 83(4):447–451
64. Brun PM, Chenaitia H, Lablanche C, Pradel AL, Deniel C, Bessereau J, Melaine R (2014) 2-point ultrasonography to confirm correct position of the gastric tube in prehospital setting. Mil Med 179(9):959–963
65. Zengin S, Yavuz E, Al B, Cindoruk S, Altunbas G, Gumusboga H, Yildirim C (2016) Benefits of cardiac sonography performed by a non-expert sonographer in patients with non-traumatic cardiopulmonary arrest. Resuscitation 102:105–109
66. Breitkreutz R, Price S, Steiger HV, Seeger FH, Ilper H, Ackermann H, Rudolph M, Uddin S, Weigand MA, Muller E, Walcher F, Emergency Ultrasound Working Group of the Johann Wolfgang Goethe-University Hospital FaM (2010) Focused echocardiographic evaluation in life support and peri-resuscitation of emergency patients: a prospective trial. Resuscitation 81(11):1527–1533
67. Salen P, Melniker L, Chooljian C, Rose JS, Alteveer J, Reed J, Heller M (2005) Does the presence or absence of sonographically identified cardiac activity predict resuscitation outcomes of cardiac arrest patients? Am J Emerg Med 23(4):459–462
68. Cureton EL, Yeung LY, Kwan RO, Miraflor EJ, Sadjadi J, Price DD, Victorino GP (2012) The heart of the matter: utility of ultrasound of cardiac activity during traumatic arrest. J Trauma Acute Care Surg 73(1):102–110
69. Aichinger G, Zechner PM, Prause G, Sacherer F, Wildner G, Anderson CL, Pocivalnik M, Wiesspeiner U, Fox JC (2012) Cardiac movement identified on prehospital echocardiography predicts outcome in cardiac arrest patients. Prehosp Emerg Care 16(2):251–255
70. Morrison LJ, Verbeek PR, Vermeulen MJ, Kiss A, Allan KS, Nesbitt L, Stiell I (2007) Derivation and evaluation of a termination of resuscitation clinical prediction rule for advanced life support providers. Resuscitation 74(2):266–275
71. Goto Y, Maeda T, Goto YN (2013) Termination-of-resuscitation rule for emergency department physicians treating out-of-hospital cardiac arrest patients: an observational cohort study. Crit Care 17(5):R235
72. Blaivas M, Fox JC (2001) Outcome in cardiac arrest patients found to have cardiac standstill on the bedside emergency department echocardiogram. Acad Emerg Med 8(6):616–621
73. Kim HB, Suh JY, Choi JH, Cho YS (2016) Can serial focussed echocardiographic evaluation in life support (FEEL) predict resuscitation outcome or termination of resuscitation (TOR)? A pilot study. Resuscitation 101:21–26
74. Holger JS, Lamon RP, Minnegan HJ, Gornick CC (2003) Use of ultrasound to determine ventricular capture in transcutaneous pacing. Am J Emerg Med 21(3):227–229
75. Perera P, Mailhot T, Riley D, Mandavia D (2010) The RUSH exam: Rapid Ultrasound in SHock in the evaluation of the critically ill. Emerg Med Clin North Am 28(1):29–56
76. Clarke JR, Trooskin SZ, Doshi PJ, Greenwald L, Mode CJ (2002) Time to laparotomy for intra-abdominal bleeding from trauma does affect survival for delays up to 90 minutes. J Trauma 52(3):420–425
77. Ruesseler M, Kirschning T, Breitkreutz R, Marzi I, Walcher F (2009) Prehospital and emergency department ultrasound in blunt abdominal trauma. Eur J Trauma Emerg Surg 35(4):341
78. Montoya J, Stawicki SP, Evans DC, Bahner DP, Sparks S, Sharpe RP, Cipolla J (2016) From FAST to E-FAST: an overview of the evolution of ultrasound-based traumatic injury assessment. Eur J Trauma Emerg Surg 42(2):119–126
79. Nunes LW, Simmons S, Hallowell MJ, Kinback R, Trooskin S, Kozar R (2001) Diagnostic performance of trauma US in identifying abdominal or pelvic free fluid and serious abdominal or pelvic injury. Acad Radiol 8(2):128–136
80. Seitz K, Reising KD (1982) Ultrasound detection of free air in the abdominal cavity. Ultraschall Med 3(1):4–6
81. Moriwaki Y, Sugiyama M, Toyoda H, Kosuge T, Arata S, Iwashita M, Tahara Y, Suzuki N (2009) Ultrasonography for the diagnosis of intraperitoneal free air in chest-abdominal-pelvic blunt trauma and critical acute abdominal pain. Arch Surg 144(2):137–141 **(discussion 42)**
82. Nazerian P, Tozzetti C, Vanni S, Bartolucci M, Gualtieri S, Trausi F, Vittorini M, Catini E, Cibinel GA, Grifoni S (2015) Accuracy of abdominal ultrasound for the diagnosis of pneumoperitoneum in patients with acute abdominal pain: a pilot study. Crit Ultrasound J 7(1):15

83. Tayal VS, Graf CD, Gibbs MA (2003) Prospective study of accuracy and outcome of emergency ultrasound for abdominal aortic aneurysm over two years. Acad Emerg Med 10(8):867–871
84. Heegaard W, Hildebrandt D, Spear D, Chason K, Nelson B, Ho J (2010) Prehospital ultrasound by paramedics: results of field trial. Acad Emerg Med 17(6):624–630
85. Saver JL, Fonarow GC, Smith EE, Reeves MJ, Grau-Sepulveda MV, Pan W, Olson DM, Hernandez AF, Peterson ED, Schwamm LH (2013) Time to treatment with intravenous tissue plasminogen activator and outcome from acute ischemic stroke. JAMA 309(23):2480–2488
86. Emberson J, Lees KR, Lyden P, Blackwell L, Albers G, Bluhmki E, Brott T, Cohen G, Davis S, Donnan G, Grotta J, Howard G, Kaste M, Koga M, von Kummer R, Lansberg M, Lindley RI, Murray G, Olivot JM, Parsons M, Tilley B, Toni D, Toyoda K, Wahlgren N, Wardlaw J, Whiteley W, del Zoppo GJ, Baigent C, Sandercock P, Hacke W, Stroke Thrombolysis Trialists' Collaborative G (2014) Effect of treatment delay, age, and stroke severity on the effects of intravenous thrombolysis with alteplase for acute ischaemic stroke: a meta-analysis of individual patient data from randomised trials. Lancet 384(9958):1929–1935
87. Ragoschke-Schumm A, Walter S, Haass A, Balucani C, Lesmeister M, Nasreldein A, Sarlon L, Bachhuber A, Licina T, Grunwald IQ, Fassbender K (2014) Translation of the 'time is brain' concept into clinical practice: focus on prehospital stroke management. Int J Stroke. 9(3):333–340
88. Lichtman JH, Watanabe E, Allen NB, Jones SB, Dostal J, Goldstein LB (2009) Hospital arrival time and intravenous t-PA use in US Academic Medical Centers, 2001–2004. Stroke 40(12):3845–3850
89. Herzberg M, Boy S, Holscher T, Ertl M, Zimmermann M, Ittner KP, Pemmerl J, Pels H, Bogdahn U, Schlachetzki F (2014) Prehospital stroke diagnostics based on neurological examination and transcranial ultrasound. Crit Ultrasound J 6(1):3
90. Schlachetzki F, Herzberg M, Holscher T, Ertl M, Zimmermann M, Ittner KP, Pels H, Bogdahn U, Boy S (2012) Transcranial ultrasound from diagnosis to early stroke treatment: part 2: prehospital neurosonography in patients with acute stroke: the Regensburg stroke mobile project. Cerebrovasc Dis 33(3):262–271
91. Lysakowski C, Walder B, Costanza MC, Tramer MR (2001) Transcranial Doppler versus angiography in patients with vasospasm due to a ruptured cerebral aneurysm: a systematic review. Stroke 32(10):2292–2298
92. Chenaitia H, Squarcioni C, Marie BP, Emgan Q, Tomislav P (2011) Transcranial sonography in prehospital setting. Am J Emerg Med 29(9):1231–1233
93. Behnke S, Becker G (2002) Sonographic imaging of the brain parenchyma. Eur J Ultrasound 16(1–2):73–80
94. Moretti R, Pizzi B (2011) Ultrasonography of the optic nerve in neurocritically ill patients. Acta Anaesthesiol Scand 55(6):644–652
95. Bergauer A, Prosen G, Flis V, Seruga T, Brvar M, Kobilica N (2012) Contrast enhanced ultrasound imaging of the optic nerve sheath diameter—what are we really measuring? Crit Ultrasound J 4(Suppl 1):A2
96. Blaivas M, Theodoro D, Sierzenski PR (2003) Elevated intracranial pressure detected by bedside emergency ultrasonography of the optic nerve sheath. Acad Emerg Med 10(4):376–381
97. Moretti R, Pizzi B, Cassini F, Vivaldi N (2009) Reliability of optic nerve ultrasound for the evaluation of patients with spontaneous intracranial hemorrhage. Neurocrit Care 11(3):406–410
98. Maissan IM, Dirven PJ, Haitsma IK, Hoeks SE, Gommers D, Stolker RJ (2015) Ultrasonographic measured optic nerve sheath diameter as an accurate and quick monitor for changes in intracranial pressure. J Neurosurg 123(3):743–747
99. Dulchavsky SA, Henry SE, Moed BR, Diebel LN, Marshburn T, Hamilton DR, Logan J, Kirkpatrick AW, Williams DR (2002) Advanced ultrasonic diagnosis of extremity trauma: the FASTER examination. J Trauma 53(1):28–32
100. Bozorgi F, Shayesteh Azar M, Montazer SH, Chabra A, Heidari SF, Khalilian A (2017) Ability of ultrasonography in detection of different extremity bone fractures; a case series study. Emergency 5(1):e15
101. Paziana K, Fields JM, Rotte M, Au A, Ku B (2012) Soft tissue foreign body removal technique using portable ultrasonography. Wilderness Environ Med 23(4):343–348
102. Kilker BA, Holst JM, Hoffmann B (2014) Bedside ocular ultrasound in the emergency department. Eur J Emerg Med 21(4):246–253
103. Blaivas M, Theodoro D, Sierzenski PR (2002) A study of bedside ocular ultrasonography in the emergency department. Acad Emerg Med 9(8):791–799
104. Whitfield DA, Portouw SJ (2012) Retinal detachment due to facial gunshot wound: the utility of ultrasonography in a medically austere environment. J Emerg Med 42(6):678–681
105. Siddiqui N, Arzola C, Friedman Z, Guerina L, You-Ten KE (2015) Ultrasound improves cricothyrotomy success in cadavers with poorly defined neck anatomy: a randomized control trial. Anesthesiology 123(5):1033–1041
106. Curtis K, Ahern M, Dawson M, Mallin M (2012) Ultrasound-guided, Bougie-assisted cricothyroidotomy: a description of a novel technique in cadaveric models. Acad Emerg Med 19(7):876–879
107. Jones PW, Moyers JP, Rogers JT, Rodriguez RM, Lee YC, Light RW (2003) Ultrasound-guided thoracentesis: is it a safer method? Chest 123(2):418–423
108. Soni NJ, Franco R, Velez MI, Schnobrich D, Dancel R, Restrepo MI, Mayo PH (2015) Ultrasound in the diagnosis and management of pleural effusions. J Hosp Med 10(12):811–816
109. Costantino TG, Parikh AK, Satz WA, Fojtik JP (2005) Ultrasonography-guided peripheral intravenous access versus traditional approaches in patients with difficult intravenous access. Ann Emerg Med 46(5):456–461
110. Maggiolini S, Gentile G, Farina A, De Carlini CC, Lenatti L, Meles E, Achilli F, Tempesta A, Brucato A, Imazio M (2016) Safety, efficacy, and complications of pericardiocentesis by real-time echo-monitored procedure. Am J Cardiol 117(8):1369–1374
111. Hughes CW (1954) Use of an intra-aortic balloon catheter tamponade for controlling intra-abdominal hemorrhage in man. Surgery 36(1):65–68
112. Qasim Z, Brenner M, Menaker J, Scalea T (2015) Resuscitative endovascular balloon occlusion of the aorta. Resuscitation 96:275–279
113. Chaudery M, Clark J, Wilson MH, Bew D, Yang GZ, Darzi A (2015) Traumatic intra-abdominal hemorrhage control: has current technology tipped the balance toward a role for prehospital intervention? J Trauma Acute Care Surg 78(1):153–163
114. Avaro JP, Mardelle V, Roch A, Gil C, de Biasi C, Oliver M, Fusai T, Thomas P (2011) Forty-minute endovascular aortic occlusion increases survival in an experimental model of uncontrolled hemorrhagic shock caused by abdominal trauma. J Trauma 71(3):720–725 **(discussion 5-6)**
115. London's Air Ambulance. World's first pre-hospital REBOA performed. 2014. https://londonsairambulance.co.uk/our-service/news/2014/06/we-perform-worlds-first-pre-hospital-reboa. Accessed 14 Nov 2017
116. Chaudery M, Clark J, Morrison JJ, Wilson MH, Bew D, Darzi A (2016) Can contrast-enhanced ultrasonography improve Zone III REBOA placement for prehospital care? J Trauma Acute Care Surg 80(1):89–94
117. Alexandrov AV, Molina CA, Grotta JC, Garami Z, Ford SR, Alvarez-Sabin J, Montaner J, Saqqur M, Demchuk AM, Moye LA, Hill MD, Wojner AW, Investigators C (2004) Ultrasound-enhanced systemic thrombolysis for acute ischemic stroke. N Engl J Med 351(21):2170–2178
118. Barlinn K, Tsivgoulis G, Barreto AD, Alleman J, Molina CA, Mikulik R, Saqqur M, Demchuk AM, Schellinger PD, Howard G, Alexandrov AV (2014) Outcomes following sonothrombolysis in severe acute ischemic stroke: subgroup analysis of the CLOTBUST trial. Int J Stroke 9(8):1006–1010
119. Schellinger PD, Alexandrov AV, Barreto AD, Demchuk AM, Tsivgoulis G, Kohrmann M, Alleman J, Howard V, Howard G, Alexandrov AW, Brandt G, Molina CA, Investigators C (2015) Combined lysis of thrombus with ultrasound and systemic tissue plasminogen activator for emergent revascularization in acute ischemic stroke (CLOTBUST-ER): design and methodology of a multinational phase 3 trial. Int J Stroke 10(7):1141–1148
120. Tsivgoulis G, Eggers J, Ribo M, Perren F, Saqqur M, Rubiera M, Sergentanis TN, Vadikolias K, Larrue V, Molina CA, Alexandrov AV (2010) Safety and efficacy of ultrasound-enhanced thrombolysis: a comprehensive review and meta-analysis of randomized and nonrandomized studies. Stroke 41(2):280–237
121. Holscher T, Dunford JV, Schlachetzki F, Boy S, Hemmen T, Meyer BC, Serra J, Powers J, Voie A (2013) Prehospital stroke diagnosis and treatment in ambulances and helicopters-a concept paper. Am J Emerg Med 31(4):743–747

122. Porter TR, Xie F, Lof J, Powers J, Vignon F, Shi W, White M (2017) The thrombolytic effect of diagnostic ultrasound-induced microbubble cavitation in acute carotid thromboembolism. Invest Radiol 52(8):477–481
123. Mehta KS, Lee JJ, Taha AA, Avgerinos E, Chaer RA (2017) Vascular applications of contrast-enhanced ultrasound imaging. J Vasc Surg 66(1):266–274
124. Saqqur M, Tsivgoulis G, Nicoli F, Skoloudik D, Sharma VK, Larrue V, Eggers J, Perren F, Charalampidis P, Storie D, Shuaib A, Alexandrov AV (2014) The role of sonolysis and sonothrombolysis in acute ischemic stroke: a systematic review and meta-analysis of randomized controlled trials and case-control studies. J Neuroimaging 24(3):209–220
125. Dickman E, Pushkar I, Likourezos A, Todd K, Hwang U, Akhter S, Morrison S (2016) Ultrasound-guided nerve blocks for intracapsular and extracapsular hip fractures. Am J Emerg Med 34(3):586–589
126. Dochez E, van Geffen GJ, Bruhn J, Hoogerwerf N, van de Pas H, Scheffer G (2014) Prehospital administered fascia iliaca compartment block by emergency medical service nurses, a feasibility study. Scand J Trauma Resusc Emerg Med 22:38
127. Lippert SC, Nagdev A, Stone MB, Herring A, Norris R (2013) Pain control in disaster settings: a role for ultrasound-guided nerve blocks. Ann Emerg Med 61(6):690–696
128. Schaeffer E, Millot I, Landy C, Nadaud J, Favier JC, Plancade D (2014) Another use of continuous transversus abdominis plane (TAP) block in trauma patient: pelvic ring fractures. Pain Med 15(1):166–167
129. Grady MV, Cummings KC 3rd (2008) The "flank bulge" sign of a successful transversus abdominis plane block. Reg Anesth Pain Med 33(4):387
130. Sarkisian AE, Khondkarian RA, Amirbekian NM, Bagdasarian NB, Khojayan RL, Oganesian YT (1991) Sonographic screening of mass casualties for abdominal and renal injuries following the 1988 Armenian earthquake. J Trauma 31(2):247–250
131. Sztajnkrycer MD, Baez AA, Luke A (2006) FAST ultrasound as an adjunct to triage using the START mass casualty triage system: a preliminary descriptive system. Prehosp Emerg Care 10(1):96–102
132. Dan D, Mingsong L, Jie T, Xiaobo W, Zhong C, Yan L, Xiaojin L, Ming C (2010) Ultrasonographic applications after mass casualty incident caused by Wenchuan earthquake. J Trauma 68(6):1417–1420
133. Shorter M, Macias DJ (2012) Portable handheld ultrasound in austere environments: use in the Haiti disaster. Prehosp Disaster Med 27(2):172–177
134. Zhang S, Zhu D, Wan Z, Cao Y (2014) Utility of point-of-care ultrasound in acute management triage of earthquake injury. Am J Emerg Med 32(1):92–95
135. Stawicki SP, Howard JM, Pryor JP, Bahner DP, Whitmill ML, Dean AJ (2010) Portable ultrasonography in mass casualty incidents: The CAVEAT examination. World J Orthop 1(1):10–19
136. Barlinn K, Barreto AD, Sisson A, Liebeskind DS, Schafer ME, Alleman J, Zhao L, Shen L, Cava LF, Rahbar MH, Grotta JC, Alexandrov AV (2013) CLOTBUST-hands free: initial safety testing of a novel operator-independent ultrasound device in stroke-free volunteers. Stroke 44(6):1641–1646
137. Kirkpatrick AW, McKee I, McKee JL, Ma I, McBeth PB, Roberts DJ, Wurster CL, Parfitt R, Ball CG, Oberg S, Sevcik W, Hamilton DR (2016) Remote just-in-time telementored trauma ultrasound: a double-factorial randomized controlled trial examining fluid detection and remote knobology control through an ultrasound graphic user interface display. Am J Surg 211(5):894–902
138. Kolbe N, Killu K, Coba V, Neri L, Garcia KM, McCulloch M, Spreafico A, Dulchavsky S (2015) Point of care ultrasound (POCUS) telemedicine project in rural Nicaragua and its impact on patient management. J Ultrasound 18(2):179–185
139. Biegler N, McBeth PB, Tiruta C, Hamilton DR, Xiao Z, Crawford I, Tevez-Molina M, Miletic N, Ball CG, Pian L, Kirkpatrick AW (2013) The feasibility of nurse practitioner-performed, telementored lung telesonography with remote physician guidance—'a remote virtual mentor'. Crit Ultrasound J 5(1):5
140. Rubin MN, Barrett KM, Freeman WD, Lee Iannotti JK, Channer DD, Rabinstein AA, Demaerschalk BM (2015) Teleneurosonology: a novel application of transcranial and carotid ultrasound. J Stroke Cerebrovasc Dis 24(3):562–565
141. Mierzwa AP, Huang SP, Nguyen KT, Culjat MO, Singh RS (2016) Wearable ultrasound array for point-of-care imaging and patient monitoring. Stud Health Technol Inform 220:241–244
142. Tsung JW, Blaivas M, Stone MB (2009) Feasibility of point-of-care colour Doppler ultrasound confirmation of intraosseous needle placement during resuscitation. Resuscitation 80(6):665–668
143. Inaba K, Chouliaras K, Zakaluzny S, Swadron S, Mailhot T, Seif D, Teixeira P, Sivrikoz E, Ives C, Barmparas G, Koronakis N, Demetriades D (2015) FAST ultrasound examination as a predictor of outcomes after resuscitative thoracotomy: a prospective evaluation. Ann Surg 262(3):512–518 **(discussion 6-8)**
144. Lamhaut L, Jouffroy R, Soldan M, Phillipe P, Deluze T, Jaffry M, Dagron C, Vivien B, Spaulding C, An K, Carli P (2013) Safety and feasibility of prehospital extra corporeal life support implementation by non-surgeons for out-of-hospital refractory cardiac arrest. Resuscitation 84(11):1525–1529
145. Lamhaut L, Hutin A, Deutsch J, Raphalen JH, Jouffroy R, Orsini JP, Baud F, Carli P (2017) Extracorporeal cardiopulmonary resuscitation (ECPR) in the prehospital setting: an illustrative case of ECPR performed in the Louvre museum. Prehosp Emerg Care. 21(3):386–389
146. Hutin A, Corrocher R, Loosli F, Mantz B, Lamhaut L. How physicians perform prehospital ECMO on the streets of Paris. 2017. http://www.jems.com/articles/print/volume-42/issue-12/features/how-physicians-perform-prehospital-ecmo-on-the-streets-of-paris.html. Accessed 11 Dec 2017
147. Vezzani A, Brusasco C, Palermo S, Launo C, Mergoni M, Corradi F (2010) Ultrasound localization of central vein catheter and detection of postprocedural pneumothorax: an alternative to chest radiography. Crit Care Med 38(2):533–538
148. Wen M, Stock K, Heemann U, Aussieker M, Kuchle C (2014) Agitated saline bubble-enhanced transthoracic echocardiography: a novel method to visualize the position of central venous catheter. Crit Care Med 42(3):e231–e233
149. King RL, Liu Y, Harris GR (2017) Quantification of temperature rise within the lens of the porcine eye caused by ultrasound insonation. Ultrasound Med Biol 43(2):476–481
150. Herman BA, Harris GR (1999) Theoretical study of steady-state temperature rise within the eye due to ultrasound insonation. IEEE Trans Ultrason Ferroelectr Freq Control 46(6):1566–1574

28

Impact of ultrasound on management for dyspnea presentations in a Rwandan emergency department

Olivier Felix Umuhire[1*], Michael B. Henry[2], Adam Carl Levine[3], Giles N. Cattermole[4] and Patricia Henwood[5]

Abstract

Background: The complexity of diagnosis for critically ill dyspnea presentations in the emergency department remains a challenge. Accurate and rapid recognition of associated life-threatening conditions is paramount for timely treatment. Point-of-care ultrasound (POCUS) has been shown to impact the diagnosis of dyspnea presentations in resource-rich settings, and may be of greater diagnostic benefit in resource-limited settings.

Methods: We prospectively enrolled a convenience sample of 100 patients presenting with dyspnea in the Emergency Department at University Teaching Hospital of Kigali (UTH-K) in Rwanda. After a traditional history and physical exam, the primary treating team listed their 3 main diagnoses and ranked their confidence accuracy in the leading diagnosis on a Likert scale (1–5). Multi-organ ultrasound scans performed by a separate physician sonographer assessed the heart, lungs, inferior vena cava, and evaluated for lower extremity deep vein thrombosis or features of disseminated tuberculosis. The sonographer reviewed the findings with the treating team, who then listed 3 diagnoses post-ultrasound and ranked their confidence accuracy in the leading diagnosis on a Likert scale (1–5). The hospital diagnosis at discharge was used as the standard in determining the accuracy of the pre- and post-ultrasound diagnoses.

Results: Of the 99 patients included in analysis, 57.6% ($n=57$) were male, with a mean age of 45 years. Most of them had high-level acuity (54.5%), the dyspnea was of acute onset (45.5%) and they came from district hospitals (50.5%). The most frequent discharge diagnoses were acute decompensated heart failure (ADHF) (26.3%) and pneumonia (21.2%). Ultrasound changed the leading diagnosis in 66% of cases. The diagnostic accuracy for ADHF increased from 53.8 to 100% ($p=0.0004$), from 38 to 85.7% for pneumonia ($p=0.0015$), from 14.2 to 85.7% for extrapulmonary tuberculosis ($p=0.0075$), respectively, pre and post-ultrasound. The overall physician diagnostic accuracy increased from 34.7 to 88.8% pre and post- ultrasound. The clinician confidence in the leading diagnosis changed from a mean of 3.5 to a mean of 4.7 (Likert scale 0–5) ($p<0.001$).

Conclusions: In dyspneic patients presenting to this Emergency Department, ultrasound frequently changed the leading diagnosis, significantly increased clinicians' confidence in the leading diagnoses, and improved diagnostic accuracy.

Keywords: Ultrasound, Dyspnea, Rwanda

*Correspondence: olivierfelixu@yahoo.fr

[1] Department of Anesthesia, Critical Care and Emergency Medicine, University of Rwanda, Kigali, Rwanda

Full list of author information is available at the end of the article

Background

Dyspnea, or shortness of breath, is one of the most common complaints in the emergency department, accounting for over three million visits yearly in the United States [1]. This medical condition requires urgent and accurate assessment by the medical practitioner in the emergency department (ED) to provide appropriate initial therapy that can improve clinical outcomes. The broad differential diagnosis for dyspnea makes it challenging to initially manage, particularly in limited-resource settings.

The surge of cardiovascular disease in Africa, combined with longstanding infectious diseases, such as human immunodeficiency virus (HIV) and tuberculosis (TB), increases the likelihood of patients presenting with acute dyspnea, especially if the underlying condition is undiagnosed or the patient is not compliant with primary care therapies [2, 3].

There is an extensive cardiopulmonary differential diagnosis for dyspnea (e.g. pulmonary embolism (PE), pneumonia, acute decompensated heart failure (ADHF), pneumothorax) with potential for evaluation by ultrasound. Even for the life-threatening conditions listed above, it is clear that there are many challenges for emergency care providers in the management of the dyspneic patient. Several studies have shown that the traditional pathway of history, physical exam and chest X-ray is not always accurate in making the diagnosis [4–6]. Moreover, resource-limited settings are challenged by the lack of readily available and accessible diagnostic tools.

Ultrasound is becoming a more widespread tool as it is non-invasive, without ionizing radiation, cost-effective, and rapid if performed by trained clinicians at the bedside [7]. Ultrasound, particularly that at the point-of-care (POCUS) is now emerging as standard practice in emergency medicine and critical care in North America and Europe, where it has been studied and described to help in diagnosing and treating several medical conditions [8–10]. The "triple scan" technique (focused heart, lung and inferior vena cava (IVC)) ultrasound evaluation has been shown to help make the diagnosis for dyspnea [10]. Several studies have proved ultrasound to be an essential tool in providing clinical information for guiding medical decisions in critically ill patients [11, 12]. Point-of-care ultrasound has shown significant diagnostic accuracy in an African context, especially when differentiating cardiac from pulmonary diseases [13].

This study aimed at incorporating ultrasound techniques as an adjunct to the history-taking and physical exam to orient critical medical decisions for dyspneic patients presenting to the ED. The primary objective of the study was to determine the proportion of cases presenting with acute dyspnea in which ultrasound changes the clinician's diagnosis for the patient. A secondary objective of this study was to determine if and how often multi-organ ultrasound exams improve the accuracy and confidence of emergency care providers' diagnosis in patients presenting with dyspnea in the Emergency Department at University Teaching Hospital-Kigali (UTH-K).

Methods

Study design and setting

This is a prospective, observational study enrolling a convenience sample of adult participants presenting with dyspnea to an urban Rwandan emergency department. We enrolled participants presenting to the Emergency Department at University Teaching Hospital of Kigali (UTH-K) over a 1-year period from January 2017 to January 2018. Ethical approval was obtained from the UTH-K Ethical Committee and the Institutional Review Board (IRB) of the College of Medicine and Health Sciences/University of Rwanda and the Partners Healthcare IRB prior to study initiation. Written consent was obtained from participants prior to participation or next of kin if the patient was too sick to consent.

UTH-K, the largest tertiary care hospital in Rwanda, is 500-inpatient bed hospital, which provides speciality surgical and medical services, emergency and critical care, as well as diagnostic services (laboratory and imaging) to approximately 2 million people of Kigali and serves as the country's main referral hospital. This emergency department receives 25,000 visits per year mostly acutely ill patients, including trauma as well as non-trauma patients. Patients at UTH-K are either directly brought in the ED from home, street, or transferred from peripheral hospitals in Rwanda. All adult patients pass through the ED and are received by either emergency and critical care residents or general practitioners. Imaging modalities including X-ray and computed tomography (CT) scans when available. The emergency department has access to ultrasound equipment immediately at the point-of-care, and ultrasound training is a formal curricular component and required competency of the emergency medicine residency-training program.

Participants

The study included a convenience sample of participants triaged as Yellow, Orange or Red according to the Triage Early Warning Score/SAT-TEWS [14] who complained of breathlessness. Participants were adults, age > 16 years. All others were excluded. Patients were only enrolled when the principal investigator (PI) was present in the department; which was mainly during daytime hours any day of the week.

Data collection

The PI, an emergency medicine physician with focused ultrasound training consistent with international recommendations [15] performed the ultrasound scans (including Heart–Lung-IVC "triple scan", FASH and DVT studies) after history and physical exam by the treating medical team, but before other diagnostic studies were completed.

Ultrasonography features of pneumonia, pneumothorax, hemothorax, DVT, pulmonary embolism, ADHF, acute COPD or asthma exacerbation, pulmonary edema, pericardial effusion, pleural effusion and extra-pulmonary tuberculosis were recorded.

After initial evaluation by ED staff, general practitioners and residents/registrars, the PI asked the clinical team to generate their top 3 presumed diagnoses, and rank their confidence in the leading diagnosis on a Likert scale (1–5) after which ultrasound was then completed by the PI. The PI did not perform an independent physical exam but some findings were evident on visual inspection during the ultrasound (tachypnea, work of breathing, diaphoresis, abdominal distention, etc.), so the PI was not overall blinded to the clinical findings. Ultrasound findings were communicated to the treating team, after which the treating team reassessed post-ultrasound presumed diagnoses, ranked their confidence in the leading diagnosis. Follow-up was done to obtain diagnosis at discharge for the enrolled participants. The hospital diagnosis at discharge was used as the standard for comparison in determining the accuracy of the pre- and post-ultrasound diagnoses. The lead sonographer received dedicated ultrasound training over a 3-year period, was enrolled in an ultrasound fellowship and had passed an ultrasound observed structured clinical skills assessment prior to leading this study. Another ultrasound-fellowship trained investigator for quality assurance purposes reviewed random samples of 5% studies and there was no discordance with interpretation. A SonoSite M-Turbo® ultrasound machine (FUJIFILM SonoSite, Inc, Bothell, WA) was utilized to scan patients, and ultrasound clips were saved on a flash drive and then stored on an external hard disk. We used REDCap (Research Electronic Data Capture), a web-based electronic capture to enter and store the data [16].

Statistical analysis

The primary objective of the study was to determine the proportion of cases presenting with acute dyspnea in which ultrasound findings change the clinician's diagnosis for the patient. Based on some prior literature and our prior experience in this setting, we estimated this to be about 40% of cases. We wanted to ensure that the margin of error around our estimate is less than 10%. We used the standard formula for calculating the sample size needed to estimate a proportion in a large population of patients: $n=(z^2_{a/2}{}^* \ p \ ^* \ (1-p))/d^2)$. In our case, using the z distribution with an alpha of 0.05, the sample size needed was calculated to be 93 patients. We planned to oversample by about 5% to allow for missing follow up data in patients.

Descriptive statistics, including proportions for categorical data and means for normally distributed continuous data, were obtained using Microsoft Excel 2011 to identify characteristics of the dyspneic patients and the accuracy of physician diagnosis. Categorical variables were compared using Pearson Chi-square or Fisher's exact test, as appropriate. Finally, student's t test was used for comparing the means for normally distributed data when appropriate (significance was set at p-value < 0.05).

Ultrasound protocols

Heart and IVC

For each patient enrolled, four cardiac views were obtained (parasternal long, parasternal short, subcostal and 4-chambers views). A visual estimate of the LV function was completed and classified as normal, decreased, or hyperdynamic. Pericardial effusion was assessed, and the quality (simple or complex) and the size of the effusion (qualitatively small or large) were noted. We defined sonographic tamponade whenever pericardial effusion was associated with RA collapse and/or RV collapse during diastole plus a plethoric IVC. The IVC was evaluated by visual estimate and recorded as "flat" and "volume responsive" when collapsing was visualized; it was recorded "plethoric" and "non-volume responsive" when it was visualized to be full without any variation during both cycles of respiration; it was reported to be "normal" when neither flat or plethoric [13].

Lungs

Lung ultrasound was performed following a 4-quadrant view protocol (Fig. 1) [11]. We started with 2 anterior views between vertical parasternal line (PSL) and the anterior axillary line (AAL). We then coupled with 2 views between the AAL and the posterior axillary line (PAL). The same protocol was applied to both the right and the left lung. Lung ultrasound was completed using a phased probe coupled with a high-frequency probe. The following features were recorded on both sides (right and left): lung sliding, pleural effusion small/large and simple/complex, B-lines focal/diffuse, subpleural/hepatization consolidation, and static/dynamic bronchograms.

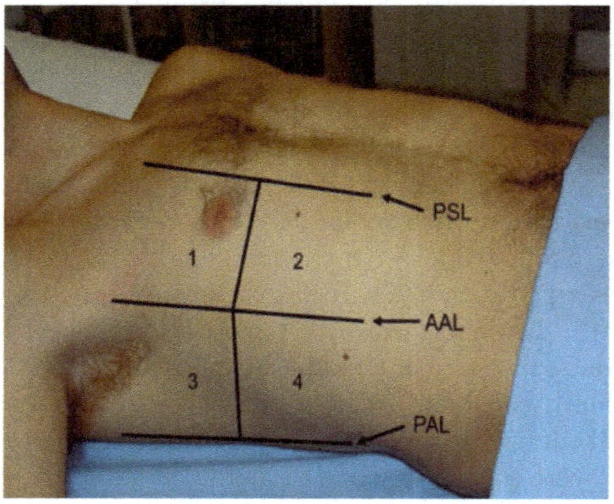

Fig. 1 The areas of lung ultrasonography considered in the study. Areas 1 and 2: upper anterior and lower anterior; areas 3 and 4: upper lateral and basal lateral. Each area was the same on right and left side. AAL, anterior axillary line; PAL, posterior axillary line [11]

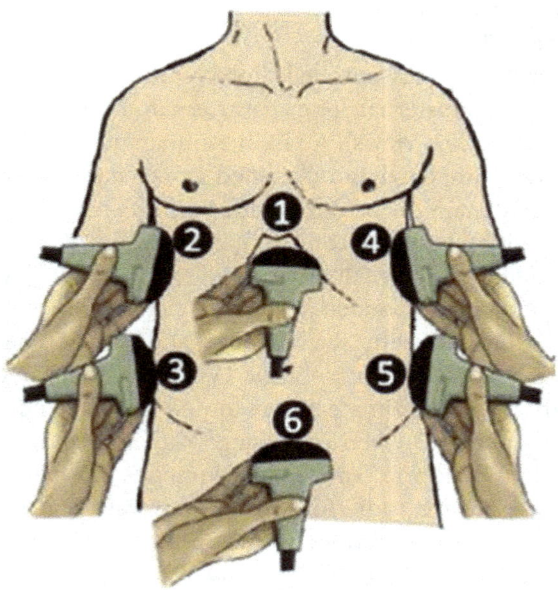

Fig. 2 Schematic drawing of the ultrasound probe positions during the FASH examination [17]

Fash

Multi-organ ultrasonography included a FASH scan evaluating 6 zones (Fig. 2) which were described to have potential significant prediction for extra-pulmonary TB in HIV patients [17, 18]. FASH was incorporated into the scan protocol considering the local TB burden and clinical presentation of extra-pulmonary TB being very non-specific and difficult to diagnose, in addition to data on para-aortic nodes predicting pulmonary TB [19]. A low frequency curvilinear and a high-frequency linear probe were used for this application. Possible positive findings were: pleural effusion, pericardial effusion, hepatic and splenic microabscesses, ascites, and para-aortic lymphadenopathies.

DVT evaluation

A bedside ultrasound was also conducted to assess for lower extremity deep venous thrombosis. We used the two-point (two zone) DVT compression examination [20]. The region of common femoral vein (CFV) and the greater saphenous vein (GSV) bifurcation and the region of popliteal vein trifurcation were scanned for compressibility; a positive DVT scan was recorded whenever the vein was not compressible with enough pressure to deform the artery.

Results

During the period of study 100 participants were enrolled. Among these, discharge data was missing for one (1%), and our analysis was conducted on the remaining 99. The study population was 57.6% ($n=57$) male with a mean age of 45 years. Most participants enrolled were of high-level acuity per the TEWS triage category (54.5%)"red". Many had dyspnea of acute onset (45.5%) as opposed to gradual or chronic and were transferred mainly from District Hospitals (50.5%) versus direct EMS

Table 1 Population characteristics ($n = 9$)

Age	45 ± 21.9 years
Gender	
Male	57 (57.6%)
Female	42 (42.4%)
Arriving from	
District Hospital (DH)	53 (53.5%)
Home	38 (38.4%)
Other	4 (4.0%)
Transport method	
DH ambulance	50 (50.5%)
Private	46 (46.5%)
EMS ambulance	3 (3.0%)
TEWS	
Red	54 (54.5%)
Orange	31 (31.3%)
Yellow	13 (13.1%)
Trauma	3 (3.0%)
Known HIV positive	17 (17.2%)
Dyspnea onset	
Acute (< 1 week)	45 (45.5%)
Gradual (1–4 weeks)	42 (42.4%)
Chronic (> 4 weeks)	12 (12.1%)

or private transport. Table 1 describes the baseline population characteristics.

Descriptive ultrasound findings

Decreased LV function was present in 28.3% of cases and hyperdynamic LV function in 33.3% of cases. The right lung ultrasound was reported to be abnormal in 80.8% of scans, whereas the left lung was reported to be abnormal in 70.7% of cases. Sonographic B-line pattern, pleural effusion, lung consolidation and air bronchograms were the most common sonographic features in abnormal lung ultrasounds among dyspneic patients. The volume responsiveness of patients was assessed by scanning the inferior vena cava (IVC); in 31.3% of cases patients were predicted volume responsive (flat IVC), 31.3% were normal and 37.4% were non-volume responsive (plethoric IVC). Positive deep venous thrombosis scans were infrequent (5.1%). Features of extrapulmonary tuberculosis were recorded 7% of the time, per the FASH protocol. Tables 2 and 3 describes the main sonographic findings.

Diagnostic accuracy

Multiorgan ultrasound was reported to change the clinician leading diagnosis in 65.7% of cases. The clinician confidence in the leading diagnosis changed from a mean of 3.5 to a mean of 4.7 (Likert scale 0–5) before and after ultrasound ($p < 0.001$).

The most common final diagnoses in this population were ADHF (26 patients, 26.3%) and pneumonia (21 patients, 21.2%). Clinicians correctly diagnosed ADHF in 14 patients (53.8%) pre-ultrasound compared to 26 patients (100%) post-ultrasound ($p = 0.0004$). The diagnosis of pneumonia was accurately made in 8 patients (38.0%) pre-ultrasound and in 18 patients (85.7%) post-ultrasound ($p = 0.0015$). Table 4 provides details of diagnostic changes pre- and post-ultrasound by final discharge diagnosis.

Prior to ultrasound, the physician leading diagnosis matched the final discharge diagnosis in only 34.3% of cases; after ultrasound, the physician leading diagnosis matched the final discharge diagnosis in 89% of cases (Fig. 3).

Discussion

This study was conducted in a low-resource setting emergency department, where patients presenting with acute dyspnea were assessed with multi-organ ultrasound, (evaluating the heart, lungs, IVC, and for features of disseminated TB or DVT) which often changed the leading clinical diagnosis, and improved the accuracy of the initial emergency clinician diagnosis relative to discharge diagnosis. In addition, physician confidence in their ED diagnosis significantly improved after ultrasound. Several

Table 2 Cardiac and lung ultrasound findings (*n* = 99)

Cardiac exam	Normal	38 (38.4%)
	Any abnormality	61 (61.6%)
	Decreased LV function	28 (28.3%)
	Hyperdynamic LV	33 (33.3%)
	RV strain	8 (8.1%)
	Pericardial effusion	
	Present	25 (25.3%)
	Simple/complex	18 (18.2%)/7(7.1%)
	Small/large	21 (21.2%)/4 (4.0%)
	Tamponde	5 (5.1%)
Right lung exam	Normal	19 (19.2%)
	Any abnormality	80 (80.8%)
	Pleural effusion	47 (47.5%)
	Simple	30 (30.3%)
	Complex	17 (17.2%)
	Small	21 (21.2%)
	Large	26 (26.3%)
	B-lines	60 (60.6%)
	Focal	35 (35.4%)
	Diffuse	25 (25.3%)
	Consolidation	41 (41.4%)
	Air bronchograms	17 (17.2%)
	Non-sliding pleura	1 (1.0%)
Left lung exam	Normal	29 (29.3%)
	Any abnormality	70 (70.7%)
	Pleural effusion	39 (39.4%)
	Simple	24 (24.2%)
	Complex	15 (15.2%)
	Small	21 (21.2%)
	Large	18 (18.2%)
	B-lines	59 (59.6%)
	Focal	33 (33.3%)
	Diffuse	26 (26.3%)
	Consolidation	35 (35.4%)
	Air bronchograms	16 (16.2%)
	Non-sliding pleura	0 (0.0%)

Table 3 Other ultrasound findings (*n* = 99)

FASH exam	Normal	74 (74.7%)
	Any abnormality	25 (25.3%)
	Hepatic microabcesses	1 (1.0%)
	Splenic microabcesses	0 (0%)
	Ascites	22 (22.2%)
	Paraaortic LNs	2 (2.0%)
DVT exam	Normal	94 (94.9%)
	Non compressible	5 (5.1%)
IVC exam	Normal	31 (31.3%)
	Flat	31 (31.3%)
	Plethoric	37 (37.4%)

Table 4 Pre- and post-POCUS diagnosis accuracy compared to discharge diagnosis

Discharge diagnosis	*N*	Pre-POCUS Correct % (*n*)	Post-POCUS Correct % (*n*)	*P* value
ADHF	26	53.8% (14)	100% (26)	*0.0004*
Pneumonia	21	38.0% (8)	85.7% (18)	*0.0015*
EPTB	7	14.2% (1)	85.7% (6)	*0.0075*
Massive PE	4	25.0% (1)	100% (4)	*0.0989*
Pleural effusion	10	10.0% (1)	100% (10)	*0.0002*
COPD	1	0% (0)	100% (1)	*0.7094*

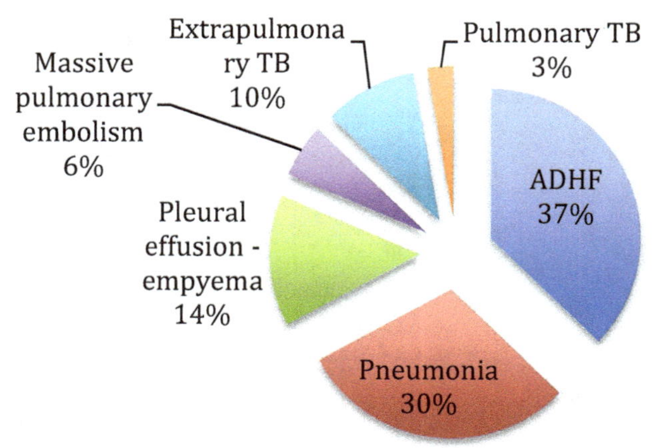

Fig. 3 Hospital discharge diagnosis

critical medical conditions were recognized with a high accuracy relative to discharge diagnosis including ADHF (100%), pneumonia (85.7%), extrapulmonary TB (85.7%) and pleural effusion (100%).

Clinicians in resource-limited settings need to make timely, urgent management decisions for dyspneic patients, often with limited radiology capacity. This study demonstrates that incorporation of point-of-care ultrasound into the evaluation of dyspneic patients changed the leading ED diagnosis in most cases. Initiating urgent treatment to cover a broad differential diagnosis may be of limited benefit and can negatively impact patients and health care resource utilization in general. Narrowing the differential and changing the leading diagnosis with ultrasound may facilitate more appropriately tailored patient care.

This study reinforces conclusions from Mantuani et al. [10], who found POCUS to have 100% sensitivity for ADHF, and Nazerian et al. [8] who highlighted the usefulness of multi-organ POCUS when clinically predicting pulmonary embolism. Shah et al. [21] worked on the educational aspect of POCUS in low resource setting and proved its reproducibility in trained clinicians treating patients with dyspnea. A previous study in similar setting by Henwood et al. showed that POCUS had a significant impact on clinical decision-making [22]. Becker et al. [13] found that up to 14% of the clinician diagnostic accuracy changed after cardiopulmonary ultrasound in a trial done in Ghana among patients who presented with dyspnea. We suspect the higher percentage in our study may be due to the multi-organ scanning protocol and the wide range of diagnosis included.

This study is unique in that in addition to the studied "triple scan" of heart-lungs-IVC, and lower extremity DVT evaluation, we incorporated the FASH protocol [17]. This widened the range of use of ultrasound in patients with dyspnea extending its use from ADHF, pulmonary edema and COPD to infectious diseases such as pulmonary TB, extrapulmonary TB, and pneumonia. In this part of East Africa, where TB and HIV are endemic, incorporating ultrasound when managing HIV patients presenting with dyspnea could be of significant value. In addition, limited local availability of CT angiogram led to the addition of DVT assessment to further management of dyspneic patients with suspected pulmonary embolism.

Some aspects of our study deserve particular attention. ADHF accounted for 26.3% of the diagnoses, taking the lead among all the patients with acute dyspnea who presented in the ED. This highlights the continuing shift in the burden of acute disease from communicable to non-communicable diseases in Rwanda and sub-Saharan Africa in general [23]. Pneumonia could also be picked up more quickly and may be treated in a more timely fashion to fight sepsis, whose mortality is a global concern [23].

This study has several significant limitations. It was conducted at a single referral hospital in Rwanda, with a small sample size, enrolled at the convenience of a single sonographer investigator, most often during daytime hours. All of these factors could have impacted the included population and subsequent results. All ultrasound interpretations were also completed by the principal investigator, which could limit external validity. In addition, the leading diagnoses or clinical impressions of the treating teams may have varied from clinician to clinician based on their clinical judgment which is also a limitation.

A major limitation is that the available standard for comparison in our study was the hospital discharge diagnosis. While this was also utilized in previous similar work [10], its accuracy is limited by available diagnostic tests in this hospital. The results of the ultrasound itself may have influenced clinical diagnosis and final discharge diagnosis due to resource and logistical barriers in obtaining other gold standard testing in the hospital.

Conclusion

Dyspnea remains a challenging clinical presentation in the emergency department, particularly in settings with limited portable or emergent diagnostic imaging modalities. Incorporating ultrasound findings with patient history and physical exam can change the initial emergency clinician diagnosis in a resource-limited setting and improve diagnostic accuracy. Further incorporation of point-of-care ultrasound into the routine management of dyspneic emergency department patients, particularly in settings with otherwise limited imaging resources, should be considered.

Abbreviations

ACEP: American College of Emergency Physicians; ADHF: acute decompensated heart failure; ARDS: acute respiratory distress syndrome; CFV: common femoral vein; CMHS: College of Medicine and Health Sciences; COPD: chronic obstructive pulmonary diseases; CT: computed tomography; CXR: chest X-ray; DVT: deep venous thrombosis; ED: emergency department; FASH: focused assessment sonography in HIV and tuberculosis; GSV: greater saphenous vein; HIV: human immunodeficiency virus; IVC: inferior vena cava; Lt: left; LV: left ventricle; PE: pulmonary embolism; PI: primary investigator; POCUS: point-of-care ultrasound; RA: right atrium; REDCAP: research electronic data capture; Rt: right; TB: tuberculosis; TEWS: Triage Early Warning Score; UR: University of Rwanda; UTH-K: University Teaching Hospital of Kigali.

Acknowledgements

Primarily go to the co-authors, the University of Rwanda, the Department of Emergency Medicine and UTH-K as well as the clinicians in the department.

Authors' contributions

OFU elaborated the protocol, obtained ethical approval, did all the scans, collected the data and participated in analysis and manuscript. PH participated in the protocol elaboration, did the ultrasound scan quality review and supervised the work. MBH participated in statistics analysis and manuscript review. GNC and ACL participated in elaborating the protocol and in manuscript review. All authors read and approved the final manuscript.

Author details

[1] Department of Anesthesia, Critical Care and Emergency Medicine, University of Rwanda, Kigali, Rwanda. [2] Columbia University Vagelos College of Physicians and Surgeons, New York, USA. [3] The Warren Alpert Medical School of Brown University, Providence, RI, USA. [4] Department of Emergency Medicine, King's College/NHS, London, UK. [5] Department of Emergency Medicine, Brigham and Women's Hospital, Boston, USA.

References

1. Rui P, Kang K. National Hospital Ambulatory Medical Care Survey: 2015 Emergency department summary tables [Internet]. Atlanta; 2015. https://www.cdc.gov/nchs/data/nhamcs/web_tables/2015_ed_web_tables.pdf. Accessed 23 Nov 2018
2. Twagirumukiza M, Nkeramihigo E, Seminega B, Gasakure E, Boccara F, Barbaro G (2007) Prevalence of dilated cardiomyopathy in HIV-infected African patients not receiving HAART: a multicenter, observational, prospective, cohort study in Rwanda. Curr HIV Res 5(1):129–137
3. Young F, Critchley JA, Johnstone LK, Unwin NC (2009) A review of co-morbidity between infectious and chronic disease in Sub Saharan Africa: TB and Diabetes mellitus, HIV and metabolic syndrome, and the impact of globalization. Global Health 5:9
4. Jang TB, Aubin C, Naunheim R, Lewis LM, Kaji AH (2012) The predictive value of physical examination findings in patients with suspected acute heart failure syndrome. Intern Emerg Med 7(3):271–274
5. Khunti K, Baker R, Grimshaw G (2000) Diagnosis of patients with chronic heart failure in primary care: usefulness of history, examination, and investigations. Br J Gen Pract 50(450):50–54
6. Logeart D, Saudubray C, Beyne P, Thabut G, Ennezat P-V, Chavelas C et al (2002) Comparative value of Doppler echocardiography and B-type natriuretic peptide assay in the etiologic diagnosis of acute dyspnea. J Am Coll Cardiol 40(10):1794–1800
7. Guttikonda SNR, Vadapalli K (2018) Approach to undifferentiated dyspnea in emergency department: aids in rapid clinical decision-making. Int J Emerg Med 11:21. https://doi.org/10.1186/s12245-018-0181-z
8. Nazerian P, Vanni S, Volpicelli G, Gigli C, Zanobetti M, Bartolucci M et al (2014) Accuracy of point-of-care multiorgan ultrasonography for the diagnosis of pulmonary embolism. Chest 145(5):950–957
9. Volpicelli G, Cardinale L, Garofalo G, Veltri A (2008) Usefulness of lung ultrasound in the bedside distinction between pulmonary edema and exacerbation of COPD. Emerg Radiol 15(3):145–151
10. Mantuani D, Frazee B, Fahimi J, Nagdev A (2016) Point-of-care multi-organ ultrasound improves diagnostic accuracy in adults presenting to the emergency department with acute dyspnea. West J Emerg Med 17(1):46–53
11. Volpicelli G, Mussa A, Garofalo G, Cardinale L, Casoli G, Perotto F et al (2006) Bedside lung ultrasound in the assessment of alveolar-interstitial syndrome. Am J Emerg Med 24(6):689–696
12. Lichtenstein DA, Mezière G, Lascols N, Biderman P, Courret J-P, Gepner A et al (2005) Ultrasound diagnosis of occult pneumothorax. Crit Care Med 33(6):1231–1238
13. Becker TK, Tafoya CA, Osei-Ampofo M, Tafoya MJ, Kessler RA, Theyyunni N et al (2017) Cardiopulmonary ultrasound for critically ill adults improves diagnostic accuracy in a resource-limited setting: the AFRICA trial. Trop Med Int Health 22(12):1599–1608
14. Rosedale K, Smith Z, Davies H, Wood D (2011) The effectiveness of the South African Triage Score (SATS) in a rural emergency department. S Afr Med J 101(8):537–540
15. Atkinson P, Bowra J, Lambert M, Lamprecht H, Noble V, Jarman B (2015) International federation for emergency medicine point of care ultrasound curriculum. Can J Emerg Med 17(02):161–170
16. Harris PA, Taylor R, Thielke R, Payne J, Gonzalez N, Conde JG (2009) Research electronic data capture (REDCap)—a metadata-driven methodology and workflow process for providing translational research informatics support. J Biomed Inform 42(2):377–381
17. Heller T, Wallrauch C, Goblirsch S, Brunetti E (2012) Focused assessment with sonography for HIV-associated tuberculosis (FASH): a short protocol and a pictorial review. Crit Ultrasound J 4:21
18. Brunetti E, Heller T, Richter J, Kaminstein D, Youkee D, Giordani MT et al (2016) Application of ultrasonography in the diagnosis of infectious diseases in resource-limited settings. Curr Infect Dis Rep 18(2):6
19. Bélard S, Heuvelings CC, Banderker E, Bateman L, Heller T, Andronikou S, Workman L, Grobusch MP, Zar HJ (2018) Utility of point-of-care ultrasound in children with pulmonary tuberculosis. Pediatr Infect Dis J 37(7):637–642. https://doi.org/10.1097/INF.0000000000001872
20. Crisp JG, Lovato LM, Jang TB (2010) Compression ultrasonography of the lower extremity with portable vascular ultrasonography can accurately detect deep venous thrombosis in the emergency department. Ann Emerg Med 56(6):601–610
21. Shah SP, Shah SP, Fils-Aime R, Desir W, Joasil J, Venesy DM et al (2016) Focused cardiopulmonary ultrasound for assessment of dyspnea in a resource-limited setting. Crit Ultrasound J 8(1):7
22. Henwood PC, Mackenzie DC, Liteplo AS, Rempell JS, Murray AF, Leo MM et al (2017) Point-of-care ultrasound use, accuracy, and impact on clinical decision making in Rwanda Hospitals. J Ultrasound Med 36(6):1189–1194
23. Vos T, Barber RM, Bell B, Bertozzi-Villa A, Biryukov S, Bolliger I et al (2015) Global, regional, and national incidence, prevalence, and years lived with disability for 301 acute and chronic diseases and injuries in 188 countries, 1990–2013: a systematic analysis for the Global Burden of Disease Study 2013. Lancet 386(9995):743–800

Permissions

All chapters in this book were first published by Springer; hereby published with permission under the Creative Commons Attribution License or equivalent. Every chapter published in this book has been scrutinized by our experts. Their significance has been extensively debated. The topics covered herein carry significant findings which will fuel the growth of the discipline. They may even be implemented as practical applications or may be referred to as a beginning point for another development.

The contributors of this book come from diverse backgrounds, making this book a truly international effort. This book will bring forth new frontiers with its revolutionizing research information and detailed analysis of the nascent developments around the world.

We would like to thank all the contributing authors for lending their expertise to make the book truly unique. They have played a crucial role in the development of this book. Without their invaluable contributions this book wouldn't have been possible. They have made vital efforts to compile up to date information on the varied aspects of this subject to make this book a valuable addition to the collection of many professionals and students.

This book was conceptualized with the vision of imparting up-to-date information and advanced data in this field. To ensure the same, a matchless editorial board was set up. Every individual on the board went through rigorous rounds of assessment to prove their worth. After which they invested a large part of their time researching and compiling the most relevant data for our readers.

The editorial board has been involved in producing this book since its inception. They have spent rigorous hours researching and exploring the diverse topics which have resulted in the successful publishing of this book. They have passed on their knowledge of decades through this book. To expedite this challenging task, the publisher supported the team at every step. A small team of assistant editors was also appointed to further simplify the editing procedure and attain best results for the readers.

Apart from the editorial board, the designing team has also invested a significant amount of their time in understanding the subject and creating the most relevant covers. They scrutinized every image to scout for the most suitable representation of the subject and create an appropriate cover for the book.

The publishing team has been an ardent support to the editorial, designing and production team. Their endless efforts to recruit the best for this project, has resulted in the accomplishment of this book. They are a veteran in the field of academics and their pool of knowledge is as vast as their experience in printing. Their expertise and guidance has proved useful at every step. Their uncompromising quality standards have made this book an exceptional effort. Their encouragement from time to time has been an inspiration for everyone.

The publisher and the editorial board hope that this book will prove to be a valuable piece of knowledge for researchers, students, practitioners and scholars across the globe.

List of Contributors

Pablo Blanco
Intensive Care Unit, Hospital Dr. Emilio Ferreyra, 4801, 59 St., 7630 Necochea, Argentina
Intensive Care Unit, Clínica Cruz Azul, 2651, 60 St., 7630 Necochea, Argentina

Giovanni Volpicelli
Emergency Medicine, San Luigi Gonzaga University Hospital, 10043 Turin, Italy

Daniel Van Kalsbeek and Karl Enroth
Department of Internal Medicine, 982055 Nebraska Medical Center, Omaha, NE 68198-2055, USA

Elizabeth Lyden
Department of Biostatistics, 984375 Nebraska Medical Center, Omaha, NE 68198-4375, USA

Mark E. Rupp
Department of Internal Medicine, Division of Infectious Diseases, 985400 Nebraska Medical Center, Omaha, NE 68198-5400, USA

Christopher J. Smith
Department of Internal Medicine, Division of Hospital Medicine, 986430 Nebraska Medical Center, Omaha, NE 68198-6430, USA

Youyou Duanmu
Department of Emergency Medicine, Stanford University School of Medicine, 900 Welch Road Suite 350, Palo Alto, CA 94304, USA

Patricia C. Henwood and Heidi H. Kimberly
Department of Emergency Medicine, Brigham and Women's Hospital, Boston, MA, USA

Sukhjit S. Takhar
Department of Emergency Medicine, Mills-Peninsula Medical Center, Burlingame, CA, USA

Wilma Chan
Department of Emergency Medicine, Hospital of the University of Pennsylvania, Philadelphia, PA, USA

Joshua S. Rempell
Department of Emergency Medicine, Cooper University Hospital, Camden, NJ, USA

Andrew S. Liteplo
Department of Emergency Medicine, Massachusetts General Hospital and Harvard Medical School, Boston, MA, USA

Viktoria Koskenoja
Department of Emergency Medicine, UP Health System-Marquette, Marquette, MI, USA

Vicki E. Noble
Department of Emergency Medicine, University Hospitals- Cleveland Medical Center, Cleveland, OH, USA

François Javaudin, François Mounier, Philippe Pes, Idriss Arnaudet, Frédéric Vignaud and Philippe Le Conte
Service des urgences, Centre Hospitalier Universitaire de Nantes, 44035 Nantes cedex, Nantes, France

Eric Frampas
Service de radiologie, Centre Hospitalier Universitaire de Nantes, Nantes, France

Bret P. Nelson, Phillip Andrus and James W. Tsung
Division of Emergency Ultrasound, Department of Emergency Medicine, Icahn School of Medicine at Mount Sinai, New York, NY, USA

Apichaya Monsomboon
Division of Emergency Ultrasound, Department of Emergency Medicine, Icahn School of Medicine at Mount Sinai, New York, NY, USA
Department of Emergency Medicine, Siriraj Hospital, Mahidol University, Bangkok, Thailand

José Muniz Pazeli Jr. and Ana Luisa Silveira Vieira
FAME - Barbacena's School of Medicina, Barbacena, Brazil
Federal University of Juiz de Fora, Juiz de Fora, Brazil

Rosimary Souza Vicentino, Bernardo Costa Lemos, Marinna Marques Rodrigues Saliba, Pedro Andrade Mello and Maurício Dutra Costa
FAME - Barbacena's School of Medicina, Barbacena, Brazil

Luisa Jabour Pazeli
SUPREMA - School of Medical Sciences and Health of Juiz de Fora, Juiz de Fora, Brazil

Charles M. LoPresti
Division of Medicine, Louis Stokes Cleveland Veterans Affairs Medical Center, 10701 East Boulevard, Cleveland, OH 44106, USA
Case Western Reserve University School of Medicine, 2109 Adelbert Rd, Cleveland, OH 44106, USA

Daniel J. Schnobrich
Department of Medicine, University of Minnesota, 401 East River Parkway, Variety Club Research Center, Suite 131, Minneapolis, MN 55455, USA

Renee K. Dversdal
Department of Medicine, Oregon Health & Science University, 3181 SW Sam Jackson Park Road, Portland, OR 97239-3098, USA

Frank Schembri
Department of Medicine, Boston Medical Center, 715 Albany St. E-113, Boston, MA 02118, USA

Bjarte Sorensen
Hjelmeland General Practice Surgery, Prestagarden 13, 4130 Hjelmeland, Norway

Steinar Hunskaar
Department of Global Public Health and Primary Care, University of Bergen, Bergen, Norway
National Centre for Emergency Primary Health Care, NORCE Norwegian Research Centre AS, Bergen, Norway

Stephanie J. Doniger
Department of Pediatric Emergency Medicine, CHOC Children's Hospital of Orange County, Orange, CA, USA

Nicholas Ng
Department of Pediatric Critical Care, Morgan Stanley Children's Hospital of New York-Presbyterian, New York, NY, USA

Matt Glogoza, Jonathan Urbach, Terry K. Rosborough and David M. Tierney
Department of Graduate Medical Education #11135, Abbott Northwestern Hospital, 800 E. 28th Street, Minneapolis, MN 55407, USA

Susan Olet
Clinical Research Informatics and Analytics, Allina Health, Minneapolis, MN, USA

Catherine A. St. Hill and Claire S. Smith
Department of Care Delivery Research, Allina Health, Minneapolis, MN, USA

Samuel L. Burleson, Christopher Greene, Courtney B. Gibson and Scott Irvine
Department of Emergency Medicine, University of Alabama at Birmingham Hospital, Old Hillman Building Suite 251, 619 19th St S, Birmingham, AL 35249, USA

Daniel Kaminstein
Department of Emergency Medicine, Augusta University, Augusta, GA, USA

Stephanie Sibley, Louise Rang, Heather White, Marco L. A. Sivilotti and Eric Bruder
Department of Emergency Medicine, Queen's University, Kingston, ON, Canada

Nathan Roth
School of Medicine, Faculty of Health Sciences, Queen's University, Kingston, ON, Canada

Charles Scott
Department of Radiology, Queen's University, Kingston, ON, Canada

Amirhosein Jahanshir
Emergency Department, Shariati Hospital, Tehran University of Medical Sciences, Tehran, Iran

Shida Mohajer Moghari
Tehran University of Medical Sciences, Tehran, Iran

Ayat Ahmadi
Knowledge Utilization Research Center, Tehran University of Medical Sciences, Tehran, Iran

Pejman Z. Moghadam
Trust ST 1/2 in Emergency Medicine, Mid Essex NHS Trust Broomfield Hospital, Chelmsford, Essex, UK

Maryam Bahreini
Department of Emergency Medicine, Sina Trauma and Surgery Research Center, Sina Hospital, Tehran University of Medical Sciences, Tehran, Iran

Eliana P. C. Giorno, Thomaz B. Couto, Sylvia C. L. Farhat, Marcela Preto-Zamperlini and Claudio Schvartsman
Emergency Department, Instituto da Criança da FMUSP, University of Sao Paulo, Av. Dr. Enéas Carvalho de Aguiar, 647, Cerqueira César, Sao Paulo, SP CEP-05403.000, Brazil

Danilo Y. Nanbu and Fernanda V. M. Sa
Emergency Department, Instituto da Criança da FMUSP, University of Sao Paulo, Av. Dr. Enéas Carvalho de Aguiar, 647, Cerqueira César, Sao Paulo, SP CEP-05403.000, Brazil
Emergency Department, Hospital Israelita Albert Einstein, Sao Paulo, Brazil

Milena De Paulis
Emergency Department, Hospital Israelita Albert Einstein, Sao Paulo, Brazil
Emergency Department, Hospital Universitario, University of Sao Paulo, Sao Paulo, Brazil

Yoshino T. Sameshima
Radiology Department, Hospital Israelita Albert Einstein, Sao Paulo, Brazil

Kirstin Weerdenburg
Dalhousie University, Halifax, NS, Canada
IWK Health Centre, Halifax, NS, Canada

Paulo Savoia
Radiology Department, Hospital Israelita Albert Einstein, Sao Paulo, Brazil
Radiology Department, Radiology Institute, University of Sao Paulo, Sao Paulo, Brazil

Werther B. Carvalho
Pediatric Intensive Care, Children's Institute, University of Sao Paulo, Sao Paulo, Brazil

T. J. Olgers, N. Azizi and J. C. ter Maaten
Dept Internal Med, Univ Groningen, Univ Med Ctr Groningen, 9700 RB Groningen, The Netherlands

H. R. Bouma
Dept Internal Med, Univ Groningen, Univ Med Ctr Groningen, 9700 RB Groningen, The Netherlands
Dept of Clinical Pharmacy and Pharmacology, Univ Groningen, Univ Med Ctr Groningen, 9700 RB Groningen, The Netherlands

Jonathan F. Swanson, Erin F. Shufflebarger, Douglas W. Wallace, Matthew A. Heimann, James C. Crosby, David C. Pigott, John P. Gullett, Maxwell A. Thompson and Christopher J. Greene
Department of Emergency Medicine, University of Alabama at Birmingham, Old Hillman Building Suite 251, 619 19th St S, Birmingham, AL 35249, USA

Frances M. Russell, Audrey Herbert and Robinson M. Ferre
Department of Emergency Medicine, Indiana University School of Medicine, 720 Eskenazi Ave, Fifth Third Faculty Office Building, 3rd Floor Emergency Medicine Office, Indianapolis, IN 46202, USA

Bita Zakeri
Education and Continuing Medical Education, Indiana University School of Medicine, Indianapolis, IN, USA

Valerie Echeverria and Dina Peterson
Indiana University School of Medicine, Indianapolis, IN, USA

Paul Wallach
Department of Internal Medicine, Office of the Dean, Indiana University School of Medicine, Indianapolis, IN, USA

Matthew G. Hanson
Division of Cardiology, Department of Medicine, Queen's University, Kingston, ON, Canada

Barry Chan
Division of General Internal Medicine, Department of Medicine, Queen's University, Kingston, ON, Canada

Kevin C. Proud, Robert Nathanson, Natalie Smith, Elizabeth K. Haro, Marcos I. Restrepo and Michael J. Mader
South Texas Veterans Health Care System, San Antonio, TX, USA
Department of Medicine, UT Health San Antonio, San Antonio, TX, USA

Jacqueline Pugh
Department of Medicine, UT Health San Antonio, San Antonio, TX, USA

Jeremy S. Boyd
Department of Emergency Medicine, Veterans Affairs - Tennessee Valley Healthcare System, Nashville, TN, USA
Department of Emergency Medicine, Vanderbilt University Medical Center, Nashville, TN, USA

Gregory Mints
Division of Hospital Medicine, Weill Cornell Medicine, New York, NY, USA

Trevor P. Jensen
Division of Hospital Medicine, University of California San Francisco Medical Center at Parnassus, San Francisco, CA, USA

Gigi Liu
Division of General Internal Medicine, Department of Medicine, Johns Hopkins School of Medicine, Baltimore, MD, USA

Benji K. Mathews
Department of Hospital Medicine, Regions Hospital, HealthPartners, St. Paul, MN, USA

Christopher K. Schott
Department of Critical Care Medicine, Veterans Affairs of Pittsburgh Health Care System, Pittsburgh, PA, USA
Departments of Critical Care Medicine and Emergency Medicine, University of Pittsburgh Medical Center, University of Pittsburgh, Pittsburgh, PA, USA

Linda Kurian
Division of Hospital Medicine, Donald and Barbara Zucker School of Medicine at Hofstra/Northwell, Hempstead, NY, USA

Phil Andrus
Department of Emergency Medicine, Donald and Barbara Zucker School of Medicine at Hofstra/Northwell, Hempstead, NY, USA

Brian P. Lucas
White River Junction VA Medical Center, White River Junction, VT, USA
Department of Medicine, Dartmouth Geisel School of Medicine, Hanover, NH, USA

Nilam J. Soni
South Texas Veterans Health Care System, San Antonio, TX, USA
Department of Medicine, UT Health San Antonio, San Antonio, TX, USA
University of Texas Health San Antonio, South Texas Veterans Health Care System, 7703 Floyd Curl Drive, MC 7982, San Antonio, TX 78229, USA

David P. Evans, Jordan Tozer, Lindsay Taylor, Michael J. Vitto and Michael Joyce
Department of Emergency Medicine, Virginia Commonwealth School of Medicine, Main Hospital 2nd floor, room 606, Suite 600, 1250 East Marshal St, Richmond, VA 23298-0401, USA

Philippe Rola
ICU Chief of Service, Santa Cabrini Hospital, Montreal, QC, Canada

Francisco Miralles-Aguiar
Anasthesia & Surgery Critical Care Service, Hospital Universitario Puerta del Mar, Cádiz, Spain

Eduardo Argaiz
Instituto Nacional de Ciencias Medicas y Nutricion Salvador, Zubiran, Tlalpan, Mexico City, Mexico

William Beaubien-Souligny
Division of Nephrology, Centre Hospitalier de L'Université de Montréal, Montreal, Canada

Korbin Haycock
Department of Emergency Medicine, Riverside University Health Systems Medical Center, Moreno Valley, CA, USA

Timur Karimov
Intensive Care, Hôpital Honoré Mercier, Ste-Hyacinthe, QC, Canada

Vi Am Dinh
Department of Emergency Medicine and Department of Internal Medicine, Division of Pulmonary and Critical Care Medicine, Loma Linda University Health, Loma Linda, CA, USA

Rory Spiegel
Department of Critical Care, Georgetown University Medstar Washington Hospital Center, Washington, DC, USA

John Cathcart and Daniel Kerr
School Health Sciences, Ulster University, Co., Antrim, UK

Victoria Vatsvåg
School Health Sciences, Ulster University, Co., Antrim, UK
Faculty of Health Sciences, Department of Quality and Health Technology, University of Stavanger, Stavanger, Norway

Kjetil Todnem
Department of Health and Working Environment, Global Business Support, Equinor ASA, Stavanger, Norway

Torvind Næsheim
Cardiovascular Research Group, Department of Clinical Medicine, Faculty of Health Sciences, UiT, The Arctic University of Norway, Tromsø, Norway
Department of Anaesthesiology, University Hospital North Norway, Tromsø, Norway

Nils Petter Oveland
Faculty of Health Sciences, Department of Quality and Health Technology, University of Stavanger, Stavanger, Norway
Department of Anaesthesiology and Intensive Care, Stavanger University Hospital, Stavanger, Norway

Claire Rimes-Stigare
Department of Perioperative Medicine and Intensive Care, Karolinska University Hospital, Solna, 171 76 Stockholm, Sweden

Mårten Renberg and Max Bell
Department of Perioperative Medicine and Intensive Care, Karolinska University Hospital, Solna, 171 76 Stockholm, Sweden
Department of Physiology and Pharmacology, Karolinska Institutet, Stockholm, Sweden

Naima Kilhamn
Department of Medicine, Karolinska Institutet, Solna, Stockholm, Sweden

Daniel Hertzberg
Department of Perioperative Medicine and Intensive Care, Karolinska University Hospital, Solna, 171 76 Stockholm, Sweden
Department of Medicine, Karolinska Institutet, Solna, Stockholm, Sweden

Kent Lund
Department of Clinical Physiology, Karolinska University Hospital, Solna, Stockholm, Sweden

Pablo Rodriguez, Igor Sviridenko, Sylvia Noveri and Ana Soca
Intensive Care Unit, Hospital Pasteur, Administración de Servicios de Salud del Estado, Montevideo, Uruguay

Christian Yic, Diego Méndez and Mario Cancela
Intensive Care Unit, Asociación Española Primera de Socorros Mutuos, Montevideo, Uruguay

José L. Díaz-Gómez
Department of Critical Care Medicine, Mayo Clinic, Jacksonville, USA

Julio Pontet
Intensive Care Unit, Hospital Pasteur, Administración de Servicios de Salud del Estado, Montevideo, Uruguay
Intensive Care Unit, Asociación Española Primera de Socorros Mutuos, Montevideo, Uruguay
Larravide 2458, Montevideo, Uruguay

Jessica Fozard, Krystle Shafer and Thompson Kehrl
WellSpan York Hospital Emergency Medicine Residency Program, WellSpan York Hospital, York, PA, USA

Christian Boßelmann
Department of Neurology and Epileptology and Hertie-Institute for Clinical Brain Research, Eberhard-Karls University of Tübingen, Hoppe-Seyler-Straße 3, 72076 Tübingen, Germany

Sven Poli
Department of Neurology and Stroke and Hertie-Institute for Clinical Brain Research, Eberhard-Karls University of Tübingen, Hoppe-Seyler-Straße 3, 72076 Tübingen, Germany

Gert Jan Scheffer
Radboud Institute for Health Sciences, Department of Anesthesiology, Pain and Palliative Medicine, Radboud university medical center, Geert Grooteplein-Zuid 10, 6525 GA Nijmegen, The Netherlands

Rein Ketelaars, Geert-Jan van Geffen and Nico Hoogerwerf
Radboud Institute for Health Sciences, Department of Anesthesiology, Pain and Palliative Medicine, Radboud university medical center, Geert Grooteplein-Zuid 10, 6525 GA Nijmegen, The Netherlands
Radboud Institute for Health Sciences, Helicopter Emergency Medical Service Lifeliner 3, Radboud university medical center, Geert Grooteplein-Zuid 10, 6525 GA Nijmegen, The Netherlands

Gabby Reijnders
Department of Intensive Care, Catharina Hospital, Michelangelolaan 2, 5623 EJ Eindhoven, The Netherlands

Olivier Felix Umuhire
Department of Anesthesia, Critical Care and Emergency Medicine, University of Rwanda, Kigali, Rwanda

Michael B. Henry
Columbia University Vagelos College of Physicians and Surgeons, New York, USA

Adam Carl Levine
The Warren Alpert Medical School of Brown University, Providence, RI, USA

Giles N. Cattermole
Department of Emergency Medicine, King's College/ NHS, London, UK

Patricia Henwood
Department of Emergency Medicine, Brigham and Women's Hospital, Boston, USA

Index